Critical Care Obstetrics for the Obstetrician and Gynecologist

Editors

CAROLYN M. ZELOP
STEPHANIE R. MARTIN

OBSTETRICS AND GYNECOLOGY CLINICS OF NORTH AMERICA

www.obgyn.theclinics.com

Consulting Editor
WILLIAM F. RAYBURN

December 2016 • Volume 43 • Number 4

ELSEVIER

1600 John F. Kennedy Boulevard • Suite 1800 • Philadelphia, Pennsylvania, 19103-2899

http://www.theclinics.com

OBSTETRICS AND GYNECOLOGY CLINICS OF NORTH AMERICA Volume 43, Number 4
December 2016 ISSN 0889-8545, ISBN-13: 978-0-323-47745-1

Editor: Kerry Holland
Developmental Editor: Kristen Helm

Obstetrics and Gynecology Clinics (ISSN 0889-8545) is published quarterly by Elsevier Inc., 360 Park Avenue South, New York, NY 10010-1710. Months of issue are March, June, September, and December. Periodicals postage paid at New York, NY, and additional mailing offices. Subscription price per year is $295.00 (US individuals), $597.00 (US institutions), $100.00 (US students), $370.00 (Canadian individuals), $754.00 (Canadian institutions), $225.00 (Canadian students), $450.00 (international individuals), $754.00 (international institutions), and $225.00 (international students). To receive student/resident rate, orders must be accompanied by name of affiliated institution, date of term, and the signature of program/residency coordinator on institution letterhead. Orders will be billed at individual rate until proof of status is received. Foreign air speed delivery is included in all *Clinics* subscription prices. All prices are subject to change without notice. POSTMASTER: Send address changes to *Obstetrics and Gynecology Clinics*, Elsevier Health Sciences Division, Subscription Customer Service, 3251 Riverport Lane, Maryland Heights, MO 63043. **Customer Service: Telephone: 1-800-654-2452 (U.S. and Canada); 314-447-8871 (outside U.S. and Canada). Fax: 314-447-8029. E-mail: journalscustomerservice-usa@elsevier.com (for print support); journalsonlinesupport-usa@elsevier. com (for online support).**

Reprints. For copies of 100 or more of articles in this publication, please contact the Commercial Reprints Department, Elsevier Inc., 360 Park Avenue South, New York, New York 10010-1710. Tel.: 212-633-3874; Fax: 212-633-3820; E-mail: reprints@elsevier.com.

Obstetrics and Gynecology Clinics of North America is also published in Spanish by McGraw-Hill Interamericana Editores S.A., P.O. Box 5-237, 06500, Mexico; in Portuguese by Reichmann and Affonso Editores, Rio de Janeiro, Brazil; and in Greek by Paschalidis Medical Publications, Athens, Greece.

Obstetrics and Gynecology Clinics of North America is covered in *MEDLINE/PubMed (Index Medicus), Excerpta Medica, Current Concepts/Clinical Medicine, Science Citation Index, BIOSIS, CINAHL,* and *ISI/BIOMED.*

Contributors

CONSULTING EDITOR

WILLIAM F. RAYBURN, MD, MBA
Associate Dean, Continuing Medical Education and Professional Development, Distinguished Professor and Emeritus Chair, Obstetrics and Gynecology, University of New Mexico School of Medicine, Albuquerque, New Mexico

EDITORS

CAROLYN M. ZELOP, MD
Director of Ultrasound and Perinatal Research, Division of Maternal-Fetal Medicine, Department of Obstetrics and Gynecology, The Valley Hospital, Ridgewood, New Jersey; Clinical Professor, Department of Obstetrics and Gynecology, New York University School of Medicine, New York, New York

STEPHANIE R. MARTIN, DO
Director, Southern Colorado Maternal Fetal Medicine; Director, Maternal Fetal Medicine Services, Centura South State, Colorado Springs, Colorado

AUTHORS

ANJALI ACHARYA, MBBS
Jacobi Medical Center, Albert Einstein College of Medicine, Bronx, New York

CYNTHIA BEAN, MD
Department of Maternal Fetal Medicine, Winfred L. Wiser Hospital for Women and Infants, The University of Mississippi Medical Center, Jackson, Mississippi

TERRI-ANN BENNETT, MD
Division of Maternal-Fetal Medicine, Department of Obstetrics and Gynecology, New York University Langone Medical Center, New York, New York

ELIZABETH A. BONNEY, MD, MPH
Professor, Department of Obstetrics, Gynecology and Reproductive Sciences, University of Vermont College of Medicine, Burlington, Vermont

STEVEN L. CLARK, MD
Department of Obstetrics and Gynecology, Texas Children's Hospital, Baylor College of Medicine, Houston, Texas

JAMIL ELFARRA, MD
Department of Maternal Fetal Medicine, Winfred L. Wiser Hospital for Women and Infants, The University of Mississippi Medical Center, Jackson, Mississippi

HOLLY ENDE, MD
Obstetric Anesthesiology Fellow, Department of Anesthesiology, Perioperative and Pain Medicine, Brigham and Women's Hospital, Boston, Massachusetts

CATHERINE EPPES, MD, MPH
Assistant Professor, Division of Maternal-Fetal Medicine, Department of Obstetrics and Gynecology, Baylor College of Medicine, Houston, Texas

MANISHA GANDHI, MD
Assistant Professor, Division of Maternal-Fetal Medicine, Department of Obstetrics and Gynecology, Associate Residency Program Director; Medical Director, Baylor Maternal Fetal Medicine Clinic, Baylor College of Medicine, Texas Children's Pavilion for Women, Houston, Texas

VERN L. KATZ, MD
Department of Obstetrics and Gynecology, Oregon Health and Science University, Portland, Oregon; Department of Human Physiology, University of Oregon, Eugene, Oregon

AMBER KHANNA, MD
Assistant Professor, Division of Cardiology, Department of Medicine, University of Colorado School of Medicine, Aurora, Colorado

GARRETT K. LAM, MD, FACOG
Chairman and Associate Professor, Department of Obstetrics and Gynecology, Regional Obstetrical Consultants, University of Tennessee College of Medicine Chattanooga, Chattanooga, Tennessee

JAMES N. MARTIN Jr, MD, FACOG, FRCOG
Department of Maternal Fetal Medicine, Winfred L. Wiser Hospital for Women and Infants, The University of Mississippi Medical Center, Jackson, Mississippi

STEPHANIE R. MARTIN, DO
Director, Southern Colorado Maternal Fetal Medicine; Director, Maternal Fetal Medicine Services, Centura South State, Colorado Springs, Colorado

TORRI D. METZ, MD, MS
Assistant Professor, Department of Obstetrics and Gynecology, University of Colorado School of Medicine, Aurora, Colorado; Department of Obstetrics and Gynecology, Denver Health Medical Center, Denver, Colorado

CHRISTY PEARCE, MD, MS
Southern Colorado Maternal Fetal Medicine; Director, Outreach Services, Centura South State, Colorado Springs, Colorado

LAUREN A. PLANTE, MD, MPH
Director, Division of Maternal-Fetal Medicine; Professor, Departments of Obstetrics & Gynecology and Anesthesiology, Drexel University College of Medicine, Philadelphia, Pennsylvania

JULIE SCOTT, MD
Associate Professor, Division of Maternal Fetal Medicine, Obstetrics and Gynecology, University of Colorado, Aurora, Colorado

AMIR A. SHAMSHIRSAZ, MD
Maternal Fetal Medicine Fellow, Division of Maternal-Fetal Medicine, Department of Obstetrics and Gynecology, Baylor College of Medicine, Texas Children's Pavilion for Women, Houston, Texas

DIRK VARELMANN, MD
Assistant Professor, Department of Anesthesiology, Perioperative and Pain Medicine, Brigham and Women's Hospital, Boston, Massachusetts

ARTHUR JASON VAUGHT, MD
Assistant Professor, Division of Maternal Fetal Medicine, Department of Gynecology and Obstetrics, The Johns Hopkins University School of Medicine, Baltimore, Maryland

CAROLYN M. ZELOP, MD
Director of Ultrasound and Perinatal Research, Division of Maternal-Fetal Medicine, Department of Obstetrics and Gynecology, The Valley Hospital, Ridgewood, New Jersey; Clinical Professor, Department of Obstetrics and Gynecology, New York University School of Medicine, New York, New York

Contents

> Obstetric hemorrhage accounts for 5% of all deliveries in the United States
> and accounts for high maternal morbidity and mortality. Many hemor-
> rhages are secondary to uterine atony and are quickly ameliorated with
> appropriate uterotonic use. However, for a subset of cases, severe hem-
> orrhage may require advanced resuscitative techniques, and innovative
> procedural and surgical techniques. This article guides a provider through
> such a resuscitation.

> Hypertensive disorders of pregnancy are among the leading preventable
> contributors of maternal and fetal adverse outcomes, including maternal
> and fetal death. Blood pressure increase has a strong association with un-
> favorable pregnancy outcomes, including stroke and pulmonary edema. A
> persistent blood pressure measurement greater than or equal to 160/110
> mm Hg lasting for more than 15 minutes, during pregnancy or postpartum,
> is considered an obstetric emergency and requires rapid appropriate treat-
> ment. Following evidence-based guidelines, implementing institutional po-
> lices, and understanding the classification and pathophysiology of
> hypertensive disorders of pregnancy are essential and can significantly
> improve the rate of preventable complications.

> Pregnant women have an increased morbidity and mortality for certain ill-
> nesses owing to the physiologic and immunologic changes in pregnancy.
> Certain infections are common during pregnancy, including urinary tract
> infections and pneumonia. Others are uncommon, but yield increased
> severity, including influenza. Human immunodeficiency virus, although it
> does not increase in pathogenesis during pregnancy, requires specific
> attention and management in the context of pregnancy.

inflammatory response syndrome. Maternal treatment is primarily supportive, whereas prompt delivery in the mother who has sustained cardiopulmonary arrest is critical for improved newborn outcome.

OBSTETRICS AND GYNECOLOGY CLINICS

Foreword

An End to Happiness...Attention to the Critically Ill Parturient

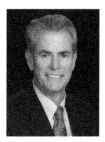

William F. Rayburn, MD, MBA
Consulting Editor

Care of the pregnant patient can be very rewarding, and safe delivery of a healthy infant brings great happiness. However, up to 1% of all pregnant women become seriously ill and require consideration for admission to an intensive care unit (ICU). Despite this very unsettling experience, the obstetrician must be prepared to identify risks, provide immediate care, understand physiologic and laboratory changes from pregnancy, and monitor maternal and, if necessary, fetal well-being.

This issue of the *Obstetrics and Gynecology Clinics of North America*, guest edited by Dr Carolyn Zelop and Dr Stephanie Martin, represents a contemporary resource on emergent conditions in obstetrics to all individuals in training as well as already established obstetricians. An endless number of medical, surgical, and obstetrical complications may be encountered during pregnancy and the puerperium. Those that are more complex and life threatening can be particularly challenging, especially when a multidisciplinary team is necessary for optimal care.

This issue addresses common morbid conditions leading to critical illness and surveys the monitoring and treatments used for those parturients. Among those admitted to an ICU, half or more have a diagnosis related to an obstetric complication such as hypertension and hemorrhage. Other common causes for admission are respiratory failure and sepsis. Common nonobstetric indications include maternal cardiac disease, trauma, drug overdose, cerebrovascular accidents, and anesthetic complications.

The authors describe in their articles some of the unique considerations when assisting in the care of the critically ill patient during pregnancy. A fundamental knowledge of pregnancy-induced physiologic changes, alterations in normal laboratory values, considerations for the fetus, and timing of any delivery is essential. The immediate postpartum period can lead to further confusion for the non-obstetrician. Fortunately, these severely ill women are usually young and in good health, so the prognosis is usually better than others admitted to the ICU.

Obstet Gynecol Clin N Am 43 (2016) xiii–xiv
http://dx.doi.org/10.1016/j.ogc.2016.08.002
0889-8545/16/© 2016 Published by Elsevier Inc.

obgyn.theclinics.com

Although the evolution of care for the critically ill parturient has generally followed developments with other aspects of medicine and surgery, there are often few specific guidelines for pregnancy. Most hospitals use a blend of concepts of all disciplines, and in general, pregnant women are placed in either medical or surgical ICUs. Intermediate care units are found beside or part of a Labor and Delivery unit at tertiary care centers where management is undertaken by obstetricians, maternal-fetal medicine specialists, and qualified anesthesiologists, but usually not for full-time care. For smaller hospitals, transfer of the patient to another larger medical center would be preferable.

Dr Zelop, Dr Martin, and the many qualified authors deserve a special thanks for their efforts in providing a very clinically useful reference for periodic review, either after or preferably before a parturient becomes critically ill. Patient safety is paramount in critical care obstetrics, and it is hoped that this issue will provide practical and timely information to reduce risk and improve outcomes.

William F. Rayburn, MD, MBA
Continuing Medical Education
and Professional Development
University of New Mexico School of Medicine
MSC 10 5580
1 University of New Mexico
Albuquerque, NM 87131-0001, USA

E-mail address:
wrayburn@salud.unm.edu

Preface

Contemporary Obstetric Intensive Care

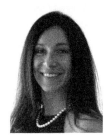 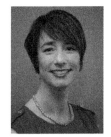

Carolyn M. Zelop, MD   Stephanie R. Martin, DO
Editors

Although pregnancy is not a disease, the 21st century has witnessed an unprecedented rise in maternal morbidity and mortality. Cardiopulmonary arrest occurs in 1/12,000 women admitted for delivery.[1] Cardiac disease, hemorrhage, hypertensive disorders, venous thromboembolism, and infection persist as the leading causes preceding maternal demise. The complexity of obstetrical clinical scenarios necessitates that contemporary obstetrical care incorporate critical care medicine. Our goal in this issue of *Obstetrics and Gynecology Clinics of North America* is to provide a comprehensive guide, using a systems-based approach of critical care medicine topics for the generalist in obstetrics or the consulting non-obstetrician specialist. Paramount to the diagnosis and treatment of critical care conditions in pregnancy is a fundamental understanding of the underlying physiologic adaptations inherent to pregnancy. This is a recurrent theme throughout this issue. Yes, pregnant women are different, and the normal physiologic changes of pregnancy often render them more susceptible to life-threatening complications and may make it more challenging for clinicians to recognize these derangements.

The authors in this issue come from a variety of specialties and represent a cross-section of the type of specialists that may be involved in caring for a critically ill pregnant or postpartum patient. We think this multispecialty approach offers a unique perspective and hope this issue is a valuable resource for the clinician at the bedside.

Carolyn M. Zelop, MD
Division of Maternal-Fetal Medicine
Department of Obstetrics and Gynecology
The Valley Hospital, Ridgewood, NJ, USA

Department of Obstetrics and Gynecology
New York University School of Medicine
New York, NY, USA

Obstet Gynecol Clin N Am 43 (2016) xv–xvi
http://dx.doi.org/10.1016/j.ogc.2016.08.001
0889-8545/16/© 2016 Published by Elsevier Inc.

obgyn.theclinics.com

Stephanie R. Martin, DO
1910 La Bellezza Grove
Colorado Springs, CO 80919, USA

E-mail addresses:
Zeloca@valleyhealth.com (C.M. Zelop)
smartin@southerncoloradomfm.com (S.R. Martin)

REFERENCE

1. Mhyre JM, Tsen LC, Einav S, et al. Cardiac arrest during hospitalization for delivery in the United States, 1998-2011. Anesthesiology 2014;120:810.

Critical Care for the Obstetrician and Gynecologist

Obstetric Hemorrhage and Disseminated Intravascular Coagulopathy

Arthur Jason Vaught, MD

KEYWORDS

- Hemorrhagic shock • Massive transfusion protocol
- Disseminated intravascular coagulopathy • Transexamic acid
- Special populations of hemorrhage

KEY POINTS

- Hemorrhage in pregnancy is common and a subset of patients succumb to hemorrhagic shock with disseminated intravascular coagulopathy.
- Massive transfusion protocol aids in complex resuscitations while avoiding acidosis and dilutional coagulopathy.
- Aside from uterotonics, there are other medications that can be used in correction of coagulopathy.

BACKGROUND

Obstetric hemorrhage accounts for 5% of all deliveries and is usually defined as greater than 500 mL and greater than 1000 mL of estimated blood loss following a vaginal delivery and cesarean section, respectively.[1] Risk factors include, but are not limited to, grand multiparity, prolonged induction, chorioamnionitis, multiple gestation, and abnormal placentation.[2]

Mostly hemorrhage is secondary to uterine atony, and this is usually resolved with medical therapies, such as oxytocin, carboprost, methergine, and misoprostol.[1,2] However, in complex hemorrhages, which can be secondary to a multitude of factors, the obstetrician must be astute in the management of hemorrhagic shock and its resultant coagulopathy and electrolyte disturbances. This article focuses on the definition, management, and therapies for such a complex hemorrhage.

Disclosure: Dr A.J. Vaught does not have any disclosures.
Division of Maternal Fetal Medicine, Department of Gynecology and Obstetrics, The Johns Hopkins University School of Medicine, 600 North Wolfe Street, Phipps 228, Baltimore, MD 21287, USA
E-mail address: Avaught2@jhmi.edu

Obstet Gynecol Clin N Am 43 (2016) 611–622
http://dx.doi.org/10.1016/j.ogc.2016.07.006
0889-8545/16/© 2016 Elsevier Inc. All rights reserved.

DEFINITION OF HEMORRHAGIC SHOCK AND DISSEMINATED INTRAVASCULAR COAGULOPATHY

Shock is state of hypoperfusion and anaerobic metabolism. In hemorrhagic, hypovolemic shock, it is further characterized into four classes (**Table 1**). Although intravascular volume increases up to 50% in the mid second trimester pregnancy, hemorrhagic classification does not change for pregnancy.[3]

As shown in **Table 1**, hemorrhagic shock is not only based on loss of blood volume, but also on clinical factors, such as mental status, heart rate, blood pressure, and urine output. In the setting of postpartum hemorrhage (PPH), which is often rapid, large-bore intravenous access should be confirmed and transition from crystalloid resuscitation to blood products should be made once the patient shows signs of class III shock.

Although defined in the nineteenth century and clinically relevant, the precise definitions of disseminated intravascular coagulation (DIC) have not been completely adopted and there have been no criteria that have shown improvement in clinical outcomes.[4–6] DIC affects 12.5 per 10,000 pregnancies and is reported to be the second most common severe maternal morbidity indicator for obstetric admissions.[7,8] The pathophysiology of clinical DIC is defined as a general inflammatory response with a release of cytokines, proteases, and hormones that leads to extensive microvascular endothelial damage.[5] This further causes vasodilation, capillary leak, and shock, which dysregulates the coagulation pathway leading to excessive thrombin generation and microthrombus formation.[5] This is clinically seen with exhaustion of both platelets and coagulation factors (ie, fibrinogen).[5] Clinically this is manifested as thrombosis of small arterial and venous vessels resulting in organ dysfunction and severe bleeding.

Outside of pregnancy, the three most common clinical conditions associated with DIC are sepsis, acute leukemia, and solid cancers.[4] However, pregnancy-related true DIC is secondary to placental abruption, preeclampsia, amniotic fluid embolism, and acute fatty liver of pregnancy (AFLP).[9] Acute hemorrhage is not as much intrinsic DIC as it is a dilutional coagulopathy. However, many times in acute hemorrhage and trauma there is a release of cytokines and proinflammatory agents that can trigger an intrinsic coagulopathy. Secondary to the lack of widely accepted guidelines, it is important for providers to treat DIC in the context of the underlying clinical disease

Table 1
Classes of hemorrhagic shock

	Class I	Class II	Class III	Class IV
Blood loss (mL)	Up to 750	750–1500	1500–2000	>2000
Blood loss (% of blood volume)	Up to 15%	15%–30%	30%–40%	>40%
Pulse rate	<100	100–120	120–140	>140
Blood pressure (mm Hg)	Normal	Normal	Decreased	Decreased
Pulse pressure (mm Hg)	Normal	Decreased	Decreased	Decreased
Respiratory rate	14–20	20–30	30–40	>35
Urine output (mL/h)	>30	20–30	5–15	Negligible
Mental status	Slightly anxious	Mildly anxious	Anxious, confused	Confused, Lethargic
Fluid replacement	Crystalloid	Crystalloid	Crystalloid + blood	Crystalloid + blood

From Advanced Trauma Life Support (ATLS) student course manual. 9th edition. Chicago (IL): American College of Surgeons; 2012.

process and laboratory abnormalities. This is further confounded by the upregulation factors, notably fibrinogen in the second and third trimester of pregnancy, and fibrinogen levels are even supranormal and range from 400 to 650 mg/dL.[10]

The clinical management of DIC is to first correct the underlying cause (ie, bleeding, infection, hypothermia) and then to resuscitate with blood products and sometimes with specific medications when necessary. Control of bleeding in obstetrics is usually the most important first step because most pregnancy-related DIC is associated with massive hemorrhage. In other cases, such as micronagiopathic hemolytic anemias, pre-eclampsia, and HELLP syndrome, specific procedural and medical pathways should be followed to correct coagulopathy and delivery when indicated. If there is ongoing bleeding, factors should be replaced with plasma, platelets, and cryoprecipitate.

MANAGEMENT AND THERAPIES FOR HEMORRHAGIC SHOCK AND DISSEMINATE INTRAVASCULAR COAGULOPATHY

The first-line management of hemorrhagic shock is assessment of the ability for the patient to maintain her airway and adequate ventilation to continue a normal acid/base status during anaerobic metabolism. In the setting of altered mental status or in the setting of severe acidosis intubation should be considered.[11] Then, adequate intravenous access should be undertaken along with intravenous resuscitation. For many large resuscitations there is initial fluid responsiveness, but it is common that blood products and intermittent vasopressor be used.

The usual first-line therapy in the setting of PPH secondary to uterine atony is uterine massage and compression, and massage is continued while other interventions are taking place. Uterotonic medications are also generally used in this setting, such as oxytocin, carboprost, and methergine, and misoprostol if there are no contraindications to these medications. Carboprost has been shown to induce asthma exacerbations, and methergine has been shown to potentiate hypertensive disease and increase the half-life of antiretroviral therapies.[12] Both rectal and buccal misoprostol have also shown benefit in the setting when other uterotonic are unavailable. However, there are no strong data that misoprostol is more effective than other uterotonics.[13-15]

In the setting of ongoing lower uterine atony, balloon tamponade and uterine packing with gauze may be a valid option. The exact mechanism of these devices remains unclear, but many believe it is secondary to a reduction in the uterine artery perfusion rather direct compression.[16] In the setting of hemodynamic stability and available staff, uterine artery embolization can be pursued. Although success rates for PPH are reportedly promising, the failure rate is 11% in some studies.[17-19] Aside from the risk of failure, there are also hypovolemia-related complications, such as cerebral infarction, acute kidney injury, lower extremity paresthesia, and postembolization syndrome.[20] Patients at the highest risk of embolization failure were those who had DIC or coagulopathy and this should be taken into consideration.[20]

If the patient is not amenable to interventional radiology, other fertility-sparing procedures, such as B-lynch and O'Leary technique, can be undertaken, but if hemorrhage persists then hysterectomy is warranted.

MASSIVE TRANSFUSION PROTOCOLS

In the setting of ongoing bleeding, many institutions with active trauma centers have protocolized rapid blood product resuscitation through massive transfusion protocols (MTP).[21] Resuscitation efforts for MTP in obstetrics are similar to that in traumatic injury where the goals are to establish rapid control of bleeding while transfusing blood products (**Table 2**) with the avoidance of DIC. The sequential transfusion of red blood

Table 2
Blood product transfusion

Product	Description	Volume	Resuscitation Change
Packed red blood cells	Derived from whole blood with removed plasma leaving a hematocrit of 60%	300 mL	Increase hemoglobin by 1 mg/dL or increase hematocrit by 3%
Fresh frozen plasma	Contains factors II, VII, IX, X; protein C; protein S; antithrombin III; ADAMTS 13	250 mL	Administer 15 mL/kg and should correct prothrombin time and partial thromboplastin time at varying rates
Cryoprecipitate	Concentrated levels of fibrinogen, factor VIII, von Willebrand factor, factor XIII	100–150 mL	Should increase fibrinogen 100–150 mg per unit
A "six pack" or "pool" of platelets	Can be from one donor or multiple donors Can be matched by HLA types	100–150 mL	Each "six pack" should increase platelets by 50,000

cells restores oxygen-carrying capacity, while plasma and platelets restore physiologic hemostasis.[22] MTP also allows for the rapid and emergency release of packaged products that can help prevent coagulopathy.

During MTP, platelets are given, which also aids in achieving hemostatic homeostasis, and are usually given to keep a platelet count above 50,000 in an actively bleeding patient. Cryoprecipitate is also used in MTP and obstetric hemorrhage. It specifically contains high concentrations of fibrinogen, factor VIII, von Willebrand factor, and factor XII with less volume of about 10 to 15 mL/U with each administration a pool of 8 to 10 U.[23] Every institution has a specific MTP protocol; however, many have adapted 1:1:1 strategy (1 U of packed red blood cells [PRBC], 1 U of fresh frozen plasma [FFP], and 1 U of platelets). The coolers are usually given in containers of 6 U of PRBC, 6 U of FFP, and one (six pack) pool of platelets. The 1:1:1 (RBC/plasma/platelets) has been adopted over a 2:1:1 (RBC/plasma/platelets) ratio secondary to significantly improved hemostasis, and less death secondary to exsanguination in the 1:1:1 group, with less use of red cell transfusion.[24]

During massive resuscitations along with medical and procedural control of bleeding, laboratory data are shown to be helpful. Laboratory studies generally consist of complete blood counts, prothrombin time, partial thromboplastin time, and fibrinogen. Aside from hematologic laboratory data, the provider should be aware of electrolyte disturbances during massive transfusion, in particular hyperkalemia and low ionized calcium levels. These electrolyte disturbances can lead to cardiac arrest or severe cardiac dysfunction. Ionized calcium levels during resuscitation less than 1.1 mmol further impairs coagulation and places patients at cardiac risk. To avoid such derangements 1 to 2 g of intravenous calcium gluconate can be given empirically for every four packed red cell transfused.[25,26] Hyperkalemia usually results from the rapid transfusion of PRBCs with lysed erythrocytes. Patients undergoing MTP should have potassium levels taken intermittently and these elevated levels can be alleviated through standard measures, such as glucose and insulin, sodium bicarbonate, and calcium gluconate or chloride.

Other laboratory tests available to guide resuscitation are thromboelastography and rotational thromboelastometry. Both thromboelastography and rotational thromboelastometry have been shown to be useful in guiding resuscitation in postpartum and obstetric hemorrhage and have been validated.[27,28] The tests provide a qualitative assessment of hemostasis in patient whole blood and are rapid and can be performed at bedside.[29] In particular they can help the provider guide factor replacement and identify fibrinogen deficiency with extended K values and active fibrinolysis prolonged lysis of clot at 30-minute values (**Table 3**).

ADJUNCTIVE MEDICAL THERAPIES TO HEMORRHAGE

In the setting of hemorrhage there are adjunctive medical therapies to help reduce the amount hemorrhage and prevent fibrinolysis and aid in factor replacement. Transexamic acid (TXA) is an antifibrinolytic drug used in such a setting as MTP or large resuscitations. TXA inhibits the activation of plasminogen to plasmin and plasmin as a synthetic lysine analogue. In the trauma literature, TXA is associated with less transfusion of products and lower all-cause mortality on early administration of medication (<3 hours in from injury). When TXA was given after 3 hours mortality actually increased.[30,31] In the obstetric literature, pilot trials of TXA have shown a decrease in continued bleeding in the setting of severe PPH defined as estimated blood loss greater than 800 mL in a vaginal delivery, change in hemoglobin of 4 g/dL, transfusion of greater than 4 U of PRBC, death, or invasive hemostatic interventions (ie, embolization, hysterectomy).[32] Larger studies are needed to determine the efficacy and risk/benefit of its use it PPH. The World Health Organization considers the use of TXA reasonable if other uterotonics have failed to stop or decrease bleeding.

Recombinant factor VIIa has been used in the setting of severe bleeding in patients with hemophilia, and in the setting of bleeding with factor VII and IX deficiencies.[33,34] It was originally contraindicated in the setting of states of possible hypercoagulability, such as DIC; however, its clinical experience in traumatic injury has led providers to believe that it is an appropriate adjunct in severe hemorrhage.[35] The case reports and studies in the literature of its use have shown that it is safe and efficacious.[36–38] In a study, women with severe PPH who failed standard oxytocin use were randomized to receiving and not receiving recombinant factor VIIa; there was a 40% reduction in the primary outcome (uterine artery embolization, uterine artery ligation, hysterectomy) in participants who received recombinant factor VIIa.[39] However, secondary to its expense and thrombotic risk, it should be considered but used with caution. It should also be noted that for recombinant factor VII to effectively clot, there needs to be components for effective clot formation. For this drug to achieve maximum effectiveness, there needs to be an adequate platelet level (preferably >50,000 mm^3), fibrinogen level (>100 mg/dL), and a hematologic environment devoid of acidosis and hypocalcemia.[40]

Prothrombin complex concentrates (PCC) have been available as FFP alternatives. PCC contains vitamin K–dependent clotting factors (factor II, VII, IX, X) and is highly concentrated. Its original indication was for reversal of vitamin K antagonist, but it has now been recently used in traumatic hemorrhage.[41,42] Advantages to PCC are avoidance of hypervolemia, decreased incidence of transfusion-related acute lung injury, and no need to thaw; however, there are disadvantages of higher cost and thrombosis. Because of no randomized control trial in pregnancy and PPH, PCC should not be considered standard therapy or practice.[43]

Table 3
Thromboelastography value interpretation

Value	Definition	Normal Value	Abnormal Value	Deficiency in or Problem with…	Treatment
R time	Time to initiate clot	5–10 min	>10 min	Coagulation factors	FFP
K time	Time to ascertain fixed clot strength	1–3 min	>3 min	Fibrinogen	Cryoprecipitate
Alpha angle	Speed of fibrin formation	53°–72°	<50°	Fibrinogen	Cryoprecipitate
Maximum amplitude	Highest vertical amplitude of thromboelastography	50–70 mm	<50 mm	Platelets	Platelet and/or DDAVP
Lysis of clot at 30 min	Percentage of maximum amplitude reduction at 30 min	0%–8%	>8%	Excessive fibrinolysis	Transexamic acid

SPECIFIC PATIENT POPULATIONS
Preeclampsia and HELLP Syndrome

Preeclampsia is a multisystem disease of the third trimester of pregnancy that affects approximately 5% to 8% of all pregnancies in the United States.[44] It generally causes hypertension and end organ damage in the form of neurologic changes, thrombocytopenia, proteinuria, acute kidney injury, hemolysis, and liver dysfunction. HELLP syndrome, which occurs in approximately 1% of all pregnancies, is thought to be a severe variant of preeclampsia that causes hemolysis, elevated liver enzymes, and low platelets. HELLP syndrome results in severe maternal morbidity with the most severe morbidities being hepatic rupture and DIC.[45] Laboratory thresholds indicate more than a 75% risk of serious maternal morbidity in the setting of lactate dehydrogenase greater than 1400 U/L, aspartate aminotransferase greater than 150 U/L, and alanine aminotransferase 100 U/L.[46,47]

In the setting of severely elevated liver enzymes and right upper quadrant pain, the clinician should be suspicious of hepatic injury and possible rupture. With such severe dysfunction, there could be coagulopathy secondary to the inability to make factors. Spontaneous rupture of a subcapsular liver hematoma in the setting of this disease is thought to occur in 1% to 2% of all cases with HELLP syndrome.[48,49] Liver hematoma and rupture are diagnosed with ultrasound, computed tomography, or MRI. In the setting of liver rupture it is important to be in a facility that has maternal fetal medicine, interventional radiology, and general or hepatic surgery for bleeding complications.

Because of the pathologic activation of endothelium and platelets with concomitant liver damage, HELLP syndrome predisposes the woman to DIC.[46] When in DIC, the manor of resuscitation is not different than outside of HELLP syndrome.

Thrombotic Thrombocytopenia Purpura

Thrombotic thrombocytopenia purpura (TTP) is defined by a severe deficiency of ADAMTS13, a von Willebrand factor cleaving protease. Although a diagnosis of TTP is made with an ADAMTS13 level less than 10, diagnosis still remains based on clinical judgment because at many institutions an ADAMTS13 result may not be available for many days.[50] The disease is hereditary and acquired as a result of inhibition of ADAMTS13 activity by an autoantibody. The disease is characterized by small vessel–rich thrombi that cause thrombocytopenia, microangiopathic hemolytic anemia, fever, and organ damage that is characterized by headache and altered mental status and kidney damage.[50] Besides appropriate laboratory information and strong suspicion, a peripheral smear with prominent shistocytes is extremely helpful in the diagnosis.

TTP is rare in pregnancy but when it does occur it closely resembles such diseases as severe preeclampsia and HELLP syndrome. Unlike HELLP syndrome or preeclampsia, TTP does not dramatically improve following delivery.[51] Secondary to severe thrombocytopenia, patients are at risk of intractable bleeding; although the initial reaction is to transfuse platelets, this can cause more thrombogenesis and exacerbate the disease process. The mainstay of therapy for TTP is plasmapharesis or plasma exchange to restore adequate levels of ADAMTS13.[52] TTP is a medical emergency and can be fatal if prompt therapy is not initiated. However, with appropriate therapy survival rates are 90%. It is imperative that these patients be transferred to a center of excellence that has appropriate resources for hematologic input and plasma exchange.

Atypical Hemolytic Uremic Syndrome

Atypical hemolytic uremic syndrome (aHUS) is a rare complement-mediated dysregulation of the alternative pathway of complement. Although aHUS can occur at any age, pregnancy along with infection, surgery, and traumatic injury can all be triggers for the disease.[53,54] Clinically the disease is also similar to HELLP syndrome with similar clinical manifestations, such as thrombocytopenia, changes in mental status, seizure, and hemolysis and kidney injury. Approximately 10% to 20% of all cases are pregnancy associated, and 20% of women diagnosed with HELLP syndrome share genetic mutations similar to aHUS.[55]

Like women with TTP, aHUS does not improve with delivery. Instead the mainstay of therapy is eculizumab, an anti-C5 monoclonal antibody that directly inhibits the alternative pathway of complement.[56] For obstetric providers, caring for these women is difficult because delineation between HELLP syndrome and aHUS is not easy. Often these women are diagnosed after delivery when there is no clinical improvement.

Secondary to low platelets and uremia, coagulopathy can certainly be an issue with delivery and postpartum and transfusion of blood products along with DDAVP may be helpful in the immediate setting. When not given the appropriate treatment morbidity and mortality is high with approximately 67% of adults either dying or progressing to end-stage renal disease.[54]

Acute Fatty Liver of Pregnancy

AFLP is a rare disorder of pregnancy that occurs in the third trimester characterized by profound hepatic failure that can result in encephalopathy, coagulopathy from hepatic synthetic dysfunction, and hypoglycemia. In AFLP, there is low antithrombin III levels, which can also predispose to DIC.[57]

Pathogenesis of AFLP is thought to be secondary to the inability to metabolize fatty acids produced by the fetus and placenta secondary to the deficiency in long-chain 3-hydroxyacyl CoA dehydrogenase.[58,59] In addition, defects in short- and medium-chain acyl-CoA dehydrogenase activity in infants have also been associated with AFLP.[60] The accumulation of long-chain 3-hydroxyacyl metabolites produced by the fetus or placenta is toxic to the liver and is thought to be the cause of the liver disease.

Patients with AFLP usually have prolonged prothrombin times and low fibrinogen levels secondary to loss of liver synthetic function.[61] Women should receive appropriate factor replacement with FFP and cryoprecipitate during heavy bleeding. Post-delivery testing for long-chain 3-hydroxyacyl CoA dehydrogenase deficiency in the mother and the fetus should be considered with prenatal or medical genetics.

HEMORRHAGE IN THE SETTING OF REFUSAL OF BLOOD PRODUCTS

Clearly, transfusion plays an important role in the setting of hemorrhagic shock. However, transfusion may not be an option for religious reasons or complex red cell antibodies. Despite optimal management by practitioners, there is still an association of increased morbidity and mortality in obstetric hemorrhage.[62] Although patients with rare blood groups and complex antibodies can still receive FFP and platelets, women who refuse blood products for cultural or religious reasons are left with fewer options.

The most well-known group of women who refuse blood products are Jehovah's Witnesses. Jehovah's Witnesses are a Christian group founded in the late 1800s. Traditionally Jehovah's Witnesses divide blood products into two groups: products they do not accept (whole blood, red cells, plasma, platelets, or white cells), and those that seem to be more individual (immunoglobins, coagulation factor preparations, albumin, vaccines, and solid organs).[63] However, these requests vary per individual, and should always be addressed and kept confidential by medical staff.

The initial steps in the process in caring for a woman where transfusion is not an option are identification, clarification of accepted blood products at initial visits, and optimization of hemoglobin through iron supplementation and vitamin B_{12} in the ante-natal period. In the setting of active hemorrhage, early definitive management, such as hysterectomy, may be life-saving and should be strongly considered.[63] Also, if avail-able and if acceptable cell savage should be used and pharmacologic antifibrinolytics, such as TXA, should be considered.

Hyperbaric oxygen has been rarely used in this setting, but there are favorable case reports in severe blood loss anemia.[64] Presumably, therapy is thought to inhibit cyto-kines and increase oxygen delivery to tissue periphery.[63]

SUMMARY

The practitioner should be aware of the different classes of hemorrhagic shock and when it is appropriate to initiate blood product transfusion. During large resuscitation, MTP aids in the administration of blood products while avoiding dilutional DIC. In the setting of DIC, the first step is to correct the underlying cause (ie, intractable bleeding, sepsis). In large resuscitations TXA and recombinant factor VIIa are viable options to aid in the cessation of obstetric hemorrhage. In the setting of abnormal coagulopathy in pregnancy not caused by acute hemorrhage, the practitioner should consider other reasons for the coagulopathy (ie, HELLP syndrome, AFLP, micronagiopathic hemolyt-ic anemias). When transfusion is not an option secondary to complex antibodies or pa-tient refusal early hysterectomy may be lifesaving and should be strongly considered.

REFERENCES

1. Lu MC, Fridman M, Korst LM, et al. Variations in the incidence of postpartum hemorrhage across hospitals in California. Matern Child Health J 2005;9(3): 297–306.
2. Sheiner E, Sarid L, Levy A, et al. Obstetric risk factors and outcome of pregnan-cies complicated with early postpartum hemorrhage: a population-based study. J Matern Fetal Neonatal Med 2005;18(3):149–54.
3. Oxford CM, Ludmir J. Trauma in pregnancy. Clin Obstet Gynecol 2009;52(4): 611–29.
4. Asakura H. Classifying types of disseminated intravascular coagulation: clinical and animal models. J Intensive Care 2014;2(1):20, 0492-2-20. [eCollection: 2014].
5. Taylor FB Jr, Toh CH, Hoots WK, et al, Scientific Subcommittee on Disseminated Intravascular Coagulation (DIC) of the International Society on Thrombosis and Haemostasis (ISTH). Towards definition, clinical and laboratory criteria, and a scoring system for disseminated intravascular coagulation. Thromb Haemost 2001;86(5):1327–30.
6. Wada H, Matsumoto T, Yamashita Y. Diagnosis and treatment of disseminated intravascular coagulation (DIC) according to four DIC guidelines. J Intensive Care 2014;2(1):15, 0492-2-15. [eCollection: 2014].
7. Creanga AA, Berg CJ, Ko JY, et al. Maternal mortality and morbidity in the United States: where are we now? J Womens Health (Larchmt) 2014;23(1):3–9.
8. Creanga AA, Berg CJ, Syverson C, et al. Pregnancy-related mortality in the United States, 2006-2010. Obstet Gynecol 2015;125(1):5–12.
9. Cunningham FG, Nelson DB. Disseminated intravascular coagulation syndromes in obstetrics. Obstet Gynecol 2015;126(5):999–1011.
10. Abbassi-Ghanavati M, Greer LG, Cunningham FG. Pregnancy and laboratory studies: a reference table for clinicians. Obstet Gynecol 2009;114(6):1326–31.
11. American College of Surgeons Committee on Trauma, editor. Advanced trauma life support: student course manual. 8th edition. Chicago: Third Impression; 2008.

12. American College of Obstetricians and Gynecologists. ACOG practice bulletin: Clinical management guidelines for obstetrician-gynecologists number 76, October 2006: postpartum hemorrhage. Obstet Gynecol 2006;108(4):1039–47.

13. Mousa HA, Cording V, Alfirevic Z. Risk factors and interventions associated with major primary postpartum hemorrhage unresponsive to first-line conventional therapy. Acta Obstet Gynecol Scand 2008;87(6):652–61.

14. Hofmeyr GJ, Gulmezoglu AM, Novikova N, et al. Misoprostol to prevent and treat postpartum haemorrhage: a systematic review and meta-analysis of maternal deaths and dose-related effects. Bull World Health Organ 2009;87(9):666–77.

15. Hofmeyr GJ, Gulmezoglu AM, Novikova N, et al. Postpartum misoprostol for preventing maternal mortality and morbidity. Cochrane Database Syst Rev 2013;7: CD008982.

16. Belfort MA, Dildy GA, Garrido J, et al. Intraluminal pressure in a uterine tamponade balloon is curvilinearly related to the volume of fluid infused. Am J Perinatol 2011;28(8):659–66.

17. Sentilhes L, Gromez A, Clavier E, et al. Predictors of failed pelvic arterial embolization for severe postpartum hemorrhage. Obstet Gynecol 2009;113(5):992–9.

18. Poujade O, Zappa M, Letendre I, et al. Predictive factors for failure of pelvic arterial embolization for postpartum hemorrhage. Int J Gynaecol Obstet 2012;117(2): 119–23.

19. Bros S, Chabrot P, Kastler A, et al. Recurrent bleeding within 24 hours after uterine artery embolization for severe postpartum hemorrhage: are there predictive factors? Cardiovasc Intervent Radiol 2012;35(3):508–14.

20. Kim YJ, Yoon CJ, Seong NJ, et al. Failed pelvic arterial embolization for postpartum hemorrhage: clinical outcomes and predictive factors. J Vasc Interv Radiol 2013;24(5):703–9.

21. Malone DL, Hess JR, Fingerhut A. Massive transfusion practices around the globe and a suggestion for a common massive transfusion protocol. J Trauma 2006;60(6 Suppl):S91–6.

22. Burtelow M, Riley E, Druzin M, et al. How we treat: management of life-threatening primary postpartum hemorrhage with a standardized massive transfusion protocol. Transfusion 2007;47(9):1564–72.

23. Callum JL, Karkouti K, Lin Y. Cryoprecipitate: the current state of knowledge. Transfus Med Rev 2009;23(3):177–88.

24. Holcomb JB, Tilley BC, Baraniuk S, et al. Transfusion of plasma, platelets, and red blood cells in a 1:1:1 vs a 1:1:2 ratio and mortality in patients with severe trauma: the PROPPR randomized clinical trial. JAMA 2015;313(5):471–82.

25. Ho KM, Leonard AD. Concentration-dependent effect of hypocalcaemia on mortality of patients with critical bleeding requiring massive transfusion: a cohort study. Anaesth Intensive Care 2011;39(1):46–54.

26. Elmer J, Wilcox SR, Raja AS. Massive transfusion in traumatic shock. J Emerg Med 2013;44(4):829–38.

27. Sharma S, Uprichard J, Moretti A, et al. Use of thromboelastography to assess the combined role of pregnancy and obesity on coagulation: a prospective study. Int J Obstet Anesth 2013;22(2):113–8.

28. Sharma SK, Philip J. The effect of anesthetic techniques on blood coagulability in parturients as measured by thromboelastography. Anesth Analg 1997;85(1):82–6.

29. Whiting D, DiNardo JA. TEG and ROTEM: technology and clinical applications. Am J Hematol 2014;89(2):228–32.

30. Roberts I, Shakur H, Coats T, et al. The CRASH-2 trial: a randomised controlled trial and economic evaluation of the effects of tranexamic acid on death, vascular

occlusive events and transfusion requirement in bleeding trauma patients. Health Technol Assess 2013;17(10):1–79.

31. Roberts I, Prieto-Merino D, Manno D. Mechanism of action of tranexamic acid in bleeding trauma patients: an exploratory analysis of data from the CRASH-2 trial. Crit Care 2014;18(6):685, 014-0685-8.

32. Ducloy-Bouthors AS, Jude B, Duhamel A, et al. High-dose tranexamic acid reduces blood loss in postpartum haemorrhage. Crit Care 2011;15(2):R117.

33. Hedner U, Ingerslev J. Clinical use of recombinant FVIIa (rFVIIa). Transfus Sci 1998;19(2):163–76.

34. Shapiro AD, Gilchrist GS, Hoots WK, et al. Prospective, randomised trial of two doses of rFVIIa (NovoSeven) in haemophilia patients with inhibitors undergoing surgery. Thromb Haemost 1998;80(5):773–8.

35. Martinowitz U, Kenet G, Segal E, et al. Recombinant activated factor VII for adjunctive hemorrhage control in trauma. J Trauma 2001;51(3):431–8 [discussion: 438–9].

36. Franchini M, Lippi G, Franchi M. The use of recombinant activated factor VII in obstetric and gynaecological haemorrhage. BJOG 2007;114(1):8–15.

37. Phillips LE, McLintock C, Pollock W, et al. Recombinant activated factor VII in obstetric hemorrhage: experiences from the Australian and New Zealand haemostasis registry. Anesth Analg 2009;109(6):1908–15.

38. Segal S, Shemesh IY, Blumenthal R, et al. Treatment of obstetric hemorrhage with recombinant activated factor VII (rFVIIa). Arch Gynecol Obstet 2003;268(4):266–7.

39. Lavigne-Lissalde G, Aya AG, Mercier FJ, et al. Recombinant human FVIIa for reducing the need for invasive second-line therapies in severe refractory postpartum hemorrhage: a multicenter, randomized, open controlled trial. J Thromb Haemost 2015;13(4):520–9.

40. Rossaint R, Bouillon B, Cerny V, et al. Management of bleeding following major trauma: an updated European guideline. Crit Care 2010;14(2):R52.

41. Samama CM. Prothrombin complex concentrates: a brief review. Eur J Anaesthesiol 2008;25(10):784–9.

42. McSwain N Jr, Barbeau J. Potential use of prothrombin complex concentrate in trauma resuscitation. J Trauma 2011;70(5 Suppl):S53–6.

43. Ekelund K, Hanke G, Stensballe J, et al. Hemostatic resuscitation in postpartum hemorrhage - a supplement to surgery. Acta Obstet Gynecol Scand 2015;94(7):680–92.

44. American College of Obstetricians and Gynecologists, Task Force on Hypertension in Pregnancy. Hypertension in pregnancy. Report of the American College of Obstetricians and Gynecologists' Task Force on Hypertension in Pregnancy. Obstet Gynecol 2013;122:1122–31.

45. Audibert F, Friedman SA, Frangieh AY, et al. Clinical utility of strict diagnostic criteria for the HELLP (hemolysis, elevated liver enzymes, and low platelets) syndrome. Am J Obstet Gynecol 1996;175(2):460–4.

46. Haram K, Svendsen E, Abildgaard U. The HELLP syndrome: clinical issues and management. A review. BMC Pregnancy Childbirth 2009;9:8, 2393-9-8.

47. Magann EF, Martin JN Jr. Twelve steps to optimal management of HELLP syndrome. Clin Obstet Gynecol 1999;42(3):532–50.

48. Merchant SH, Mathew P, Vanderjagt TJ, et al. Recombinant factor VIIa in management of spontaneous subcapsular liver hematoma associated with pregnancy. Obstet Gynecol 2004;103(5 Pt 2):1055–8.

49. Pauzner R, Dulitzky M, Carp H, et al. Hepatic infarctions during pregnancy are associated with the antiphospholipid syndrome and in addition with complete or incomplete HELLP syndrome. J Thromb Haemost 2003;1(8):1758–63.

50. George JN. Clinical practice. Thrombotic thrombocytopenic purpura. N Engl J Med 2006;354(18):1927–35.

51. Martin JN Jr, Bailey AP, Rehberg JF, et al. Thrombotic thrombocytopenic purpura in 166 pregnancies: 1955-2006. Am J Obstet Gynecol 2008;199(2):98–104.

52. McCarthy LJ, Dlott JS, Orazi A, et al. Thrombotic thrombocytopenic purpura: yesterday, today, tomorrow. Ther Apher Dial 2004;8(2):80–6.

53. Fakhouri F, Roumenina L, Provot F, et al. Pregnancy-associated hemolytic uremic syndrome revisited in the era of complement gene mutations. J Am Soc Nephrol 2010;21(5):859–67.

54. Noris M, Caprioli J, Bresin E, et al. Relative role of genetic complement abnormalities in sporadic and familial aHUS and their impact on clinical phenotype. Clin J Am Soc Nephrol 2010;5(10):1844–59.

55. Salmon JE, Heuser C, Triebwasser M, et al. Mutations in complement regulatory proteins predispose to preeclampsia: a genetic analysis of the PROMISSE cohort. PLoS Med 2011;8(3):e1001013.

56. Legendre CM, Licht C, Muus P, et al. Terminal complement inhibitor eculizumab in atypical hemolytic-uremic syndrome. N Engl J Med 2013;368(23):2169–81.

57. Castro MA, Goodwin TM, Shaw KJ, et al. Disseminated intravascular coagulation and antithrombin III depression in acute fatty liver of pregnancy. Am J Obstet Gynecol 1996;174(1 Pt 1):211–6.

58. Treem WR, Rinaldo P, Hale DE, et al. Acute fatty liver of pregnancy and long-chain 3-hydroxyacyl-coenzyme a dehydrogenase deficiency. Hepatology 1994;19(2):339–45.

59. Wilcken B, Leung KC, Hammond J, et al. Pregnancy and fetal long-chain 3-hydroxyacyl coenzyme a dehydrogenase deficiency. Lancet 1993;341(8842):407–8.

60. Browning MF, Levy HL, Wilkins-Haug LE, et al. Fetal fatty acid oxidation defects and maternal liver disease in pregnancy. Obstet Gynecol 2006;107(1):115–20.

61. Nelson DB, Yost NP, Cunningham FG. Hemostatic dysfunction with acute fatty liver of pregnancy. Obstet Gynecol 2014;124(1):40–6.

62. Currie J, Ridout AE, Bhangu N, et al. Maternal mortality and serious maternal morbidity in Jehovah's witnesses in the Netherlands. BJOG 2009;116(13):1822–3 [author reply: 1823].

63. Kidson-Gerber G, Kerridge I, Farmer S, et al. Caring for pregnant women for whom transfusion is not an option. a national review to assist in patient care. Aust N Z J Obstet Gynaecol 2016;56(2):127–36.

64. Graffeo C, Dishong W. Severe blood loss anemia in a Jehovah's witness treated with adjunctive hyperbaric oxygen therapy. Am J Emerg Med 2013;31(4):756.e3-4.

Management of Hypertensive Crisis for the Obstetrician/Gynecologist

 CrossMark

Jamil ElFarra, MD*, Cynthia Bean, MD,
James N. Martin Jr, MD, FRCOG

KEYWORDS

- Hypertension • Pregnancy • Hypertensive crisis • Hypertensive urgency/emergency
- Preeclampsia • Eclampsia • HELLP syndrome • Pregnancy safety bundles

KEY POINTS

- Systolic blood pressure greater than 160 mm Hg is associated with many adverse maternal outcomes, such as stroke and pulmonary edema.
- Blood pressure measurements greater than or equal to 160/110 mm Hg lasting longer than 15 minutes warrant immediate medical therapy.
- Hydralazine, labetalol, and nifedipine are currently considered first-line treatment options for the emergent reduction of blood pressure in pregnancy.
- Early maternal warning signs, such as a systolic blood pressure greater than 160 mm Hg, tachycardia, and oliguria, allow timely diagnostic and therapeutic interventions.
- Health care providers taking care of obstetric patients should familiarize themselves with the most updated classifications and management of hypertensive disorders of pregnancy.

INTRODUCTION

Hypertensive disorders of pregnancy are considered among the leading causes of maternal and fetal morbidity and mortality. Complicating approximately 10% of pregnancies, they are responsible for an estimated 50,000 to 60,000 preeclampsia-related deaths per year worldwide, many of which are preventable.[1–7]

In pregnancy, irrespective of the underlying cause, a blood pressure measurement greater than or equal to 160/110 mm Hg persisting for more than 15 minutes is considered an obstetric emergency. This condition warrants immediate attention and prompt appropriate therapy.[1,5,8] Medical professionals taking care of obstetric patients must

Disclosure: The authors have nothing to disclose.
Department of Maternal Fetal Medicine, Winfred L. Wiser Hospital for Women and Infants, The University of Mississippi Medical Center, 2500 N State Street, Jackson, MS 30216, USA
* Corresponding author.
E-mail address: jelfarra@umc.edu

Obstet Gynecol Clin N Am 43 (2016) 623–637
http://dx.doi.org/10.1016/j.ogc.2016.07.005
0889-8545/16/© 2016 Elsevier Inc. All rights reserved.

have a good understanding of maternal physiology, as well as the classification and management of hypertensive disorders encountered during pregnancy and the puerperium. They should also be familiar and comfortable with the most up-to-date and evidence-based guidelines. Adherence to these guidelines is of paramount importance, because it has been shown in numerous studies to reduce the incidence of adverse maternal and fetal outcomes. The improvement in maternal outcomes is mainly secondary to a reduction in cerebral and respiratory complications.[1,5,7–11] Prompt medical treatment is extremely important in cases of hypertensive urgency/ crisis because the timing of initiation of therapy can alter morbidity and mortality risk.

WHY ARE HYPERTENSIVE DISORDERS IN PREGNANT AND POSTPARTUM PATIENTS IMPORTANT?

Hypertensive disorders are a leading cause of preventable maternal and fetal morbidity and mortality. Hypertensive disorders in pregnancy are often complex, and usually involve multiple organ systems and may be related to the secondary causes. Optimizing blood pressure remains of paramount importance, especially the control of systolic pressure, given its direct association with stroke and pulmonary edema.[1,5,7,11] However, treatment and management go beyond controlling the blood pressure. The entire disease spectrum needs to be taken into consideration to achieve desired outcomes and avoidance of complications. Optimal delivery timing needs to be considered as well as the treatment of any underlying disorder when applicable. Treatment with other necessary medications, such as betamethasone and magnesium sulfate, to prepare the fetus for delivery or to stabilize the mother must also accompany blood pressure control.[1,5]

COMMON COMPLICATIONS ASSOCIATED WITH HYPERTENSIVE DISORDERS OF PREGNANCY

These complications can be divided into maternal and fetal types and include[1,2,5,12–16]:

Maternal
- Increased risk of:
  - Hemorrhagic stroke
  - Pulmonary edema
  - Acute renal failure or accelerated end-organ damage
  - Gestational diabetes
  - Heart failure/cardiopulmonary decompensation
  - Hypertensive encephalopathy
  - Retinopathy
  - Cesarean delivery
  - Postpartum hemorrhage
  - Maternal mortality

Fetal
- Increased risk of:
  - Abruptio placenta
  - Fetal growth restriction (intrauterine growth restriction [IUGR])
  - Preterm delivery
  - Intrauterine fetal demise
  - Perinatal mortality
  - Complications of prematurity
  - Potential teratogen exposure from hypertensive medications

DEFINITION OF HYPERTENSION IN PREGNANCY

Hypertensive disorders in pregnancy can be classified according to the degree of blood pressure increase (**Table 1**).[1,2,5]

CLASSIFICATION OF HYPERTENSIVE DISORDERS OF PREGNANCY

Hypertensive disorders of pregnancy can either precede pregnancy or be pregnancy specific (first encountered during pregnancy) and are classified as follows[1]:

Pregnancy specific
- Gestational hypertension:
  - Increase of blood pressure that is first encountered in pregnancy with absence of the diagnostic criteria for preeclampsia.
- Preeclampsia:
  - Increase of blood pressure with proteinuria or evidence of multisystem involvement fulfilling the diagnostic criteria for preeclampsia.
  - Preeclampsia is further divided into:
    - Preeclampsia without severe features
    - Preeclampsia with severe features
- Superimposed preeclampsia:
  - A chronic hypertensive patient who at some point in pregnancy has an escalation of the disease process fulfilling the diagnostic criteria for preeclampsia.
- Hemolysis, elevated liver enzymes, low platelet (HELLP) syndrome:
  - Specific form of preeclampsia/eclampsia that is characterized by the presence of:
    - Hemolysis
    - Increased liver enzyme level
    - Low platelet level
- Eclampsia:
  - The occurrence of new-onset grand mal seizures in a pregnant woman that cannot be attributed to another cause.

Gestational trophoblastic diseases and mirror syndrome are rare pregnancy-specific causes of hypertensive disorders of pregnancy. Usually they occur in the first

Table 1
Mild versus severe hypertension in pregnancy

Mild	Severe
Systolic blood pressure	Systolic blood pressure
• ≥140- <160 mm Hg	• ≥160 mm Hg
Or	Or
Diastolic blood pressure	Diastolic blood pressure
• ≥90 to <110 mm Hg.	• ≥110 mm Hg
Or increase in both	Or increase of both
• At least 2 increased blood pressure measurements	• Two severe blood pressure values taken 15–60 min apart
• Taken correctly	• Taken correctly
• At least 4 h apart	• Severe values do not need to be consecutive
	• Persistent hypertension can occur antepartum, intrapartum, or postpartum
	• Treatment is recommended if severe-range blood pressure lasts more than 15 min

2 trimesters of pregnancy. Ultrasonography and human chorionic gonadotropin levels help differentiate them from other possible causes.[1,2]

Non–pregnancy specific
- Essential hypertension:
  - Blood pressure increase identified before pregnancy with no identifiable underlying cause.
- Secondary hypertension: (potentially curable):
  - Blood pressure increase with an identifiable secondary cause.
  - Includes conditions such as[1,2,17]:
    - Renal disease
    - Obstructive sleep apnea
    - Cushing syndrome
    - Renal artery stenosis
    - Pheochromocytoma
    - Coarctation of the aorta
    - Primary aldosteronism
    - Thyroid dysfunction
    - Lupus flare
    - Illicit drugs and medications
    - Cardiac causes
    - Adrenal disease

DEFINITIONS OF HYPERTENSIVE URGENCY/EMERGENCY/CRISIS IN NONPREGNANT VERSUS PREGNANT PATIENTS

The definition and diagnostic parameters of hypertension are similar in both pregnant and nonpregnant patients. However, a major difference lies in what constitutes a hypertensive crisis/urgency. In pregnancy and in the postpartum period (up to 6 weeks) asymptomatic or symptomatic increase of blood pressure greater than or equal to 160/110 mm Hg is considered an emergency that requires immediate evaluation and treatment.[1,5] Before pregnancy and beyond 6 weeks postpartum, when to immediately treat an asymptomatic patient with increased blood pressure remains a topic of controversy. However, most authorities agree that a systolic blood pressure of greater than 180 to 200 mm Hg and a diastolic blood pressure greater than 110 to 120 mm Hg warrants treatment. The major difference between hypertensive urgency and emergency is the symptoms and the susceptibility to intracranial hemorrhage at lower systolic blood pressures than nonpregnant and nonpostpartum patients. Patients with hypertensive emergency are usually symptomatic and have multisystem involvement with evidence of end-organ damage.[18]

WHAT IS THE PATHOPHYSIOLOGY OF HYPERTENSIVE CRISIS IN PREGNANT PATIENTS WITH PREECLAMPSIA?

The exact pathophysiology of hypertensive disorders and their interaction with various organ systems and blood biomarkers is complex and remains elusive. The disease process is thought to originate from some form of placental insult that leads to placental ischemia, which many clinicians consider the trigger for the disease process.[19–21]

Ischemia results in the release of a variety of placental factors, such as the soluble fms-like tyrosine kinase-1 (sFlt-1), the angiotensin II type-1 receptor autoantibody, and cytokines such as tumor necrosis factor alpha. These placental factors are thought to trigger widespread maternal vascular dysfunction.[19–21] The circulating levels of sFlt-1 have been shown to be proportionately increased in relation to maternal hypertension.[19–21]

BASIC EMERGENT LABORATORY EVALUATION AND IMAGING

New-onset hypertension in pregnancy, or worsening hypertension in a known hypertensive patient, is of great concern and warrants immediate attention and bedside evaluation. Once the initial evaluation is performed, appropriate laboratory evaluation and imaging as needed are initiated to determine the disease severity and diagnosis. Correct management is then guided based on the classification of the hypertensive disorder and its severity.

Initial laboratory evaluation includes[1,2]:

- Quantitative assessment of urine protein (ie, 12-hour or 24-hour urine collection or a protein/creatinine ratio)
- Renal function tests
- Complete blood count with platelet count
- Glucose
- Electrolytes
- Uric acid
- Liver enzymes

Depending on the degree of blood pressure increase, clinical assessment, symptoms, and laboratory evaluation, further laboratory tests or diagnostic imaging may be warranted, including[1,2]:

- Chest radiograph
  - Recommended in the presence of shortness of breath, decreased oxygen saturation, or abnormal pulmonary examination.
- Electrocardiogram (ECG) and possible echocardiogram
  - Recommended in presence of shortness of breath, decreased oxygen saturation, or abnormal cardiac examination.
  - If chest pain is present, cardiac enzymes may need to be checked.
- Thyroid-stimulating hormone
- Head imaging
  - Evaluation for intracranial hemorrhage, cerebral thrombosis, or posterior reversible encephalopathy syndrome.
  - MRI and computed tomography scan are usually the modalities of choice.
- Abdominal imaging
  - Recommended in the presence of persistent abdominal pain.
  - Useful in the diagnosis of liver hematoma.

TARGETS OF TREATMENT

The ultimate goal of treatment is to minimize both maternal and fetal risk, while safely guiding both the mother and fetus through pregnancy and beyond. Management decisions are altered based on the following factors[1,2,5,8,12]:

- Type of hypertensive disorder and underlying cause
- Gestational age
- Disease severity
- Severity of hypertension
- Maternal and fetal clinical status

- Maternal response to intervention
- Maternal comorbidities

Factors that can influence the occurrence of complications are varied and include[1,2,5,8,12]:

- Achieving the correct diagnosis
- Early identification of the highest risk patients
- Prompt and appropriate administration of medications
- Timing of delivery
- Compliance with prenatal care
- Correct and accurate gestational age
- Disease severity
- Other comorbidities (eg, diabetes mellitus, obesity)

The treatment targets should focus on the following areas:

1. Blood pressure control
2. Maternal well-being
3. Fetal well-being and delivery preparation

Blood Pressure Control

Blood pressure targets differ slightly for postpartum patients compared with undelivered mothers. A brief overview is summarized here:

Antepartum[1]:
- Reduce blood pressure to achieve ranges consistently below the severe range (<160/110 mm Hg) as so-called high-normal levels.
- Therapy should be given within 1 hour of persistent severe-range blood pressures (ideally within 15 minutes).
- Blood pressure should be reduced to approximately 140 to 150 over 90 to 100 mm Hg and not any lower to avoid hypoperfusion of the fetus and maternal organs.

Postpartum[1]:
- Therapy should be given within 1 hour of persistent severe-range blood pressures.
- Reduce blood pressure to achieve levels consistently less than 150/90 mm Hg.
- Blood pressure should be monitored closely for the first 72 hours postpartum.
- Outpatient surveillance should be considered for those discharged before 72 hours (eg, home nursing visit).
- Reevaluate the patient within 7 to 10 days of discharge.
- Avoid nonsteroidal antiinflammatory drugs in the hypertensive postpartum patient.

Blood pressure control is extremely important to reduce the adverse outcomes seen in hypertensive disorders in pregnancy and the postpartum period. One element of particular interest is the association between systolic blood pressure severity and stroke. In a study involving 28 patients who had strokes associated with hypertensive disorders of pregnancy, all but 1 had a systolic blood pressure in the severe range. In that same study, baseline maternal pulse pressure (the difference between systolic and diastolic pressure in millimeters of mercury) was doubled just before the occurrence of stroke.[11] The association between stroke and systolic hypertension has also been shown in studies outside of pregnancy.[22]

Maternal Well-Being

Maternal well-being is of utmost importance and outcomes can be improved by appropriate and timely intervention. Listed here are some key points that need to be taken into consideration when caring for hypertensive pregnant patients:

- Close observation of maternal vital signs, including oxygen saturation.
- Appropriate and timely treatment of hypertension.
- Appropriate laboratory evaluation and treatment as needed.
- Appropriate and timely administration of magnesium sulfate for seizure prophylaxis (magnesium sulfate is not used for blood pressure control).
- Strict input and output documentation.
- Appropriate use of imaging modalities.
- Appropriate transfer to the intensive care unit (ICU) when indicated.
- Transfer to a facility that has the necessary and appropriate level of care (adequate maternal and neonatal intensive care resources).
- Safe transport should be arranged when higher level of care is needed.
- Involvement of subspecialists when indicated.

Fetal Well-Being and Delivery Preparation

It is desirable to prolong the pregnancy as much as the maternal and fetal conditions allow in preterm patients. However, there are certain conditions when pregnancy prolongation is not possible. Fetal well-being needs to be periodically assessed using fetal surveillance tools such as the nonstress test and/or the biophysical profile. Once the maternal condition allows, detailed ultrasonography should be performed to help assess whether pregnancy prolongation is an option.

In order to potentially optimize neonatal outcomes, the following should be administered based on gestational age and likelihood of delivery within the next 72 hours[1]:

- Magnesium sulfate to help decrease the incidence of moderate to severe cerebral palsy if the gestational age is less than 32 weeks.[23,24]
- Corticosteroids from 24 to 34 weeks of gestation (may be considered at 23 weeks) to help enhance fetal lung maturity.[25]

ANTIHYPERTENSIVE MEDICATIONS IN PREGNANCY

In the continued absence of reliable noninvasive tests or biomarkers to identify hypertensive patients at immediate risk of adverse outcomes, blood pressure remains the most commonly gauged parameter and is the cornerstone that guides treatment.

The choice of antihypertensive medication in pregnancy depends on[1]:

- Pregnancy safety profile
- Urgent control versus long-term control
- Evidence-based guidelines/institutional policies
- Medicine availability
- Clinical scenario
- Patient-specific comorbidities and contraindications to certain medications
- Comfort level of provider
- Availability of intravenous (IV) access

There is a lack of quality pregnancy literature evaluating racial and ethnic variations in response to antihypertensive therapy. However, some literature outside of pregnancy suggests that ethnicity may play a role in response to treatment. For example, some studies have shown that African Americans are less responsive to β-blockers than white people. This finding should be taken in consideration when choosing therapy.[18,26]

Blood pressure control in pregnancy is divided into 2 stages. The first is directed at acute blood pressure control. The second is directed at long-term blood pressure control throughout the remainder of the pregnancy.

Immediate Control

- First-line pharmacologic therapy used in pregnancy for immediate/urgent control of blood pressure includes (**Fig. 1**)[1,5,27]:
  ○ Labetalol (IV)
  ○ Hydralazine (IV)
  ○ Nifedipine (oral)
- Second-line pharmacologic therapy used in pregnancy for immediate/urgent control of blood pressure includes[5,28]:
  ○ Esmolol
  ○ Nicardipine (infusion pump)
  ○ Labetalol (infusion pump)
  ○ Sodium nitroprusside

Sodium nitroprusside should be used as a last resort and for the shortest time possible because it can worsen maternal cerebral edema. There is also concern for maternal and fetal cyanate and thiocyanate toxicity.[5]

When second-line therapy is needed, it should be done in conjunction with a specialist (maternal-fetal medicine, anesthesia, internal medicine, or critical care).

Long-Term Control

- First-line pharmacologic therapy used in pregnancy for long-term control of hypertension in pregnancy[1,2]:
  ○ Methyldopa (oral)
  ○ Labetalol (oral)
  ○ Nifedipine (oral)
- Second-line therapy and ancillary medications:
  ○ Diuretics (thiazide diuretics)

Thiazide diuretics are generally considered safe to use in pregnancy. However, they should be used with caution secondary to the potential concern for intravascular volume depletion and hypokalemia.[1]

Drugs to Avoid in Pregnancy

1. Angiotensin-converting enzyme inhibitors[1,2,29]
2. Angiotensin receptor blockers

These drugs are known teratogens and are associated with fetal renal agenesis and dysfunction.

Commonly used antihypertensive medications include:

Methyldopa[1,30–32]
- Mechanism of action: central-acting alpha-2 adrenergic agonist.
- Use in pregnancy: long term only, not for immediate control of blood pressure (used for gradual blood pressure control).
- Dose: 0.5 to 3 g/d by mouth 2 to 3 times daily. Maximum dose 3 g/d.

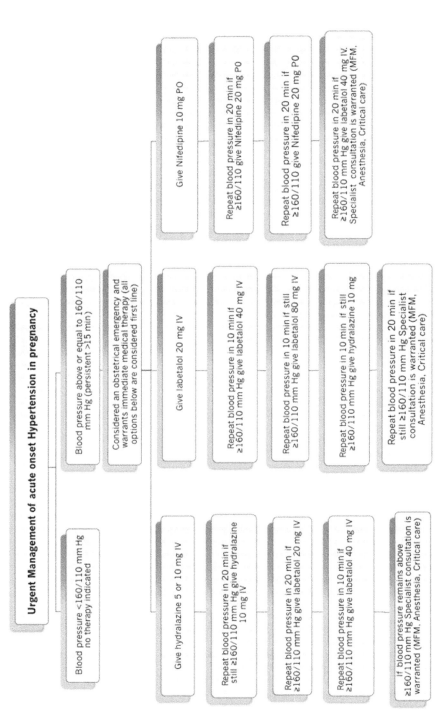

Fig. 1. Acute management of severe pregnancy-associated hypertension. MFM, maternal fetal medicine specialist. (*Data from* American College of Obstetrics and Gynecology Committee opinion no. 623: emergent therapy for acute-onset, severe hypertension during pregnancy and the postpartum period. Obstet Gynecol 2015;125(2):521–5.)

- Side effects:
  - Fetal: no known fetal adverse effects. There are long-term postdelivery data up to 7 years of age.
  - Maternal: hepatic dysfunction and necrosis, hemolytic anemia.
- Comments:
  - May be less effective in controlling severe-range blood pressures than the other commonly used medications.

Labetalol[1,2,5,27,33–36]

- Mechanism of action: combined α-blocker and β-blocker.
- Use in pregnancy: can be used for both immediate and long-term control of blood pressure.
- Dose:
  - Immediate control: 20, 40, 80 mg IV given every 10 minutes as needed over a 20-minute period (maximum dose, 300 mg IV). Can give 200 mg orally if unable to achieve IV access. Can also be used as an infusion at a rate of 1 to 2 mg/min IV (second line).
  - Long-term control: 2 to 3 doses divided daily with a daily maximum of 2400 mg.
- Side effects:
  - Fetal: possible concern of IUGR (contradictory and inconclusive evidence).
  - Maternal: bronchoconstriction, heart block, orthostatic hypotension, sleep disturbances, fatigue, bradycardia.
- Comments:
  - Avoid in patients with asthma, heart disease, congestive heart failure, or if the maternal heart rate is less than 60 beats/min.

Nifedipine[1,5,27,37]

- Mechanism of action: calcium channel blocker.
- Use in pregnancy: can be used for immediate and long-term control of blood pressure.
- Dose:
  - Immediate control: 10, 20, 20 mg orally respectively every 20 minutes if blood pressure is still in the severe range (see **Fig. 1**).
  - Long-term control: 30 to 120 mg daily dose of the extended release preparation.
- Side effects: hypotension, headache, reflex tachycardia.
- Comments: should be used with caution in patients receiving magnesium sulfate because there is a theoretic risk of hypotension and neuromuscular blockade when combined.

Hydralazine[1,2,5,13,27,36]

- Mechanism of action: peripheral vasodilator.
- Use in pregnancy: urgent control of blood pressure.
- Dose: 5 to 10 mg IV over 2 minutes repeated every 20 minutes with a single cumulative dose of a maximum of 20 mg (after that, switching to another agent is recommended).
- Side effects: maternal hypotension, reflex tachycardia, vomiting, headache, and aggravation of angina pectoris.

MATERNAL EARLY WARNING CRITERIA

The National Partnership for Maternal Safety defined a list of abnormal parameters (**Box 1**) that require immediate bedside evaluation by a health care provider. The

> **Box 1**
> **Maternal early warning criteria**
>
> - Systolic blood pressure of less than 90 or greater than 160 mm Hg
>
> - Diastolic blood pressure of greater than 100 mm Hg
>
> - Heart rate less than 50 or greater than 130 beats per minute
>
> - Oxygen saturation on room air, at sea level less than 95%
>
> - Oliguria (<35 mL/h for 2 hours or more)
>
> - Maternal agitation, confusion, or unresponsiveness (changed mental status)
>
> - Nonremitting headache in patients with hypertensive disease of pregnancy
>
> - Shortness of breath
>
> *Modified from* Mhyre JM, D'Oria R, Hameed AB, et al. The maternal early warning criteria: a proposal from the National Partnership for Maternal Safety. J Obstet Gynecol Neonatal Nurs 2014;43(6):773; with permission.

aim of these early warning parameters is to provide timely diagnostic and therapeutic interventions and enhance quality of care.[38,39]

STRATEGIES TO IMPROVE MATERNAL AND FETAL OUTCOMES

Early recognition, timely and appropriate intervention, and adherence to guidelines serve as the foundation for achieving optimal and quality care for mothers and fetuses. Implementation of nationwide or institutional guidelines in the United States, United Kingdom, and Canada has shown a decline in complication rates caused by hypertensive disorders.[7,40–43] Some suggested strategies for consideration to reduce the rate of potential preventable complications are as follows[8,39]:

- Introduction of hospital-wide early warning criteria (including the emergency department) for obstetric patients.
- Guidelines to mandate immediate bedside assessment by an appropriate health care provider if any of the early warning criteria are met (any team member taking care of the patient should be able to escalate).
- Staff training regarding the proper measurement of blood pressure in patients.
- Administration of appropriate antihypertensive medication in a timely fashion in patients with persistent severe-range blood pressures (≥160/110 mm Hg).
- Establish institution-wide/hospital-wide evidence-based guidelines and protocols for management of hypertensive disorders of pregnancy.
- Introducing checklists or order sets to standardize management by all providers.
- Periodic drills and simulations for all members of the obstetric team with debriefings and feedbacks.
- Debriefings and team meetings after poor/adverse outcomes or near misses to help avoid these events in the future.
- Early and appropriate involvement of subspecialist care, including maternal-fetal medicine specialists, anesthesia, internal medicine, nephrology, hematology, critical care, and so forth, as needed.

MANAGEMENT BEYOND BLOOD PRESSURE CONTROL

Once the blood pressure has been reduced to target range, a more thorough and detailed evaluation can be undertaken. Management is dictated by the information obtained and ultimately the final diagnosis.

Transfer to the ICU may be indicated in certain patients with a hypertensive disorder of pregnancy either in the antenatal or postpartum period. Such decisions are made collectively as a team and are based on the stability of the patient, physical examination, vital signs, laboratory values, imaging, and degree of anticipated level of care needed. Another determining factor is the level of care available at a local level. If clinically possible, fetal monitoring should be undertaken in certain ICU patients. In the presence of any of the following factors, strong consideration should be given to critical care transfer for the patient to receive a higher level of care.[44,45]

- Need for respiratory support and possible intubation.
- Vital sign abnormalities, such as a heart rate greater than 150 beats/min or less than 40 beats/min.
- Tachypnea (respiratory rate >35/min).
- Patients with acid-base imbalance or severe electrolyte abnormalities.
- Need for pressor support or other forms of cardiovascular support.
- Need for more invasive monitoring, such as pulmonary artery catheterization.
- Abnormal ECG findings, especially patients who require further intervention, such as cardioversion or defibrillation.
- Patients refractory to first-line hypertensive medications who require a drip.

Once a diagnosis is made, management is tailored to that specific diagnosis, including the use of other medications. Optimal timing of delivery is decided by multiple factors, including fetal well-being, gestational age, and type of hypertensive disorders. Some hypertensive disorders of pregnancy can potentially be managed expectantly, like preeclampsia, without severe features, whereas others, like eclampsia, require delivery soon after maternal stabilization.

The following points are reemphasized as critically important concepts and components of high-risk pregnancy and postpartum care for hypertensive patients:

- Maternal hypertensive disorders are among the leading causes of maternal and fetal morbidity and mortality.
- Systolic blood pressure greater than 160 mm Hg is associated with many adverse maternal outcomes, such as stroke and pulmonary edema.
- Early recognition and prompt appropriate treatment are essential.
- Blood pressure measurements greater than or equal to 160/110 mm Hg lasting longer than 15 minutes warrant immediate medical therapy.
- Hydralazine, labetalol, and nifedipine are currently considered first-line treatment options for the emergent reduction of blood pressure in pregnancy.
- Methyldopa is not used for urgent reduction of blood pressure.
- Magnesium sulfate is not recommended for use as an antihypertensive agent.
- If first-line treatments fail to reduce blood pressure, then consultation with a specialist is warranted.
- Early maternal warning signs, such as a systolic blood pressure greater than 160 mm Hg, tachycardia, and oliguria, allow timely diagnostic and therapeutic interventions.
- Following evidence-based guidelines has shown a reduction in the incidence of preventable morbidity and mortality.

Health care providers taking care of obstetric patients should familiarize themselves with the most updated classifications and management of hypertensive disorders of pregnancy.

REFERENCES

1. American College of Obstetricians and Gynecologists, Task Force on Hypertension in Pregnancy. Hypertension in pregnancy. Report of the American College of Obstetricians and Gynecologists' Task Force on hypertension in pregnancy. Obstet Gynecol 2013;122(5):1122–31.
2. Creasy RK, et al. Creasy and Resnik's maternal-fetal medicine: principles and practice. p. 1 online resource.
3. World Health Organization. The world health report: 2005: make every mother and child count. Geneva (Switzerland): WHO; 2005. Available at: http://www.who.int/whr/2005/whr2005_en.pdf.
4. Duley L. Maternal mortality associated with hypertensive disorders of pregnancy in Africa, Asia, Latin America and the Caribbean. Br J Obstet Gynaecol 1992;99(7):547–53.
5. Committee on Obstetric Practice. Committee opinion no. 623: emergent therapy for acute-onset, severe hypertension during pregnancy and the postpartum period. Obstet Gynecol 2015;125(2):521–5.
6. Stevens TA, Swaim LS, Clark SL. The role of obstetrics/gynecology hospitalists in reducing maternal mortality. Obstet Gynecol Clin North Am 2015;42(3):463–75.
7. Cantwell R, Clutton-Brock T, Cooper G, et al. Saving mothers' lives: reviewing maternal deaths to make motherhood safer: 2006-2008. The eighth report of the Confidential Enquiries into Maternal Deaths in the United Kingdom. BJOG 2011;118(Suppl 1):1–203.
8. Martin JN Jr. Severe systolic hypertension and the search for safer motherhood. Semin Perinatol 2016;40(2):119–23.
9. Menzies J, Magee LA, Li J, et al. Instituting surveillance guidelines and adverse outcomes in preeclampsia. Obstet Gynecol 2007;110(1):121–7.
10. von Dadelszen P, Sawchuck D, McMaster R, et al. The active implementation of pregnancy hypertension guidelines in British Columbia. Obstet Gynecol 2010;116(3):659–66.
11. Martin JN Jr, Thigpen BD, Moore RC, et al. Stroke and severe preeclampsia and eclampsia: a paradigm shift focusing on systolic blood pressure. Obstet Gynecol 2005;105(2):246–54.
12. Sibai BM. Chronic hypertension in pregnancy. Obstet Gynecol 2002;100(2):369–77.
13. Alexander JM, Wilson KL. Hypertensive emergencies of pregnancy. Obstet Gynecol Clin North Am 2013;40(1):89–101.
14. Sibai BM, Anderson GD. Pregnancy outcome of intensive therapy in severe hypertension in first trimester. Obstet Gynecol 1986;67(4):517–22.
15. Zetterstrom K, Lindeberg SN, Haglund B, et al. Maternal complications in women with chronic hypertension: a population-based cohort study. Acta Obstet Gynecol Scand 2005;84(5):419–24.
16. Vanek M, Sheiner E, Levy A, et al. Chronic hypertension and the risk for adverse pregnancy outcome after superimposed pre-eclampsia. Int J Gynaecol Obstet 2004;86(1):7–11.
17. Viera AJ, Neutze DM. Diagnosis of secondary hypertension: an age-based approach. Am Fam Physician 2010;82(12):1471–8.
18. Izzo JL, Sica DA, Black HR. Hypertension primer [the essentials of high blood pressure: basic science, population science, and clinical management]. Philadelphia: Lippincott Williams & Wilkins; 2008. p. 1 [online resource (xxix, 610 p)].

19. LaMarca BD, Alexander BT, Gilbert JS, et al. Pathophysiology of hypertension in response to placental ischemia during pregnancy: a central role for endothelin? Gend Med 2008;5(Suppl A):S133–8.

20. Murphy SR, LaMarca BB, Cockrell K, et al. Role of endothelin in mediating soluble fms-like tyrosine kinase 1-induced hypertension in pregnant rats. Hypertension 2010;55(2):394–8.

21. LaMarca BD, Gilbert J, Granger JP. Recent progress toward the understanding of the pathophysiology of hypertension during preeclampsia. Hypertension 2008; 51(4):982–8.

22. Lindenstrom E, Boysen G, Nyboe J. Influence of systolic and diastolic blood pressure on stroke risk: a prospective observational study. Am J Epidemiol 1995; 142(12):1279–90.

23. Committee opinion no 652: magnesium sulfate use in obstetrics. Obstet Gynecol 2016;127(1):e52–3.

24. American College of Obstetricians and Gynecologists Committee on Obstetric Practice, Society for Maternal-Fetal Medicine. Committee opinion no. 455: magnesium sulfate before anticipated preterm birth for neuroprotection. Obstet Gynecol 2010;115(3):669–71.

25. American College of Obstetricians and Gynecologists, Society for Maternal-Fetal Medicine. ACOG obstetric care consensus no. 3: periviable birth. Obstet Gynecol 2015;126(5):e82–94.

26. ALLHAT Officers and Coordinators for the ALLHAT Collaborative Research Group, The Antihypertensive and Lipid-Lowering Treatment to Prevent Heart Attack Trial. Major outcomes in high-risk hypertensive patients randomized to angiotensin-converting enzyme inhibitor or calcium channel blocker vs diuretic: The Antihypertensive and Lipid-Lowering Treatment to Prevent Heart Attack Trial (ALLHAT). JAMA 2002;288(23):2981–97.

27. Rezaei Z, Sharbaf FR, Pourmojieb M, et al. Comparison of the efficacy of nifedipine and hydralazine in hypertensive crisis in pregnancy. Acta Med Iran 2011; 49(11):701–6.

28. Too GT, Hill JB. Hypertensive crisis during pregnancy and postpartum period. Semin Perinatol 2013;37(4):280–7.

29. Rosa FW, Bosco LA, Graham CF, et al. Neonatal anuria with maternal angiotensin-converting enzyme inhibition. Obstet Gynecol 1989;74(3 Pt 1):371–4.

30. Redman CW, Beilin LJ, Bonnar J. Treatment of hypertension in pregnancy with methyldopa: blood pressure control and side effects. Br J Obstet Gynaecol 1977;84(6):419–26.

31. Ounsted M, Cockburn J, Moar VA, et al. Maternal hypertension with superimposed pre-eclampsia: effects on child development at 71/2 years. Br J Obstet Gynaecol 1983;90(7):644–9.

32. American Society of Hospital Pharmacists. AHFS drug information. Bethesda (MD): Authority of the Board of Directors of the American Society of Hospital Pharmacists; 1989.

33. Plouin PF, Breart G, Maillard F, et al. Comparison of antihypertensive efficacy and perinatal safety of labetalol and methyldopa in the treatment of hypertension in pregnancy: a randomized controlled trial. Br J Obstet Gynaecol 1988;95(9): 868–76.

34. Pickles CJ, Symonds EM, Broughton Pipkin F. The fetal outcome in a randomized double-blind controlled trial of labetalol versus placebo in pregnancy-induced hypertension. Br J Obstet Gynaecol 1989;96(1):38–43.

35. Magee LA, von Dadelszen P. The management of severe hypertension. Semin Perinatol 2009;33(3):138–42.
36. Magee LA, Cham C, Waterman EJ, et al. Hydralazine for treatment of severe hypertension in pregnancy: meta-analysis. BMJ 2003;327(7421):955–60.
37. Magee LA, Miremadi S, Li J, et al. Therapy with both magnesium sulfate and nifedipine does not increase the risk of serious magnesium-related maternal side effects in women with preeclampsia. Am J Obstet Gynecol 2005;193(1): 153–63.
38. D'Alton ME, Main EK, Menard MK, et al. The National Partnership for Maternal Safety. Obstet Gynecol 2014;123(5):973–7.
39. Mhyre JM, D'Oria R, Hameed AB, et al. The maternal early warning criteria: a proposal from the National Partnership for Maternal Safety. J Obstet Gynecol Neonatal Nurs 2014;43(6):771–9.
40. Magee LA, Helewa M, Moutquin JM, et al. Diagnosis, evaluation, and management of the hypertensive disorders of pregnancy. J Obstet Gynaecol Can 2008;30(3 Suppl):S1–48.
41. Magee LA, Pels A, Helewa M, et al. Diagnosis, evaluation, and management of the hypertensive disorders of pregnancy: executive summary. J Obstet Gynaecol Can 2014;36(7):575–6.
42. Clark SL, Christmas JT, Frye DR, et al. Maternal mortality in the United States: predictability and the impact of protocols on fatal postcesarean pulmonary embolism and hypertension-related intracranial hemorrhage. Am J Obstet Gynecol 2014;211(1):32.e1-9.
43. Clark SL, Hankins GD. Preventing maternal death: 10 clinical diamonds. Obstet Gynecol 2012;119(2 Pt 1):360–4.
44. Practice bulletin no. 158: critical care in pregnancy. Obstet Gynecol 2016;127(1): e21–8.
45. Guidelines for intensive care unit admission, discharge, and triage. Task Force of the American College of Critical Care Medicine, Society of Critical Care Medicine. Crit Care Med 1999;27(3):633–8.

Management of Infection for the Obstetrician/ Gynecologist

Catherine Eppes, MD, MPH

KEYWORDS

• Pregnancy • Infection • HIV • Influenza • Congenital infection

KEY POINTS

- Pregnant women have an increased morbidity and mortality for certain illnesses owing to the physiologic and immunologic changes in pregnancy.
- Certain infections are common during pregnancy, including urinary tract infections and pneumonia. Others are uncommon, but yield increased severity, including influenza.
- Human immunodeficiency virus, although it does not increase in pathogenesis during pregnancy, requires specific attention and management in the context of pregnancy.

INTRODUCTION

Pregnant women have an increased morbidity and mortality for certain illnesses owing to the physiologic and immunologic changes in pregnancy. These changes include alterations in the cardiopulmonary system, acid–base physiology, and immunologic response.

Immune System Changes

Immune system changes include a shift from T helper type 1 cell–mediated immunity, in favor of T helper type 2 humeral immunity.[1] This change creates susceptibility to certain type of infections, including intracellular pathogens such as viral infections or toxoplasmosis.

Cardiopulmonary Changes

Owing to changes in the elevation of the diaphragm related to the gravid uterus, pregnant women's total lung capacity, expiratory residual volume, and residual volume are decreased. They also have an increase in inspiratory capacity, and decreased total lung capacity. There is an increase in minute ventilation. And finally, there are cardiovascular changes that include increased heart rate, stroke volume, cardiac output,

The author has no disclosures.
Division of Maternal Fetal Medicine, Department of Obstetrics and Gynecology, Baylor College of Medicine, 1504 Taub Loop, 3rd Floor OB/Gyn, Houston, TX 77030, USA
E-mail address: Catherine.Eppes@bcm.edu

Obstet Gynecol Clin N Am 43 (2016) 639–657
http://dx.doi.org/10.1016/j.ogc.2016.07.009
0889-8545/16/© 2016 Elsevier Inc. All rights reserved.

and oxygen demand. All of these changes make women more susceptible to certain infections, obscure the diagnosis of sepsis, and decrease a pregnant women's ability to appropriately combat sepsis.[2]

Acid–Base Changes

The changes in the CO_2 baroreceptor lead to a respiratory alkalosis, and therefore a compensatory change in bicarbonate. Changes such as tissue ischemia or increase in acids such as lactate are poorly tolerated in gravidas owing to this decreased acid-buffering capacity.

HISTORICAL BACKGROUND

Studies have illustrated this increased susceptibility and morbidity found in pregnant women in relation to infectious diseases. Hartert and colleagues[3] looked at 297 pregnant women hospitalized for respiratory disease during 8 influenza seasons. The majority of these women have comorbid conditions, predominantly asthma. Seven women required intensive care unit admissions and 3 pregnancies resulted in fetal deaths. Cox and colleagues[4] looked 21,447 respiratory hospitalizations during influenza season, and found 3.4 in 1000 pregnancy hospitalizations were for respiratory illness. Of these hospitalizations, 30% included deliveries, and high-risk comorbidities such as cardiac or pulmonary disease were present in 23.5% of hospitalization. Those hospitalized with a respiratory illness had an odds ratio of 4.08 for preterm delivery, and 2.48 for fetal distress compared with pregnant women hospitalized for nonrespiratory illnesses.

Although these physiologic changes have an impact on maternal health and susceptibility, infections during this time also carry the novel risk of fetal or neonatal infections. Certain maternal illnesses, such as varicella, exist with only rare infectious risk to the fetus. However, others such as syphilis frequently cause congenital infections when not treated. Maternal infections can also lead to pregnancy complications, such as fetal growth restriction, preterm labor and/or delivery, and developmental abnormalities.

Recent infectious disease outbreaks have illustrated that pregnant women represent a unique subset of the population, for which specific attention and planning is necessary (**Fig. 1**). In 2000, one-fourth of those with laboratory confirmed severe respiratory distress syndrome in the United States were pregnant women, and those infected had high rates of mechanical ventilation, intensive care unit admissions, renal failure, disseminated intravascular coagulopathy, and death.[5] During the 2009 H1N1 pandemic, pregnant women represented 6% of cases of mortality, despite only making up 1% of the population.[6] Approximately 10% of pregnant women hospitalized with influenza-like illness were admitted to the intensive care unit.[7] The 2009 influenza pandemic was not a novel finding; previous influenza outbreaks including the pandemics of 1918 and 1957 demonstrated mortality rates from 27% to 51%.[8,9]

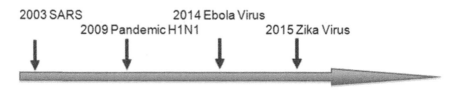

Fig. 1. Timeline with recent public health infectious disease outbreaks affecting pregnant women.

In 2014, West Africa drew international attention owing to the largest Ebola outbreak in history. During that outbreak 28,616 individuals were infected with Ebola.[10] Pregnant women and their fetuses seemed to have increased mortality compared with others affected, with 88% to 95% mortality noted.[11,12] Neonates born to women with Ebola virus have a near-lethal prognosis. In addition, the conditions surrounding labor and delivery, including high exchanges of potentially contaminated body fluids, make specific precautions an important consideration. Recently, the effect of Zika, an arbovirus leading to birth defects in infants, has further drawn attention on the unique maternal–fetal unit during pregnancy.[13] The Centers for Disease Control and Prevention now has an entire division devoted to emergency preparedness for pregnant women and infants.[14–19]

Specific infections are common in pregnancy (**Box 1**). Others, although uncommon, carry high rates of morbidity and mortality (**Box 2**). Last, certain infections may not have significant maternal effects, but are associated with in utero infection, teratogenicity, or congenital infections (**Box 3** and **Table 1**).

COMMON INFECTIONS IN PREGNANCY
Influenza

Influenza is one of the more common infections in pregnancy, and also is associated with higher rates of hospitalization, intensive care admission, and death during pregnancy.[6,7] The focus of influenza in this article covers prevention, diagnosis, treatment, and complications.

Box 1
Common infections in pregnancy

Urinary Tract infections

Cystitis

Pyelonephritis

Respiratory infections

Pneumonia

Influenza

"Common cold"

Group B streptococcal

Colonization

Urinary tract

Intraamniotic

Endometritis

Sexually transmitted infections

Gonorrhea

Chlamydia

Syphilis

Hepatitis A, B, and C

Human immunodeficiency virus

Box 2
Infections that carry severe morbidity and mortality in pregnancy

Uncommon but severe infections

Legionella

Listeria

Group A streptococcus

Ebola

Hepatitis E virus

Septic abortion

Prevention of influenza

Since 2004, the Centers for Disease Control and Prevention, the American college of Obstetrics and Gynecology, and the Advisory Committee on Immunization Practices all routinely endorse universal influenza vaccination during pregnancy. Numerous studies have demonstrated the safety and benefits of influenza vaccination. A large study in Bangladesh demonstrated a 63% reduction in laboratory-proven respiratory illness in infants and mothers.[20,21] Despite these features, historical vaccine uptake rates have remained low. Before 2009, reported rates during pregnancy

---

Box 3
Infections that lead to congenital infection

Cytomegalovirus

Mumps

Parvovirus B19

Rubella

Varicella

Coxsackie

Herpes simplex virus

Listeria monocytogenes

Rubeola

Vaccinia

Hepatitis C

Human immunodeficiency virus

Mycoplasma tuberculosis

Salmonella typhi

Borrelia burgdorferi

Toxoplasmosis

Lymphocystic choriomeningitis

Smallpox

Poliovirus

Hepatitis B

Table 1 Infections with known in utero infections or teratogenic effects	
Etiology	**Fetal Effect**
Cytomegalovirus	Hepatosplenomegaly, jaundice, pneumonitis petechiae or purpura, meningoencephalitis, hydrocephalus, microcephaly, intracranial calcifications, hearing deficits, chorioretinitis or retinopathy, optic atrophy
Toxoplasmosis	Hepatosplenomegaly, jaundice, pneumonitis petechiae or purpura, meningoencephalitis, hydrocephalus, maculopapular exanthems, microcephaly, intracranial calcifications, hearing deficits, chorioretinitis or retinopathy
Parvovirus B19	Nonimmune hydrops fetalis
Rubella	Hepatosplenomegaly, jaundice, pneumonitis petechiae or purpura, meningoencephalitis, hydrocephalus, adenopathy, hearing deficits, myocarditis, bone lesions, glaucoma, chorioretinitis, cataracts, microphthalmia
Syphilis	Hepatosplenomegaly, jaundice, pneumonitis petechiae or purpura, meningoencephalitis, adenopathy, maculopapular exanthems, bone lesions, glaucoma, chorioretinitis or retinopathy, uveitis
Herpes simplex virus	Hepatosplenomegaly, jaundice, pneumonitis petechiae or purpura, meningoencephalitis, hydrocephalus, microcephaly, maculopapular exanthems, vesicles, myocarditis, chorioretinitis or retinopathy, cataracts, conjunctivitis
Zika virus	Microcephaly, intracranial calcifications, ventriculomegaly, absence of the corpus callosum, hypogyrations, poorly developed brain stem

were 2% to 15%.[22,23] This rate peaked at 80% to 85% during the 2009 pandemic, and has decreased thereafter.[24–26]

Numerous factors seem to be associated with these low uptake rates, including patient and provider features. Studies have shown that greater provider knowledge about influenza leads to greater patient vaccine acceptance.[25] Several common patient perceptions have been shown to lead to decreased vaccination uptake.[27,28] These include lack of knowledge of the vaccine importance, lack of perception of self-risk, and concerns for fetal effects.

Diagnosis and treatment

Although little research has been done specific to the evaluation of influenza-like illness in pregnant women, it is reasonable to assume it is similar to the evaluation in nonpregnant women. Certain factors have been associated with increased rates of hospitalization, including medical comorbidities such as asthma, cardiac disease, diabetes, and HIV infection.[28] Some symptoms indicate severe infection, and therefore should prompt a higher level of care. A triage algorithm to determine whether pregnant women should be evaluated over the phone or in person has been suggested by researchers at Northwestern, and is shown in **Fig. 2**.[29] Similarly, these authors evaluated a triage protocol and criteria for admission, and this process seems to be efficient without increased influenza-related morbidity (**Fig. 3**). Criteria for admission are similar for that proposed in other respiratory conditions.[30]

Diagnostic testing for influenza

Most facilities have 1 of 2 options available for testing for influenza, rapid influenza diagnostic tests (RIDTs) and reverse transcription polymerase chain reactions (PCR)

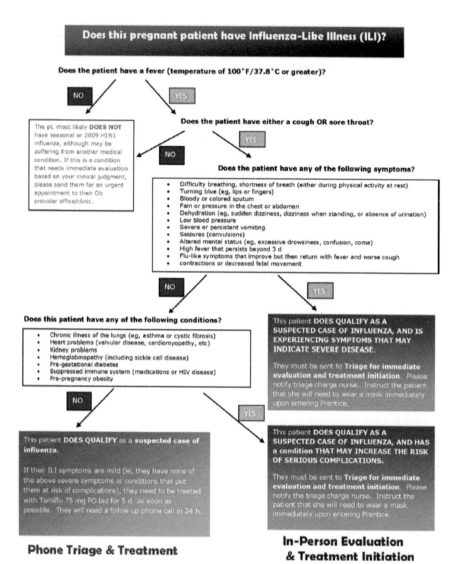

Fig. 2. Influenza telephone triage protocol. PO, by mouth. (*From* Eppes CS, Garcia PM, Grobman WA. Telephone triage of influenza-like illness during pandemic 2009 H1N1 in an obstetric population. Am J Obstet Gynecol 2012;207(1):4; with permission.)

testing. Benefits of the RIDTs testing include rapid turn around time (typically <30 minutes). However, they have limited sensitivity and specificity, particularly in the clinically applied method of specimen collection (ie, nasal vs nasopharyngeal). RIDTs do not give specific information about the type of virus (eg, H3N2 vs H1N1). Therefore, if influenza is suspected clinically in pregnant women, treatment decisions should not involve RIDT testing. Specifically, any pregnant women with clinically suspected influenza during a known period of influenza activity should be treated with an antiviral medication.[31] Reverse transcription PCR testing has a higher sensitivity and specificity; however, it is not as readily available at all hospitals, and has a longer turn

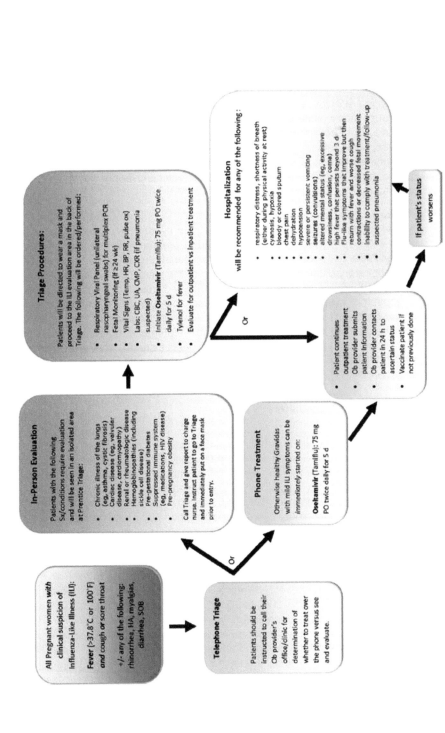

Fig. 3. Influenza evaluation unit triage protocol. BP, blood pressure; CBC, complete blood cell count; CMP, comprehensive metabolic profile; HA, headache; HR, heart rate; Ob, obstetrician; PCR, polymerase chain reaction; PO, by mouth; SOB, shortness of breath; Sx, symptoms; UA urinalysis. (*From* Eppes CS, Garcia PM, Grobman WA. Telephone triage of influenza-like illness during pandemic 2009 H1N1 in an obstetric population. Am J Obstet Gynecol 2012;207(1):5; with permission.)

around time and a higher cost. The Centers for Disease Control and Prevention recommend consideration for reverse transcription PCR testing in all hospitalized patients.

Treatment of influenza in pregnancy

Numerous studies have demonstrated increased incidence of death, admission to critical care units, and severe illness in pregnant women were antiviral treatment is delayed.[32,33] There are 2 classes of antiviral influenza treatment, M2 ion channel inhibitors and neuraminidase inhibitors. M2 ion channel inhibitors include amantadine and rimantadine, and are effective for treatment of influenza A. These medications have increasingly recognized rates of resistance.[34] Neuraminidase inhibitors include osteltamivir and zanamivir; these are effective against influenza A and B. Since 2009, increasing data are available regarding the safety of osteltamivir in pregnancy, with no adverse outcomes reported in the literature.[34]

Severe complications with influenza in pregnancy

Historically, the mortality of acute respiratory distress syndrome in pregnancy has been high (30%–60%).[35] This diagnosis increased in pregnant women surrounding the pandemic in 2009. Extracorporeal membrane oxygenation therapy has been studied for acute respiratory distress syndrome, owing to the small tidal volumes limiting the maximal plateau pressure. A small review analyzed cases of pandemic 2009 H1N1 and respiratory failure in pregnancy who were then placed on extracorporeal membrane oxygenation therapy. Despite their serious diagnosis, the authors concluded that women in this review had acceptable maternal and neonatal survival outcomes. However, owing to the lack of larger prospective studies, they were unable to conclude whether these outcomes were better than those achieved with standard of care ventilation.[36]

HUMAN IMMUNODEFICIENCY VIRUS
Epidemiology

The worldwide prevalence of HIV makes it one of the most common, and most deadly, diseases worldwide. In 2014, the World Health Organization global summary of the AIDS epidemic included 36.9 million people living with HIV, of whom 17.4 million were women and 2.6 million were children under 15 years of age.[37]

Of all maternal deaths worldwide, 6% to 20% are related to HIV.[38] HIV-positive women have a 2 to 10 times higher chance of dying than HIV-negative women, and many of the causes of death involve infectious complications such as AIDS, tuberculosis, malaria, pneumonia, puerperal sepsis, and sepsis related to abortion. Although there is no evidence that HIV disease accelerates during pregnancy, there is the suggestion that it may accelerate postpartum.[38]

In the United States, the number of HIV-infected women delivering infants increases annually, with a 30% increase from 2000 to 2006.[39] Despite this occurrence, our rates of prenatal infections seem to be decreasing. There are significant disparities noted in those women living with HIV, with African American women representing a statistically greater number of cases as compared with Caucasian or Hispanic women.[40] Last, HIV is a complex disease, with many social determinants of health often relating to disproportionate exposure, delayed disease diagnosis, and lack of health care access in those who are infected.

Diagnosis of Human Immunodeficiency Virus and Disease Severity

Owing to the state laws mandating HIV testing during pregnancy, many women are diagnosed with HIV for the first time during pregnancy. In 2013, the US Preventive

Services Task Force recommended routinely screening adolescents and adults aged 15 to 65 and all pregnant women.[41] Patients should be notified that testing will be performed, but given the option of declining (ie, opt-out testing). Data from the National Institutes of Health–sponsored trials indicate a clear advantage to having HIV status recognized and early treatment initiated. The Centers for Disease Control and Prevention recommended testing algorithm was amended in 2013. The currently recommended first line test is a fourth-generation antibody/antigen test. This test can become positive within 14 days of an acute infection (**Fig. 4**). This is of particular importance, because those with acute HIV often have very increased viral loads and are therefore highly infectious. If the initial screening test is positive, the follow-up test should be an antibody differentiation test, which can distinguish between HIV 1 and HIV 2. If this test is positive, a diagnosis of HIV is confirmed. If this test is negative, the discordant results should be resulted as indeterminate and either a qualitative nucleic acid test or a HIV viral load test should be performed. Importantly, this algorithm can allow a positive test result in approximately 2 hours, which is dramatically shorter than the older Western blot confirmation. However, a positive fourth-generation HIV test and negative antibody differentiation test is an indeterminate result and will need a nucleic acid test or viral load test for further evaluation, and these tests require additional time for a final result.[42]

Disease activity is monitored with serum viral load and CD4 counts. AIDS is diagnosed when CD4 counts are less than 200 cells or opportunistic infections are present (**Table 2**).

Treatment

Acute HIV often presents with viral-type symptoms, including fever, malaise, myalgias, and lymphadenopathy. Individuals with untreated and longer standing HIV infection may present with AIDS and opportunistic infections, and be seriously ill. Therefore, certain presentations should prompt HIV testing, including any patient with a newly

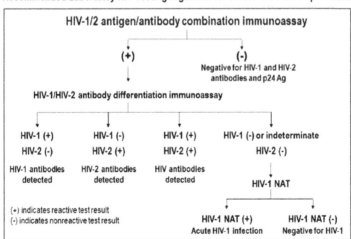

Fig. 4. Testing algorithm for human immunodeficiency virus (HIV). NAT, nucleic acid test. (*Adapted from* Centers for disease control and prevention. Quick reference guide—laboratory testing for the diagnosis of HIV infection: updated recommendations. 2014. Available at: https://stacks.cdc.gov/view/cdc/23446. Accessed June 5, 2016.)

Table 2
CD4 count levels and opportunistic infection prophylaxis

CD4 Count Below Which to Offer Prophylaxis	Organisms	Preferred Prophylaxis
<200 cells/mm^2	Pneumocystis pneumonia[a]	TMP-SMX DS daily or TMP-SMX SS daily
<100 cells/μL	*Toxoplasma gondii* encephalitis[b]	TMX-SMX DS daily
<50 cells/μL	Disseminated *Mycobacterium avium* complex	Azithromycin 1200 mg once weekly
Screening test for TB positive without active TB	*Mycobacterium tuberculosis*	INH 300 mg plus pyridoxine 25 mg for 9 mo

Abbreviations: INH, isoniazid; TB, tuberculosis; TMP-SMX DS, trimethoprim-sulfamethoxazole double strength.

[a] It is also recommended to offer prophylaxis against pneumocystis pneumonia with oropharyngeal candidiasis, a CD4 count of less than 14%, or a history of AIDS-defining illness.

[b] Those who are toxoplasma IgG positive it is recommended to offer prophylaxis with a CD4 count of less than 100 cells/μL. Additionally, those who seroconvert for toxoplasma antibodies should be offered treatment with a CD4 count of less than 100 cells/μL.

diagnosed sexually transmitted infection. Last, individuals with acute HIV are highly infectious; therefore, diagnosis serves the dual role of benefit to the individual and their potential sexual partners.

Coinfections are common with HIV, because many of the factors that predispose individuals to HIV are risk factors for other illnesses. Importantly, the co-relation of HIV with many other infections may increase the risk of maternal to child transmission of HIV and the coinfection. This has been noted in retrospective studies of syphilis,[43] hepatitis B and C,[44,45] and tuberculosis.[46,47]

When patients have HIV, most commonly with AIDS, treatment with antiretroviral (ARV) drugs can lead to a rapid increase in CD4 count and concurrent exaggerated inflammatory reaction to other infections. These infections may have been present, but the suppressed immune system failed to mount a response. This exaggerated immune response, or immune reconstitution inflammatory syndrome, can occur in 2 forms, either an unmasking of an underlying, previously undiagnosed infection soon after ARV therapy or a paradoxic worsening of a previously treated infection after ARV therapy is started.[48] Previously, the timing of initiation of ARV therapy in those with a low CD4 count and disorders such as tuberculosis was controversial. However, recent studies indicate that early initiation of ARV therapy may improve survival; therefore, delaying beyond 2 to 4 weeks is likely inadvisable.[49–52] Additionally, the timing of pregnancy and the ability to delay therapy and still optimally decrease viral load is a difficult balance, without specific trials to guide recommendations for pregnancy.

It is highly recommended that all pregnant women with HIV receive ARV therapy with the goal of maximal viral suppression during pregnancy. Numerous studies have demonstrated the linear relationship between viral load and vertical transmission of HIV.[53] Women will often present for obstetric care in one of 3 scenarios:

1. Already receiving ARV therapy,
2. Newly diagnosed HIV without previous ARV therapy, or
3. Previously diagnosed HIV without current ARV therapy but previous exposure.

Each scenario requires different considerations.

Women Entering Pregnancy with Diagnosed Human Immunodeficiency Virus and Currently Taking Antiretroviral Therapy

Women can present for pregnancy care already receiving ARV therapy at various gestational ages. For all times in pregnancy, assessment of the degree of viral suppression, CD4 count, medications compliance, and tolerability are important. The importance of optimal viral suppression on reduction of maternal to child transmission is a key talking point. Contemporary studies indicate a less than 2% risk of vertical transmission of HIV with antepartum antiviral treatment and viral suppression, in addition to postpartum neonatal treatment.[54] Conversations between a woman and her physician should also reaffirm:

- The importance of treatment on maternal health,
- The importance of adherence to avoid resistance, and
- The known data for infants after in utero drug exposure for specific medications the patient maybe taking.

If women have a suppressed viral load, continuation of their therapy is likely to improve compliance and is highly recommended. Only rare medications have potential teratogenicity, including efavirenz, which has been linked potentially to neural tube defects in the first trimester.[55] The US Preventive Services Task Force recommends that efavirenz can often be continued in women who present for antenatal care, because the risk of neural tube defects is restricted to the first 5 to 6 weeks of pregnancy. Pregnancy is rarely recognized before 5 to 6 weeks, and unnecessary changes in ARV drugs during pregnancy may be associated with loss of viral control and increased risk of perinatal transmission. Women on efavirenz should be counseled about the potential teratogenicity, and anatomic survey via ultrasound examination is recommended at 18 to 20 weeks gestation.

Women Diagnosed in Pregnancy

Because of the universal recommendations for HIV testing during pregnancy, many women are diagnosed for the first time when they seek prenatal care. In this situation several factors are of key importance:

- Assessing their degree of immune suppression via CD4 count and history of AIDS defining illnesses.
- Discussing the importance of disclosure of their HIV status to sexual partners.
- Determining whether their current partner is aware of their HIV status, and encouraging HIV testing if needed.
- Evaluating the social determinant of health in the woman's environment to assist with medication compliance. This includes transportation to visits, funding to cover medications, housing, domestic abuse, drug abuse, and concomitant psychiatric illness.
- Determining the most appropriate ARV regimen to begin.

Specific guidance regarding the ARV regimen is complex and should balance the woman's medical history, aid in compliance, and focus on recommended regimens in pregnancy. The US Preventive Services Task Force Guidelines are an excellent resource.[56]

Women with Human Immunodeficiency Virus Entering Pregnancy Not Taking Medications

Women with known HIV and not on medications before pregnancy are often those who face the greatest challenges to optimal therapy. Although previous recommendation did not including initiating therapy until specific CD4 counts, evidence largely now indicates that early ARV therapy leads to increase life expectancy and decreased morbidity.[57,58] Providers are encouraged to assess what previous barriers to ARV therapy occurred and work together with their patients to decrease these factors. Comorbidities such as substance abuse and psychological conditions are common, and difficult to combat. Models such as Nesheim's framework for elimination of maternal to child transmission of HIV highlight the complex nature of avoiding a case of neonatal infection (**Fig. 5**).[57]

Owing to ARV therapy, women who become pregnant with HIV often have relatively good immune function. However, those who have had long-standing HIV or AIDS, and are not on ARV therapy can present for evaluation extremely ill. Overall mortality rates

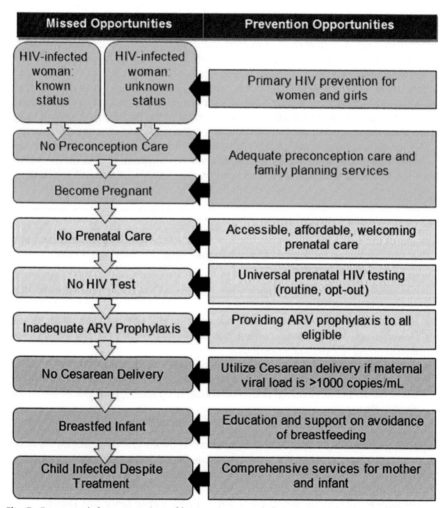

Fig. 5. Framework for prevention of human immunodeficiency virus (HIV). ARV, antiretroviral. (*From* Centers for disease control and prevention. Pregnant women, infants and children. Elimination of mother-to-child HIV transmission (EMCT) in the United States. Available at: http://www.cdc.gov/hiv/group/gender/pregnantwomen/emct.html. Accessed June 5, 2016.)

for HIV infected patients requiring intensive care in the present era is 30% to 40%, which has improved dramatically since from 70% in the 1980s.[59] The following section outlines severe illnesses that clinicians caring for HIV-positive women may encounter.

Respiratory
Acute respiratory failure is the most common reason for admission to the intensive care unit among HIV-positive patients, with *Pneumocystis jiroveci* (formerly referred to as *Pneumocystis carinii*) representing the primary pathogen.[59] Unfortunately, the mortality of pneumocystis pneumonia condition remains around 15% to 25%.[60–63] Patients often present with cough without sputum, fever, and dyspnea that has worsened over time.

Evaluation of patients presenting with respiratory complaints should include a history and physical examination, laboratory evaluations, and chest radiograph.[62] Oxygen saturation often reveals hypoxemia. Laboratory evaluations can include a complete blood count with differential, evaluation of the patients HIV viral load, and CD4 cell count if this is not known from recent values, lactate dehydrogenase. Bronchiolar lavage with demonstration of *P jirovecii* cysts is the gold standard in diagnosing pneumocystis pneumonia. The sensitivity for induced sputum detecting *P jirovecii* is variable, with studies reporting 50% to 90%.[64]

Chest radiographs will often reveal bilateral diffuse granular opacities, which may include pneumatoceles or pneumothoraces. However, 20% may have a negative radiograph, but computed tomography scans are typically positive in this setting.[64]

Treatment regimens are in **Table 3**. The preferred regimen is sulfamethoxazole trimethoprim (TMX/SMX) 5 mg/kg every 8 hours orally or intravenously for 21 days. Corticosteroids are recommended with Pao_2 less than or equal to 70 mg Hg or an A-a gradient of greater than 35 mm Hg.[65]

The second most common cause of respiratory complaints is bacterial pneumonia. Diagnosis of bacterial pneumonia is similar to that in HIV-negative women. Because of the medical comorbidity of HIV, inpatient admission and treatment is recommended.[30] Empiric therapy should provide coverage for methicillin-resistant *Staphylococcus aureus* and *Pseudomonas*.

Neurologic
Specific severe illness should be considered for pregnant women with HIV presenting will neurologic complaints. These include:

- Primary cerebral lymphoma,
- Toxoplasmosis,

Table 3 Treatment for *Pneumocystis jiroveci* pneumonia	
Medication	**Dose and Route**
TMX/SMX	5mg/kg q8h oral or IV
Dapsone plus trimethoprim	100 mg orally daily 5mg/kg q8h orally
Clindamycin	600 mg IV q6-8h
Clindamycin plus primaquine	300–450 mg orally q6h 15–30 mg base/d orally
Atovaquone	750 mg orally with food twice daily
Pentamadine	3–4 mg/kg/d IV

Abbreviations: IV, intravenous; TMX/SMX, trimethoprim-sulfamethoxazole.

- Cryptococcus,
- Progressive multifocal leukoencephalopathy, and
- Herpes simplex encephalitis.

Of these conditions, toxoplasmosis is the most common and has an high associated mortality.[60] *Toxoplasma gondii* is a protozoal infection, and neurologic disease is often related reactivation of infection. The primary manifestation is encephalitis and patients often have fevers, confusion, headache, seizures, and focal neurologic signs. Toxoplasmosis should be considered in any patient with a CD4 of less than 50 presenting with neurologic complaints. Evaluation should include:

- History and physical examination,
- Lumbar puncture with toxoplasma PCR testing of the cerebrospinal fluid, and
- Computed tomography scan.

The lumbar puncture often shows normal to increased protein and mononuclear pleocytosis. Computed tomography scanning will show multiple ring-enhancing lesions in the basal ganglia and corticomedullary junction. Brain biopsy is the gold standard, and may be required to exclude lymphoma if toxoplasmosis directed therapy is not successful. The recommended treatment regimen is pyrimethamine 200 mg orally once, followed by 75 mg/d. Alternative regimens are in **Table 4**. Adjunctive therapies include corticosteroids if mass-effect is present, anticonvulsants for seizures, and initiation of opportunistic infection prophylaxis for other conditions.

Gastrointestinal

The most common gastrointestinal presentation requiring critical care admission in HIV positive patients include gastrointestinal bleeding, esophagitis and diarrhea. Mild presentations of diarrhea are common, and can be related to infectious complications or medications. Several HIV-related conditions can cause gastrointestinal bleeding, including:

- Kaposi's sarcoma,
- Lymphoma,
- Cytomegalovirus enteritis,
- Mycobacteria, and
- AIDS cholangiopathy.

If a patient presents with diarrhea, the following organisms/evaluations should be performed based on the patients clinical history, and treatment directed as appropriate:

- Guiac testing
- Clostridium difficile testing
- Acid fast stain to assess

Table 4 Treatment for toxoplasmosis encephalitis	
Medication	**Dose and Route**
Pyrimethamine	200 mg orally once, followed by 75 mg/d
Pyrimethamine Plus sulfaziadine Plus leucovorin	200 mg orally once, followed by pyrimethamine 50 mg orally daily plus sulfadiazine 1 mg orally 4 times daily plus leucovorin 10–20 mg orally daily

- o Isosporidia
- o Cyclospora
- o Cryptosporidium
- o Microsporidium
- o Cystoisospora
- Bacterial culture
- Ova and parasites

Therapy should be aimed at the organism identified.

Failure of Viral Suppression and Resistance

The goal of ARV therapy is early initiation to allow reaching an undetectable viral load as early as possible in pregnancy. Contemporary studies highlight the risk of in utero transmission with delayed viral suppression.[66] Women who have not reached viral suppression by the third trimester should be assessed for potential mechanisms. This often includes viral resistance, which can be determined with an HIV genotype or resistance panel. The viral load must be greater than 500 to 1000 depending on the laboratory to determine the resistance profile. Poor compliance is a common etiology of failed viral suppression, but difficult to tackle. Strategies such as directly observed therapy (inpatient or outpatient) may lead to improved compliance, but this strategy has not been proven in peer-reviewed publications, likely because of the issues of patient self-selection for this strategy. Recent evidence indicates that the addition of integrate inhibitors such raltegravir may lead to a more rapid decline in viral load, and therefore this medication may offer rapid viral suppression.[67]

Labor Management

The previous mantra for HIV-positive women in labor included cesarean delivery, avoidance of rupture of membranes, and intravenous zidovudine. Currently, the US Preventive Services Task Force recommendations stratify the most appropriate management of labor for women with HIV based on viral load (**Table 5**).

Postnatal Treatment

The recommended postnatal treatment for infants is stratified based on the patient's antenatal and intrapartum HIV status and management. For infants born to mothers on antenatal ARV this includes zidovudine for 4 to 6 weeks. Infants born to mothers without antepartum ARV prophylaxis should also receive 3 doses of nevirapine. Expanded treatments are currently experimental, and further studies are currently underway.[68]

Table 5 Viral load and route of delivery plus zidovudine		
Viral Load	Recommended Route of Delivery	IV Zidovudine?
>1000 cells/µL	Prelabor cesarean	Yes
Detectible-1000 cell/µL	Vaginal delivery Individualized conversation	No
Undetectable	Vaginal delivery	No

Abbreviation: IV, intravenous.

SUMMARY

Pregnant women and their infants are a unique subgroup of our population, who have risks factors for illness acquisition and acuity. Certain illnesses such as influenza and HIV are commonly encountered during pregnancy, and therefore physicians caring for pregnant women should be aware of the common presentations, diagnostic approaches, and therapies.

REFERENCES

1. Remington J, Klein J, Wilson C, et al. Infectious diseases of the fetus and newborn infant. 7th edition. Elsevier; 2011.
2. Belfort M, Dildy GA, Saade GR, et al. Critical care obstetrics. 5th edition. Wiley-Blackwell; 2010.
3. Hartert T, Meuzil K, Shintani A, et al. Maternal morbidity and perinatal outcomes among pregnant women with respiratory hospitalizations during influenza season. Am J Obstet Gynecol 2008;189(6):1705–12.
4. Cox S, Posner SF, McPheeters M, et al. Hospitalizations with respiratory illness among pregnant women during influenza season. Obstet Gynecol 2006;107(6):1315–22.
5. Lam CM, Wong SF, Leung TN, et al. A case-controlled study comparing clinical course and outcomes of pregnant and non-pregnant women with severe acute respiratory syndrome. BJOG 2004;111(8):771–4.
6. Callaghan W, Chu S, Jamieson J. Deaths from seasonal influenza among regnant women in the United States, 1998-2005. Obstet Gynecol 2010;115(5):919–24.
7. Varner MW, Rice MM, Anderson B, et al. Influenza-like illness in hospitalized pregnant and postpartum women during the 2009-2010 H1N1 pandemic. Obstet Gynecol 2011;118(3):593–601.
8. Phillippe M. Pandemic influenza: what obstetricians need to know. Obstet Gynecol 2009;114(2 Pt 1):206–8.
9. Neuzil K, Reed G, Mitchel E, et al. Impact of influenza on acute cardiopulmonary hospitalizations in pregnant women. Am J Epidemiol 1998;148(11):1094–102.
10. Centers for Disease Control and Prevention (CDC). Ebola outbreak in West Africa - case counts. 2014. Available at: https://www.cdc.gov/vhf/ebola/outbreaks/2014-west-africa/case-counts.html. Accessed June 2, 2016.
11. Mupapa K, Mukundu W, Bwaka MA, et al. Ebola hemorrhagic fever and pregnancy. J Infect Dis 1999;179(Suppl 1):S11–2.
12. Jamieson DJ, Uyeki TM, Callaghan WM, et al. What obstetrician-gynecologists should know about Ebola. A perspective from the center for disease control and prevention. Obstet Gynecol 2014;124(5):1005–10.
13. Brasil P, Pereira J, Raja Gabaglia C, et al. Zika virus infection in pregnant women in Rio de Janeiro – preliminary report. N Engl J Med 2016. [Epub ahead of print].
14. Centers for Disease Control and Prevention (CDC). Emergency preparedness and response: pregnant women and newborns. Available at: http://www.cdc.gov/reproductivehealth/emergency/. Accessed June 2, 2016.
15. Zotti ME, Tong VT, Kieltyka L, et al. Making evacuation decisions: the case of high risk pregnant and postpartum women. In: David E, Enarson E, editors. The women of Katrina: how gender, race, and class matter in an American disaster. Nashville: Vanderbilt University Press; 2012. p. 90–104.
16. Tong VT, Zott ME, Hsia J. Impact of the 1997 Red River catastrophic flood on women giving birth in North Dakota. Matern Child Health J 2010;15:281–8.
17. Zotti ME, Williams AM, Robertson M, et al. Post-disaster reproductive health outcomes. Matern Child Health J 2012;17(5):783–96.

18. Callaghan WM, Rasmussen SA, Jamieson DJ, et al. Health concerns of women and infants in times of natural disasters: lessons learned from Hurricane Katrina. Matern Child Health J 2007;11(4):307–11.

19. Horney J, Zotti ME, Williams AM, et al. Cluster sampling with referral to improve the efficiency of estimating unmet needs among pregnant and postpartum women after disasters. Womens Health Issues 2012;22(3):253–7.

20. Zaman K, Roy E, Arifeen S, et al. Effectiveness of maternal influenza immunization in mothers and infants. N Engl J Med 2008;359:1554–64.

21. Schatz M, Chambers CD, Jones KL, et al. Safety of influenza immunization and treatment during pregnancy: the vaccine and medications in pregnancy surveillance system. Am J Obstet Gynecol 2011;204(6 Suppl 1):S64–8.

22. Beigi RH, Switzer GE, Meyn LA. Acceptance of a pandemic avian influenza vaccine in pregnancy. J Reprod Med 2009;54(6):341–6.

23. Tong A, Biringer A, Ofner-Agostini M, et al. A cross-sectional study of maternity care providers and women's knowledge, attitudes, and behaviors towards influenza vaccination during pregnancy. J Obstet Gynaecol Can 2008;30(5):404–10.

24. Eppes C, Wu A, Cameron K, et al. Does obstetrician knowledge regarding influenza increase H1N1 vaccine uptake among their pregnancy patients? Vaccine 2012;30:5782–4.

25. Goldfarb I, Panda B, Wylie B, et al. Uptake of influenza vaccine in pregnant women during the 2009 H1N1 influenza pandemic. Am J Obstet Gynecol 2011; 204:S112–5.

26. Eppes C, Wu A, You W, et al. Barriers to influenza vaccination among pregnant women. Vaccine 2013;31(27):2874–8.

27. Fischer B, Scott J, Hart J, et al. Behaviors and perceptions regarding seasonal and H1N1 influenza vaccination during pregnancy. Am J Obstet Gynecol 2011; 204(6 Suppl 1):S107–11.

28. Jamieson DJ, Honein MA, Rasmussen SA, et al. H1N1 2009 influenza virus infection during pregnancy in the USA. Lancet 2009;374:451–8.

29. Eppes CS, Garcia PM, Grobman WA. Telephone triage of influenza-like illness during pandemic 2009 H1N1 in an obstetric population. Am J Obstet Gynecol 2012;207(1):3–8.

30. Yost NP, Bloom SL, Richey SD, et al. An appraisal of treatment guidelines for antepartum community-acquired pneumonia. Am J Obstet Gynecol 2000;183(1): 131–5.

31. Centers for Disease Control and Prevention (CDC). Influenza testing. Guidance for clinicians on the use of rapid influenza diagnostic tests. Available at: http://www.cdc.gov/flu/professionals/diagnosis/clinician_guidance_ridt.htm#figure1. Accessed June 2, 2016.

32. Louie J, costa M, Jamieson J, et al. Severe 2009 H1N1 influenza in pregnant and postpartum women in California. N Engl J Med 2010;362(1):27–36.

33. Siston AM, Rasmussen SA, Honein MA, et al. Pandemic 2009 influenza A(H1N1) virus illness among pregnant women in the United States. JAMA 2010;303(15): 1517–25.

34. Greer L, Sheffield J, Rogers V, et al. Maternal and neonatal outcomes after antepartum treatment of influenza with antiviral medications. Obstet Gynecol 2010; 115(4):711–7.

35. Cole DE, Taylor TL, McCullough DM, et al. Acute respiratory distress syndrome in pregnancy. Crit Care Med 2005;33(10 Suppl):S269–78.

36. Saad A, Rahman M, Maybauer DM, et al. Extracorporeal membrane oxygenation in pregnant and postpartum women with H1N1-related acute respiratory distress

syndrome: a systematic review and meta-analysis. Obstet Gynecol 2016;127(2): 241–7.

37. World Health Organization (WHO). HIV/AIDS. Data and statistics. Available at: http://www.who.int/hiv/data/en/. Accessed June 2, 2016.

38. Lathrop E, Jamieson DJ, Danel I. HIV and maternal mortality. Int J Gynaecol Obstet 2014;127(2):213–5.

39. Whitmore SK, Zhang X, Taylor AW, et al. Estimated number of infants born to HIV-infected women in the United States and five dependent areas, 2006. J Acquir Immune Defic Syndr 2011;57(3):218–22.

40. Centers for Disease Control and Prevention (CDC). Racial/ethnic disparities among children with diagnoses of perinatal HIV infection - 34 states, 2004-2007. MMWR Morb Mortal Wkly Rep 2010;59(4):97–101.

41. Available at: http://www.cdc.gov/hiv/testing/. Accessed June 2, 2016.

42. Branson BM, Ginocchio CC. Introduction to 2013 Journal of Clinical Virology supplement on HIV testing algorithm. J Clin Virol 2013;58(Suppl 1):e1.

43. Mwapasa V, Rogerson SJ, Kwiek JJ, et al. Maternal syphilis infection is associated with increased risk of mother-to-child transmission of HIV in Malawi. AIDS 2006;20(14):1869–77.

44. Polis CB, Shah SN, Johnson KE, et al. Impact of maternal HIV coinfection on the vertical transmission of hepatitis C virus: a meta-analysis. Clin Infect Dis 2007; 44(8):1123–31.

45. Landes M, Newell ML, Barlow P, et al. Hepatitis B or hepatitis C coinfection in HIV-infected pregnant women in Europe. HIV Med 2008;9(7):526–34.

46. Mofenson LM, Laughon BE. Human immunodeficiency virus, mycobacterium tuberculosis, and pregnancy: a deadly combination. Clin Infect Dis 2007;45(2): 250–3.

47. Thillagavathie P. Current issues in maternal and perinatal tuberculosis: impact of the HIV-1 epidemic. Semin Neonatol 2000;5(3):189–96.

48. Panel on Opportunistic Infections in HIV-Infected Adults and Adolescents. Guidelines for the prevention and treatment of opportunistic infections in HIV-infected adults and adolescents: recommendations from the Centers for Disease Control and Prevention, the National Institutes of Health, and the HIV Medicine Association of the Infectious Diseases Society of America. Available at: http://aidsinfo.nih.gov/contentfiles/lvguidelines/adult_oi.pdf. Accessed June 2, 2016.

49. Abdool Karim SS, Naidoo K, Grobler A, et al. Timing of initiation of antiretroviral drugs during tuberculosis therapy. N Engl J Med 2010;362(8):697–706.

50. Abdool Karim SS, Naidoo K, Grobler A, et al. Integration of antiretroviral therapy with tuberculosis treatment. N Engl J Med 2011;365(16):1492–501.

51. Blanc FX, Sok T, Laureillard D, et al. Earlier versus later start of antiretroviral therapy in HIV-infected adults with tuberculosis. N Engl J Med 2011;365(16): 1471–81.

52. Havlir DV, Kendall MA, Ive P, et al. Timing of antiretroviral therapy for HIV-1 infection and tuberculosis. N Engl J Med 2011;365(16):1482–91.

53. Garcia PM, Kalish LA, Pitt J, et al. Maternal levels of plasma human immunodeficiency virus type 1 RNA and the risk of perinatal transmission. Women and Infants Transmission Study Group. N Engl J Med 1999;341(6):394–402.

54. European Collaborative Study. Mother-to-child transmission of HIV infection in the era of highly active antiretroviral therapy. Clin Infect Dis 2005;40(3):458–65.

55. Ford N, Mofenson L, Shubber Z, et al. Safety of efavirenz in the first trimester of pregnancy: an updated systematic review and meta-analysis. AIDS 2014; 28(Suppl 2):s123–31.

56. Panel on Treatment of HIV-Infected Pregnant Women and Prevention of Perinatal Transmission. Recommendations for Use of Antiretroviral Drugs in Pregnant HIV-1-Infected Women for Maternal Health and Interventions to Reduce Perinatal HIV Transmission in the United States. Available at: http://aidsinfo.nih.gov/contentfiles/lvguidelines/PerinatalGL.pdf. Accessed June 5, 2016.

57. Panel on Antiretroviral Guidelines for Adults and Adolescents. Guidelines for the use of antiretroviral agents in HIV-1-infected adults and adolescents. Department of Health and Human Services. Available at: http://aidsinfo.nih.gov/contentfiles/lvguidelines/AdultandAdolescentGL.pdf. Accessed June 5, 2015.

58. Nesheim S, Taylor A, Lampe MA, et al. A framework for elimination of perinatal transmission of HIV in the United States. Pediatrics 2012;130(4):738–44.

59. Avidan MS, Jones N, Pozniak AL. The implications of HIV for the anaesthetist and intensivist. Anaesthesia 2000;55:344–54.

60. Crothers K, Huang L. Critical care of patients with HIV. HIV InSite Knowledge Base Chapter. 2003. Available at: http://hivinsite.ucsf.edu/InSite?page=kb-03-03-01. Accessed June 5, 2016.

61. Kaplan JE, Benson C, Holmes KK, et al. Guidelines for prevention and treatment of opportunistic infections in HIV-infected adults and adolescents: recommendations from the CDC, the National institutes of Health and the HIV medicine association of the IDSA. MMWR Recomm Rep 2009;58:1.

62. Huang L, Cattamanchi A, Davis JL, et al. HIV associated pneumocystis pneumonia. Proc Am Thorac Soc 2011;8:294.

63. Moon SM, Kim T, Sung H, et al. Outcomes of moderate-to-severe Pneumocystis pneumonia treated with adjunctive steroids in non-HIV infected patients. Antimicrob Agents Chemother 2011;55:4613.

64. Cruciani M, Marcati P, Malena M, et al. Meta-analysis of diagnostic procedures for PCP in HIV-1 infected patients. Eur Respir J 2002;20:982.

65. Benfield T, Atzori C, Miller RF, et al. Second-line salvage treatment of AIDS-associated pneumocystis jirovecii pneumonia: a case series and systematic review. J Acquir Immune Defic Syndr 2008;49:63.

66. Birkhead GS, Pulver WP, Warren BL, et al. Acquiring human immunodeficiency virus during pregnancy and mother to child transmission in New York City. Obstet Gynecol 2010;115(6):1247–55.

67. Rahangdale L, Cates J, Potter J, et al. Integrase inhibitors in late pregnancy and rapid HIV viral load reduction. Am J Obstet Gynecol 2016;214(3):385.e1-7.

68. Panel on Antiretroviral Therapy and Medical Management of HIV-Infected Children. Guidelines for the use of antiretroviral agents in pediatric HIV infection. Available at: http://aidsinfo.nih.gov/contentfiles/lvguidelines/pediatricguidelines.pdf. Accessed June 5, 2016.

Management of Sepsis and Septic Shock for the Obstetrician–Gynecologist

Lauren A. Plante, MD, MPH

KEYWORDS

• Sepsis • Septic shock • Pregnancy • Puerperium

KEY POINTS

- Sepsis is a syndrome, not a disease, and no diagnostic test exists. Sepsis is defined as life-threatening organ dysfunction caused by a dysregulated host response to infection.
- The 2 categories are sepsis and septic shock. The clinical criteria is summarized in the quick Sequential Organ Failure Assessment score.
- Specific criteria for pregnancy should be developed; rates of sepsis in pregnancy are increasing, with approximately 10 cases per 10,000 deliveries.
- Early recognition, early antimicrobial treatment, and early correction of organ dysfunction are essential for optimizing outcomes.

INTRODUCTION

Despite an explosion of information about sepsis during the last 2 or 3 decades, much remains uncertain or evolving. Specific knowledge about sepsis in the particular setting of pregnancy and the puerperium still lags behind, although in recent years we have advanced, at least, from single-center case series and expert opinion; nevertheless, there is much still unknown and much work to do.

Sepsis must be understood as distinct from either infection or bacteremia. It is best conceptualized as a life-threatening condition in which the host's own response to an infectious insult results in damage to organs or tissues.[1] Furthermore, it must be appreciated as a syndrome rather than a disease. No diagnostic test exists.

Clinical criteria for sepsis have gone through several different iterations in the last few decades. In 1991, a consensus conference was convened by the American College of Chest Physicians and the Society of Critical Care Medicine in an effort to

Division of Maternal-Fetal Medicine, Department of Obstetrics & Gynecology, Drexel University College of Medicine, 245 North 15th Street, MS 495, Philadelphia, PA 19102, USA
E-mail address: Lauren.Plante@drexelmed.edu

Obstet Gynecol Clin N Am 43 (2016) 659–678
http://dx.doi.org/10.1016/j.ogc.2016.07.010   obgyn.theclinics.com
0889-8545/16/© 2016 Elsevier Inc. All rights reserved.

create a conceptual and practical framework to define the systemic inflammatory response to infection, a process that was subsumed under the generalized term "sepsis."[2] This represented the first attempt to categorize sepsis as a syndrome, and to distinguish it from both infection (defined as a microbial phenomenon characterized by an inflammatory response to microorganisms, or the invasion of normally sterile host tissue by such organisms) and bacteremia (defined as the presence of viable bacteria in blood). Four entities, along a progression of severity, were described (**Box 1**):

1. The systemic inflammatory response syndrome (SIRS), which may be produced by noninfectious causes (eg, burns, pancreatitis)
2. Sepsis (SIRS owing to infection)

Box 1
1991 definitions for sepsis

Systemic Inflammatory Response Syndrome

The systemic inflammatory response to certain clinical insults, not limited to infection (eg, burns, pancreatitis produce same response).

Manifested by 2 or more of the following:
 Temperature greater than 38°C or less than 36°C
 Heart rate greater than 90 bpm
 Respiratory rate greater than 20/min, or $Paco_2$ less than 32 torr
 WBC greater than 12,000 cells/mm^3 or less than 4000 cells/mm^3 or greater than 10% immature forms (bands)

Sepsis

The systemic response to infection. Manifested by 2 or more of the following as a result of infection:

Temperature greater than 38°C or less than 36°C

Heart rate greater than 90 bpm

Respiratory rate greater than 20/min, or $Paco_2$ less than 32 torr

WBC greater than 12,000 cells/mm^3 or less than 4000 cells/mm^3 or greater than 10% immature forms (bands)

Severe Sepsis

Sepsis associated with organ dysfunction, hypotension, or hypoperfusion (including lactic acidosis, oliguria, or acute change in mental status)

Septic shock

Sepsis with hypotension despite adequate fluid resuscitation, along with perfusion abnormalities such as lactic acidosis, oliguria, or acute change in mental status. (Note: patients on vasopressors may still exhibit hypoperfusion though hypotension is no longer present)

Adapted from Bone RC, Balk RA, Cerra FR, et al; Members of the American College of Chest Physicians/Society of Critical Care Medicine Consensus Conference Committee. American College of Chest Physicians/Society of Critical Care Medicine Consensus Conference: definitions for sepsis and organ failure and guidelines for the use of innovative therapies in sepsis. Crit Care Med 1992;101(6):1646; with permission.

3. Severe sepsis (sepsis with organ dysfunction)
4. Septic shock

These concepts characterized research on sepsis during the last decade of the 20th century. In 2001, however, recognizing that it is difficult to provide elegant definitions for a syndrome in the absence of an underlying diagnostic test, a second conference revised terminology and offered new directions for investigation.[3] The SIRS concept was retained, despite a professed distaste for its lack of specificity, and hopes were raised that biomarkers for SIRS could be found in the future. Diagnostic criteria for sepsis multiplied (**Box 2**) and laboratory testing featured more prominently. Severe sepsis and septic shock were not redefined.

Shortly after this, the Surviving Sepsis Campaign (SSC) was launched by the Society for Critical Care Medicine, the European Society for Intensive Care Medicine, and the

---

Box 2
2001 diagnostic criteria for sepsis (adults)

Infection, documented or suspected, and some of the following:

- General variables
  - Fever (core temperature >38.3°C)
  - Hypothermia (temperature <36°C)
  - Heart rate greater than 90 bpm
  - Tachypnea
  - Altered mental status
  - Significant edema or positive fluid balance (>20 mL/kg over 24 hours)
  - Hyperglycemia (plasma glucose >120 mg/dL) in the absence of diabetes

- Inflammatory variables
  - Leukocytosis (WBC >12,000/mm^3)
  - Leukopenia (WBC <4000/mm^3)
  - Normal WBC but greater than 10% immature forms
  - Plasma C-reactive protein greater than 2 standard deviations above normal
  - Plasma procalcitonin greater than 2 standard deviations above normal

- Hemodynamic variables
  - Hypotension
    - Systolic BP less than 90 mm Hg
    - Mean arterial pressure less than 70 mm Hg
    - Decrease in systolic BP of greater than 40 mm Hg
  - Mixed venous oxygen saturation greater than 70%
  - Cardiac index greater than 3.5 L/min/m^2

- Organ dysfunction variables
  - Arterial hypoxemia (Pao$_2$/Fio$_2$ <300)
  - Oliguria (urine output <0.5 mL/kg/h for at ≥hours)
  - Increase in serum creatinine of greater than 0.5 mg/dL
  - Coagulation abnormalities (INR >1.5 or aPTT >60 s)
  - Ileus (clinically, absent bowel sounds)
  - Thrombocytopenia (platelet count <100,000/mm^2)
  - Hyperbilirubinemia (plasma total bilirubin >4 mg/dL)

- Tissue perfusion variables
  - Hyperlactatemia (>1 mmol/L)
  - Decreased capillary refill or mottling

Abbreviations: aPTT, activated partial thromboplastin time; BP, blood pressure; INR, international normalized ratio; WBC, white blood cell count.
Adapted from Levy MM, Fink MP, Marshall JC, et al. 2001 SCCM/ESICM/ACCP/ATS/SIS International Sepsis Definitions Conference. Intensive Care Med 2003;29:533; with permission.

International Sepsis Forum, with a goal of reducing sepsis mortality by 25% in 5 years. The SSC has since made extensive efforts to create and implement guidelines for care of patients with sepsis, including bundles for clinical care. It has been very successful in raising awareness of sepsis among clinicians and patients. SSC recommendations are reviewed elsewhere in this article.

By 2014, with the expansion of critical care services, increased awareness of sepsis, and a developing understanding of the pathophysiology underpinning sepsis, a third consensus task force (Sepsis-3) was constituted to update definitions once again[a] (**Box 3**).[4–6] The system is now much simpler. The previous SIRS criteria have been discarded as unhelpful, and laboratory assessment for sepsis has been downplayed: the focus is once again on clinical findings, because the task force acknowledged the difficulty of defining a syndrome for which there remains no diagnostic test. Only categories of sepsis and septic shock have been retained.

Sepsis is now defined as "life-threatening organ dysfunction caused by a dysregulated host response to infection."[6] The best clinical criteria which correlate with sepsis,

---

Box 3
The Third International Consensus Definitions for Sepsis and Septic Shock (Sepsis-3)

- Sepsis is defined as life-threatening organ dysfunction caused by a dysregulated host response to infection.

- Organ dysfunction is defined as an acute change in SOFA score of ≥ 2 points, consequent to infection.
  - Baseline SOFA score is assumed to be zero in patients not known to have preexisting organ dysfunction.
  - SOFA score of ≥ 2 reflects overall mortality risk $\sim 10\%$ in general adult population with infection. Even modest dysfunction at presentation can deteriorate.

- Patients with suspected infection who are likely to have significant morbidity (prolonged ICU stay or in-hospital death) can be identified at the bedside with quick SOFA (qSOFA), if any 2 are present:
  - Alteration in mental status
  - Systolic BP less than or equal to 100 mm Hg
  - Respiratory rate greater than 22/min

- Septic shock is a subset of sepsis in which underlying circulatory/cellular/metabolic abnormalities are profound enough to substantially increase mortality (>40%).

- Patients with septic shock can be identified by:
  - Sepsis with persisting hypotension, requiring vasopressors to maintain mean arterial pressure of ≥ 65 mm Hg, and
  - Serum lactate level of greater than 2 mmol/L (18 mg/dL) despite adequate fluid resuscitation

Abbreviations: BP, blood pressure; ICU, intensive care unit; SOFA, Sequential Organ Failure Assessment; qSOFA, quick Sequential Organ Failure Assessment.

Adapted from Singer M, Deutschman CS, Seymour CW, et al. The Third International Consensus definitions for sepsis and septic shock (Sepsis-3). JAMA 2016;315(8):80; with permission.

---

[a] Centers for Medicare and Medicaid Services (CMS) still using old classification system as of 2016, which affects coding, billing, reimbursement. See SEP-1 at CMS (required reporting) and National Quality Foundation (NQF) measure 0500.

in infected patients not already in the intensive care unit (ICU), are any 2 of the following criteria:

- Systolic BP of less than of equal to 100 mm Hg
- Respiratory rate of greater than or equal to 22/min
- Altered mental status

Together, these constitute the quick Sequential Organ Failure Assessment (SOFA) score. Septic shock is redefined as "a subset of sepsis in which underlying circulatory and cellular metabolism abnormalities are profound enough to substantially increase mortality."[6] Operationally, this equates to persistent hypotension (mean arterial pressure [MAP] $\leq$65 mm Hg), requiring vasopressors, with a serum lactate level of greater than 2 mmol/L despite adequate volume resuscitation. For patients already in ICU, an increase of at least 2 points in the full SOFA score (**Table 1**) suggests sepsis.

These criteria may be used without modification when the obstetrician–gynecologist is dealing with gynecology patients. None of these definitions or redefinitions, however, were ever validated in pregnant and postpartum women, whose underlying physiology differs from that of other adults. That having been said, it will almost certainly be easier to apply the third consensus definitions, rather than the earlier iterations, in an obstetric population. At the time of this writing, however, no publications have yet addressed their usefulness in obstetric care.

Table 1
SOFA score (sepsis-related organ failure assessment, also called the sequential organ failure assessment)

SOFA Score	1	2	3	4
Respiration: Pao$_2$/Fio$_2$	<400	<300	<200, with respiratory support	<100, with respiratory support
Coagulation: platelets	<150,000/mm^3	<100,000/mm^3	<50,000/mm^3	<20,000/mm^3
Liver: bilirubin (mg/dL)	1.2–1.9	2.0–5.9	6.0–11.9	>12.0
Cardiovascular: hypotension	MAP <70 mm Hg	Dopamine $\leq$5 μg/kg/min, or Dobutamine (any dose)	Dopamine >5 μg/kg/min, or Epinephrine $\leq$0.1 μg/kg/min, or Norepinephrine $\leq$0.1 μg/kg/min	Dopamine >15 μg/kg/min, or Epinephrine >0.1 μg/kg/min, or Norepinephrine >0.1 μg/kg/min
CNS: Glasgow Coma Score	13–14	10–12	6–9	<6
Renal: serum creatinine or urine output	1.2–1.9 mg/dL	2.0–3.4 mg/dL	3.5–4.9 mg/dL, or Output <500 mL/d	>5.0 mg/dL or Output <200 mL/d

Abbreviations: CNS, central nervous system; MAP, mean arterial pressure.
Total SOFA score at admission to the intensive care unit performs well in obstetric patients as a predictor of mortality; sensitivity 87%, specificity 90%, and area under the curve of 0.95 using a cutoff of 9.[56]
Adapted from Vincent J-L, Moreno R, Takala J, et al. The SOFA (Sepsis-Related Organ Failure Assessment) score to describe organ dysfunction/failure. On behalf of the Working Group on Sepsis-Related Problems of the European Society of Intensive Care Medicine. Intensive Care Med 1996;22:707–10; with permission.

PATHOPHYSIOLOGY

Only a small number of infections end in sepsis. Even bacteremia does not necessarily lead to sepsis: among 135 bacteremic women identified in a Paris hospital during pregnancy or puerperium, only 5 were sick enough to be admitted to an ICU.[7]

The innate immune system of humans and other mammals contains pattern-recognition receptors (such as Toll-like receptors [TLRs]). These pattern-recognition receptors are keyed to identify pathogen-associated molecular patterns and the host's own danger-associated molecular patterns (also known as alarmins). Inflammatory signals are released by pattern-recognition receptors and packaged into complexes known as inflammasomes. Activated inflammasomes, along with other molecular packages, mediate the release of interleukins, initiate apoptosis, and prompt the expression of genes that code for cytokines.[8] All of these responses are, obviously, proinflammatory. In concert, the host must activate an antiinflammatory systemic response, which involves epigenetic modification, immune cells, cytokine receptors, interference with TLR signaling, and a vagally mediated cholinergic pathway.[8-10] A host response balanced between proinflammatory and antiinflammatory response clears infection without destroying its own organs and tissues. An overly proinflammatory response produces collateral damage to the host's tissues, death of necrotic cells with further release of danger-associated molecular patterns, and a feedback loop that continues to escalate the process; an exaggerated antiinflammatory response fails to contain infection and microbial replication, in addition to leaving the host vulnerable to secondary infection. Sepsis results when immune system homeostasis fails.

Both host and pathogen factors are involved in activation of the immune system, not just in isolation, but even in cross-talk. Pathogen virulence varies by quorum and inoculum, and certain molecules produced by a stressed or compromised mammalian host can be identified by a bacterial quorum sensing system, which then preferentially turns on replication and virulence genes. In addition to obvious host factors (age, comorbidities) affecting susceptibility to infection, genetic differences play a role. For example, specific polymorphisms in cytokine and TLR genes have been identified that increase host susceptibility to certain pathogens, and polymorphisms in interleukin-8, protein C, and others increase the risk of organ failure and mortality when sepsis is present.[11]

Organ dysfunction or failure may manifest in many ways. The respiratory and cardiovascular systems are commonly affected, in the form of acute respiratory distress syndrome, or hypotension or hyperlactatemia. Acute kidney injury is seen as oliguria or increasing serum creatinine; brain dysfunction as altered mental status; the gastrointestinal system may be affected, for example, ileus or hepatic injury, with increasing transaminases; endocrinologic disturbances may occur, such as adrenal or thyroid dysfunction, or dysregulated glucose control; and hematologic derangement is common, specifically, thrombocytopenia or coagulopathy.[12] Among 4158 cases of (severe) maternal sepsis in the United States, respiratory dysfunction was seen in 34%, coagulopathy in 19%, renal dysfunction in 16%, cardiovascular dysfunction in 12%, hepatic dysfunction in 10%, and central nervous system alteration in 8%.[13]

EPIDEMIOLOGY
Epidemiology of Sepsis in the General Adult Population

Classic work by Angus and colleagues[14] in 1995 calculated 3.0 cases of severe sepsis per 1000 population and estimated 751,000 cases per year in the United States. The age-specific incidence rate was lower among women than among men, although the predilection for source of infection varied by gender: women were more likely to have genitourinary and less likely to have respiratory sources than men. Adjusted for age, comorbidity, and site of original infection, the likelihood of dying from sepsis was the same, with in-hospital mortality of 29%. The probability of death correlated with the number of failing organ systems, increasing from 21% with single-organ failure, to 44% with 2 organ systems having failed, to 76% for failure of 4 or more. More recently, in a general (not pregnant) population drawn from the National Inpatient Sample, the proportion of hospital discharges coded for severe sepsis more than doubled, from 1.0% in 2000 to 2.4% in 2007,[15] an increase that could not be accounted for by population aging. Whereas the incidence of severe sepsis increased over the time period studied, in-hospital mortality decreased significantly, from 40% in 2000 to 27% in 2007. It is impossible to tell whether this reflects a true evolution in patterns of sepsis, an improvement in care, or a different threshold to diagnose sepsis in different years. Differences in coding and reimbursement may have played a role. Both incidence and mortality increase with advancing age; specifically, in the age groups most commonly perceived as reproductive age, incidence of severe sepsis in this study was 35 per 100,000 at age 18 to 24, increasing to 78 per 100,000 at 35 to 39. Survival to hospital discharge did not necessarily equate to normal quality of life; only 20% were discharged to home outright, 35% were discharged to a skilled nursing facility and another 12% to some type of home care.

Epidemiology of Sepsis in Pregnancy and the Puerperium

Previous and recent changes in sepsis definitions, as well as questionable case ascertainment, leave questions of epidemiology somewhat unsettled. Furthermore, the decision about what constitutes the denominator varies: researchers have used live births, delivery hospitalizations, and total pregnancies. Until recently, information about sepsis in pregnancy was limited to case series, usually single institution.

Fortunately, there are now a number of population-based studies available on sepsis related to pregnancy and the puerperium. In the Netherlands, between 2004 and 2006, sepsis was reported in 2.1 per 10,000 deliveries.[16] The United Kingdom Obstetric Surveillance System (UKOSS) estimated the incidence of severe sepsis, including septic shock, as 4.7 per 10,000 maternities in a prospective case-control study from 2011 to 2012.[17] Because less than one-third of these were admitted to ICU, however, one might question the severity of sepsis.

Rates of sepsis seem to be increasing in obstetric populations. Between 1991 and 2003, the incidence of "septicemia" was calculated at 2.2 per 10,000 delivery hospitalizations in the United States.[18] By comparison, in California between 2005 and 2007, rates of "uncomplicated sepsis," including "septicemia," were 5.0 per 10,000; another 4.5 per 10,000 were coded as "severe sepsis," including septic shock.[19] Even allowing for differences in case ascertainment, this estimate of nearly 10 cases per 10,000 delivery hospitalizations would represent a doubling in incidence of maternal sepsis. Using data from 5 million births derived from the US National Inpatient Sample, Al-Ostad and colleagues[20] demonstrated a steady increase in maternal sepsis between 2003 and 2008, from approximately 2 cases per 10,000 to approximately 4 per 10,000. Other researchers using the National Inpatient Sample reported that the overall rate of sepsis during hospitalization for delivery remained stable at 3 in 10,000 from 1998 to 2008, but the incidence of severe sepsis and deaths from sepsis increased by 10% each year: by the end of the 10-year period, rates of severe sepsis and sepsis-related deaths had more than doubled.[13] In a careful analysis of 4 million pregnancy hospitalizations and 5 million estimated pregnancies across a decade, Oud and Watkins[21] found that the rate of pregnancy-associated severe sepsis associated with delivery hospitalizations in Texas rose from 6 per 10,000 live births in 2001 to 12 per 10,000 live births in 2010. These researchers also pointed out that studying the incidence of severe sepsis associated only with delivery hospitalization will severely underestimate the burden of disease in an obstetric population. In this study, only about one-third of pregnancy-associated severe sepsis hospitalizations occurred at the delivery hospitalization. Analyzing total estimated pregnancies (livebirths, abortions, and fetal losses), they calculated the incidence of pregnancy-associated severe sepsis as 11 per 10,000 pregnancies in 2001 and 26 per 10,000 pregnancies in 2010. Although the absolute numbers are greater than those reported by others, the increasing trend is in line.

Many of these population-based studies do not separate antepartum from postpartum cases when describing sources of infection and microbiology. Antepartum cases make up less than one-half of the total recognized maternal sepsis.[16,17,21] Generally, in antepartum sepsis, major contributors are the urinary tract, the genital tract, and pneumonia. Postpartum sepsis is most often attributed to genital tract sources, followed by wound and urinary tract infections (**Table 2**). Other sources include abdomen (appendicitis was surprisingly common in the Dutch study), central nervous system, endocarditis, and medical devices such as intravenous cannulas. A significant percentage (>20%) is described as "unknown."

A full accounting of microorganisms associated with sepsis in the obstetric population is difficult; in many studies, these were not recorded, not reported, or there was no laboratory confirmation. In Acosta and coworkers'[17] meticulous case control study, the clinical laboratory was able to identify the inciting organism in only 64% of cases, and the clinician could identify the source in only 74%; in 16%, neither the source nor the organism was known. These figures are not out of line with the larger experience of sepsis: in general (nonpregnant) adult populations, blood cultures are negative in two-thirds of patients with sepsis, and in another one-third all cultures from all sites are negative.[12] A summary of pathogens is presented in **Table 3**.

Various clinical factors have been evaluated for associations with sepsis or severe sepsis in obstetric patients. Not all factors have been assessed in all studies, and evidence conflicts among others. The best-supported associations with sepsis in high-income countries are surgical procedures (cerclage, cesarean, curettage), multiple pregnancy, maternal comorbidities (cardiovascular, hepatic, renal disease, human immunodeficiency virus infection), and African ancestry/ethnicity.[13,16,17,19–21] Various researchers have pointed to obesity, parity, or maternal age as risk factors, but these are not universally borne out.

CASE FATALITY/MORTALITY

Mortality from sepsis has decreased over time in the general population. In a large American population-based dataset, mortality among (nonpregnant) adults decreased from nearly 40% in 2000 to 27% in 2007.[14] Using data from both administrative data sets and the control arm of clinical trials, Stevenson showed that mortality from severe sepsis decreased from 47% in 1991 to 1995 to 29% in 2006 to 2009, and calculated an annual percentage decrease of 3% per year.[22]

Sepsis mortality, like incidence, is heavily dependent on age, so these figures cannot be directly compared with the (much younger) pregnant and postpartum group. It does seem that the mortality rate from sepsis in the obstetric population is lower. Kramer and associates[16] calculated the overall case fatality rate as 7.7% in the Netherlands. This is a rare study in that it breaks down outcome by source and timing of septic insult: 8% for "obstetric sepsis" and 12% for "nonobstetric sepsis,"

Table 2
Sources of sepsis (pregnant and postpartum)

	Temporal Distribution (%)	Pneumonia (%)	Urinary (%)	Genital Tract (%)	Genitourinary (%)	Pyelonephritis (%)	Chorioamnionitis (%)	Endometritis (%)	Wound	Endocarditis	Meningitis	Central Line or Device-Related	Abdominal Source (Not Uterus)
Antepartum	43.6 and 10.3 intrapartum[16]	9[17]	33.6[16]	20.2[17]	—	—	—	—	—	—	—	—	—
Postpartum	46.2[16]	3.5[17]	11.7[16]	37.2[17]	—	—	—	—	14.3[17]	—	—	—	—
Obstetric	58[16]	—	—	—	—	—	—	—	—	—	—	—	—
Nonobstetric	44[16]	8[16]	14[16]	—	—	—	—	—	—	—	—	—	6 appendicitis[16]
Timing not specified: Pregnant + postpartum	—	29.7[20] 24.8[21]	33.3[21]	—	29.7[13]	5.8[13]	18.4[13]	8.6[13]	4.7[13]	2.3[13]	<1[13]	<1[13] 3.6[21]	—

Categorization schemes vary by study.

Table 3
Organisms identified in maternal sepsis

	Antepartum (%)	Postpartum (%)	"Obstetric" Causes (%)[16]	Timing Not Specified (%)
Gram positive	—	—	—	11.7[21]
Streptococcus	—	—	—	20.1[13]
Group A streptococcus	1.5[17]	13.0[17]	31.8[16]	—
Group B streptococcus	9.7[17]	7.4[17]	~2[16]	—
Other streptococcus	4.5[17]	6.5[17]	~2[16]	—
Pneumococcus	—	—	—	3.8[13]
Staphylococcus	1.5[17]	9.1[17]	—	22.2[13]
Gram negative	—	—	—	18.3[21]
E coli	24.6[17]	19.1[17]	11.4[16]	26.7[13]
Citrobacter	—	—	~2[16]	—
Pseudomonas	—	—	—	2.4[13]
H influenzae	—	—	—	1.1[13]
Serratia	—	—	—	<1[13]
Anaerobes	—	—	—	2[13] 1[21]
Fusobacterium	—	—	~2[16]	—
Mixed	3.7[17]	6.1[17]	—	—
Fungal	—	—	—	1.3[21]
Candida	—	—	—	1.8[13]
No growth in laboratory	41.8[17]	32.9[17]	—	—

11% for antenatal onset of sepsis, versus less than 3% for postpartum sepsis. In this paper, group A streptococcus–associates sepsis was particularly deadly, with the case fatality rate calculated at 14%.

Mortality was much lower in the UKOSS, being 1.5% in antepartum and 1.3% in postpartum cases.[17] As mentioned, the UKOSS report probably includes less severe forms of sepsis, because fewer than one-third of cases were admitted to ICU. Case fatality estimates for maternal septic shock in the United States range from 3.2%[13] to 4.4%.[20] Oud and Watkins' data[21] for pregnancy-associated severe sepsis in Texas, in which organ failure or shock were inclusion criteria, put the mortality risk for severe sepsis at 9.7% in 2001 to 2002, increasing to 12% in 2009 to 2010.

Survival is not the only outcome of interest, of course. Many sepsis survivors have a profoundly altered quality of life. Both functional and cognitive impairments are common.[22,23] The extent of this dysfunction is unknown among survivors of pregnancy-associated sepsis, but may be inferred from the Texas data, in which only 74% of survivors were discharged home without provision for additional care (eg, skilled nursing facility, home nursing, etc). More subtle challenges for these survivors, such as how they cope with the challenges of caring for themselves and their newborns, are entirely unmapped.

SUSPICION AND DIAGNOSIS OF SEPSIS IN PREGNANCY

The definitions for sepsis have been drawn from nonpregnant individuals, and do not take into account the alterations in normal physiology that accompany pregnancy. If nonpregnant norms are used, either overdiagnosis or underdiagnosis of sepsis may occur. Bauer and colleagues[24] analyzed the literature on maternal physiologic parameters with reference to the 1992 sepsis criteria (see **Box 1**). Tachypnea, tachycardia, $Paco_2$, and leukocytosis cutoffs for SIRS and sepsis overlapped with normal ranges for pregnancy, labor, and/or early puerperium, which would render them useless for diagnosing sepsis in obstetrics. In addition to the high false-positive rate, there is potential for the obstetrician, who commonly sees these findings in normal pregnancy, to miss the signal of sepsis for the background noise.

Dissatisfaction with existing scoring systems to predict morbidity in pregnant patients continues. Attempts have been made to devise a pregnancy-specific scoring system for sepsis. One such score, the "Sepsis in Obstetrics Score" evaluated a combination of temperature, blood pressure, heart rate, respiratory rate, peripheral oxygen saturation, white blood cell count, percentage of bands, and lactic acid as a predictor of ICU admission for sepsis.[25] Parameters were modified to account for known changes in pregnancy (**Table 4**). Among a group of women presenting to an obstetric triage unit with a clinician's suspicion of sepsis, the positive predictive value of the "Sepsis in Obstetrics Score" was higher than that of its comparators, the Rapid Emergency Medicine Score and the Modified Early Warning Score, but was still only 16.7% for this surrogate endpoint of ICU admission, with no information about clinically relevant endpoints such as significant morbidity or death.

The previous SIRS criteria have been uniformly deemed "unhelpful" in identifying sepsis by the Sepsis-3 task force, which suggests that the problem of sepsis determination extends to more than just the obstetric population. The 2016 Sepsis-3 criteria[6] recommend that sepsis be considered if any 2 of these criteria are present:

- Altered mentation
- Respiratory rate of greater than or equal to 22/min
- Systolic blood pressure of less than or equal to 100 mm Hg

This is the quick SOFA score. An abnormal quick SOFA should then prompt the physician to investigate whether organ dysfunction is present and to either initiate or escalate therapy, as appropriate. (For a patient already in ICU, use the full SOFA score instead; consider sepsis if SOFA score increases by ≥2 points.) The cornerstone of management in sepsis is early recognition with early treatment. In the absence of a diagnostic test, the clinician should consider sepsis as a possibility if there are either signs of infection or signs of organ dysfunction. The most recent triennial report on maternal death in the United Kingdom explicitly states: "'Think Sepsis' at an early stage when presented with an unwell pregnant or recently pregnant woman."[26] It is important not to rely too greatly on temperature. Fever is not necessarily present in sepsis, as shown by the Michigan series of maternal deaths: 73% of women who died of sepsis were afebrile at presentation and 25% never mounted a fever during the hospital course.[27]

MANAGEMENT

If sepsis is recognized or suspected, it is crucial to assess and correct perfusion, look for organ dysfunction, and begin appropriate antimicrobials. Cultures should be obtained, including blood cultures, but initiation of antibiotics should not be delayed to do so.

Management guidelines have been promulgated by the SSC.[28] For the gynecology patient, no modifications are necessary. In the absence of evidence-based pregnancy-specific management recommendations for sepsis, it is probably advisable

Table 4
Sepsis in obstetrics score

Variable					Normal				
Score	+4	+3	+2	+1	0	+1	+2	+4	+4
Temperature (°C)	>40.9	39–40.9	—	38.5–38.9	36–38.4	34–35.9	32–33.9	30–31.9	<30
Systolic BP (mm Hg)	—	—	—	—	>90	—	70–90	—	<70
Heart rate (bpm)	>179	150–179	130–149	120–129	≤119	—	—	—	—
Respiratory rate/min	>49	35–49	—	25–34	12–24	10–11	6–9	—	≤5
S_pO_2	—	—	—	—	>92%	90%–91%	—	85%–89%	<85%
WBC (/µL)	>39.9	—	25–39.9	17–24.9	5.7–16.9	3–5.6	1–2.9	—	<1
% Immature neutrophils	—	—	≥10%	—	<10%	—	—	—	—
Lactic acid (mmol/L)	—	—	≥4	—	<4	—	—	—	—

Abbreviations: BP, blood pressure; WBC, white blood cell count.

Score ≥6, 16.7% admitted to intensive care unit (ICU); Score >6, 0.1% admitted to ICU.

Adapted from Albright CM, Ali TN, Lopes TN, et al. The sepsis in obstetrics score: a model to identify risk of morbidity from sepsis in pregnancy. Am J Obstet Gynecol 2014;211:39.e2; with permission.

to follow general management guidelines. These were first published by the SSC in 2003, updated in 2008, and revised again in 2012. Guidelines, care bundles and other resources are available online at www.survivingsepsis.org. Recommendations for initial resuscitation, screening for sepsis, diagnosis, antimicrobial treatment, source control, and infection prevention are included; some are addressed herein.

Antimicrobial Therapy

Delay in implementing appropriate antimicrobial therapy has been associated with worse outcome. In a cohort study of more than 2700 adults (nonpregnant) admitted with septic shock, the interval between onset of hypotension and administration of effective antibiotic treatment was inversely proportional to survival: each hour of delay lowered the risk of survival by about 7%. In other words, when antibiotics were begun within the first hour of hypotension in septic shock, nearly 80% of patients survived to hospital discharge, compared with 70% when antimicrobial therapy began at 1 to 2 hours, 42% when it was delayed to 5 to 6 hours, and only 25% if treatment was delayed to 9 to 12 hours after the onset of hypotension.[29] The effect of treatment delay is seen even in the absence of overt shock; in a smaller study, adults with severe sepsis who were receiving goal-directed fluid resuscitation and whose time from initial triage to antibiotic initiation was 1 hour or less had a 81% probability of in-hospital survival, compared with the 67% probability they incurred when antibiotics were given at more than 1 hour after triage.[30] A multicenter study analyzing nearly 18,000 patients with severe sepsis or septic shock showed an increase in mortality of about 5% to 7% per hour as time increased between recognition of sepsis and first administration of antibiotic.[31]

Delays in recognition or management have been recorded in more than 70% of cases of maternal septic shock and septic death.[27,32] This suggests there is plenty of room for improvement. Interestingly, gender disparity affects sepsis care; on average, women with a diagnosis of sepsis receive antibiotics about one-half of an hour later than men.[33]

The initial choice of antibiotic will be empiric and broad. If the source is known, specific antimicrobial regimens can be used per guideline or hospital protocol (eg, treatment for community-acquired pneumonia, methicillin-resistant *Staphylococcus aureus*, influenza, etc). The source may not, however, be clear. Because group A streptococcus and *Escherichia coli* are the most common contributors to sepsis in pregnancy and responsible for a significant fraction of deaths, coverage should include these organisms. Group A streptococcus remains widely sensitive to beta-lactams at the time of this writing. Local patterns of resistance should be accounted for; an infectious disease consultant or the local or state department of health can often provide assistance in developing the antibiotic pathway. Single-agent coverage will not be sufficient. Common combinations in septic obstetric patients include a penicillin plus aminoglycoside plus clindamycin, or vancomycin plus piperacillin-tazobactam.[28] If the source or organism is known, antibiotic therapy can be focused more tightly. Within a few days of presentation, culture results will often dictate a change in therapy; antibiotics should be narrowed once cultures are back.

Source Control

Source control is an important component of sepsis management. This ranges from minor or peripheral (removing a catheter) to major (draining an intraabdominal abscess, removing an infected organ). Although there is sparse literature delineating the optimal time for achieving source control, most believe that sooner is better, as long as the patient is stable enough to tolerate the intervention. Diagnostic imaging is helpful in confirming clinical suspicion. The intervention with the least potential for physiologic derangement is preferable, for example, percutaneous drainage of an abdominal or pelvic abscess rather than laparotomy.[34] Many cases of obstetric sepsis are amenable to source control, because the source can often be identified (eg, uterus, surgical site) and is often accessible to drainage or evacuation. Source control is especially crucial in septic abortion.

Early Goal-directed Therapy

The concept of early goal-directed therapy (EGDT) in the management of septic shock refers to treatment guided by central venous monitoring, predicated on aggressive fluid resuscitation, transfusion, vasopressors and inotropes to achieve a central venous pressure (CVP) of 8 to 12 mm Hg and a central venous oxygenation saturation of 70% or greater. In a small randomized controlled trial in 2001, Rivers and co-workers[35] demonstrated a benefit in mortality: in-hospital mortality was 46% in the usual care group and 30% in the EGDT group, and the 60-day mortality 57% versus 43%. This management strategy was quickly adopted elsewhere, and has been recommended in the obstetric population as well,[36–38] although, as usual, data specific to pregnancy have been lacking.

Support for EGDT has waned, however, with the publication of 3 larger randomized, controlled trials (totaling >3000 patients), which have shown no benefit at all, and suggest more organ failure, more interventions, longer hospital stays, and higher cost when EGDT is used in sepsis, compared with standard care or other protocol-based management.[39–41] Notably, survival in all 3 of these large trials—carried out between 2010 and 2014—was much better than in Rivers's original paper, being about 20% at 60 days, which suggests that even if EDGT does not provide a benefit, something about the management of septic shock has improved in a 15-year span. New care bundles from SSC, acknowledging the lack of benefit of a central venous catheter in sepsis and septic shock, have been revised so that volume status and tissue perfusion may be assessed with either focused clinical examination, or 2 of the following: CVP, $ScvO_2$, bedside cardiac ultrasound imaging, or dynamic assessment of fluid responsiveness via passive leg raising or fluid challenge.[42,43] The preponderance of evidence, then, is marshaled against any recommendation for EGDT in sepsis in pregnancy: it was never tested in pregnant patients in the first place, and is largely discredited outside of pregnancy.

Fluid Therapy

Sepsis is associated with vasodilation and, often, with myocardial dysfunction. Fluid resuscitation, or a fluid challenge, is proposed as a way to restore preload in the veno-dilated septic patient. Unfortunately, not all hemodynamically unstable patients are fluid responders, and in those who are not, aggressive fluid resuscitation will only worsen diastolic dysfunction and tissue edema.[44] SSC guidelines[28] recommend crystalloid at 30 mL/kg for hypotension or for lactate of 4 mmol/L or greater in nonpregnant adults. This may be overly aggressive, however, in pregnancy, when colloid oncotic pressure is lower and the potential for pulmonary edema is greater. A quick and reversible way to assess a patient's responsiveness to a fluid challenge is to passively raise the legs and look for hemodynamic improvement. Fluid responders—about 50% of critically ill patients—are good candidates for bolus IV fluids, whereas those who do not show hemodynamic improvement with passive leg raising should be approached more cautiously; aggressive fluid resuscitation will probably not improve blood pressure significantly and has the potential to cause organ failure. As ever, neither of these strategies has been formally tested in pregnancy. When choosing a crystalloid solution, balanced salt solutions (Ringer's lactate, Isolyte, Normosol, Plasmalyte) are associated with lower mortality in sepsis, compared with isotonic saline.[44] SSC prioritizes crystalloid over colloid. Peripheral or central access is acceptable.[39–41] A central venous catheter does provide a measurement of CVP, but this is a poor stand-in for intravascular volume in general,[45] even less valid in pregnancy,[46] and the optimal CVP is not known. Targeting of central venous oxygen saturation to 65% to 70%, once recommended by SSC,[28] confers no survival benefit.[39–41]

Vasopressors

The purpose of vasopressors is to constrict a pathologically dilated peripheral circulation and thereby maintain adequate perfusion. SSC[28] recommends norepinephrine as the first-line drug and suggests individualizing the target for MAP. Although the usual recommendation is a MAP target of 65 mm Hg, this will often be too high for a previously healthy young patient, and is almost certainly too high in pregnancy. Fortunately, many pregnant patients have another measure of perfusion readily available, in the form of the fetal heart rate tracing: this is exquisitely sensitive to placental perfusion. Rather than aiming for a prespecified MAP of 65 mm Hg, the MAP should be interpreted with reference to organ perfusion, including (although not limited to) fetal heart rate tracing.

Norepinephrine has been used to maintain blood pressure under regional anesthesia for cesarean delivery[47] and, at least at low doses, seems to be safe for fetuses, in contrast with ongoing maternal shock, which is demonstrably unsafe. Some additional reassurance on its safety profile comes from a dual-perfused single-cotyledon model of human placenta, in which norepinephrine did not affect perfusion on the fetal side[48] The clinician should not hesitate to administer norepinephrine to a septic pregnant patient when indicated.

Dobutamine, which is not a vasopressor but an inotrope, is recommended by SSC when myocardial dysfunction or ongoing hypoperfusion exists despite adequate intravascular MAP and intravascular volume. There is little use for this outside the Rivers EGDT protocol, which, as discussed, is outdated. In the recent ProCESS (A Randomized Trial of Protocol-Based Care for Early Septic Shock) trial,[39] only 1% of patients with septic shock not randomized to EGDT were treated with dobutamine. It is unlikely to be called for in septic pregnant patients. Dobutamine does decrease blood flow to the gravid uterus in pregnant ewes,[49] although there are no data in human pregnancy.

Adjunctive and Supportive Therapy (Discussed in the Surviving Sepsis Campaign Guidelines)

- Corticosteroids are no longer recommended (except in rare cases of septic shock refractory to fluids and vasopressors).[28] No data are available in pregnancy. Many pregnant patients will have received dexamethasone or betamethasone for fetal lung maturity. Animal data suggest that there may be a benefit of dexamethasone in improving hemodynamics and reversing shock in sepsis.[50]
- Blood products
  - SSC recommends red cell transfusion in sepsis if the hemoglobin concentration decreases to less than 7.0 g/dL, targeting a value of 7.0 to 9.0 g/dL. No data are available in pregnancy.
  - Fresh frozen plasma should not be given to correct laboratory values, unless bleeding is present or an invasive procedure is planned.
  - Platelets
    - Prophylactic, even without bleeding, if the platelet count is 10,000/mm^3 or less.

- Prophylactic, even without bleeding, if platelet count is 20,000/mm^3 or less and the patient has a significant risk of bleeding (temperature >38°C, recent hemorrhage, even if minor, rapid decrease in platelet count, or other coagulation abnormalities).
  - Higher platelet count (≥50,000/mm^3) advisable if actively bleeding or surgery is planned.
- Recombinant activated protein C (drotrecogin alfa) was withdrawn from the market in 2011 after the PROWESS (Recombinant Human Activated Protein C Worldwide Evaluation in Severe Sepsis) trial showed no effect on mortality in septic shock.[51]
- Mechanical ventilation for sepsis-induced acute respiratory distress syndrome, (See Briggs H, Varelmann D: Respiratory considerations including airway and ventilation issues in critical care obstetric patients, in this issue).
- Glucose control: In general critical care populations, intensive insulin therapy and tight glucose control (targeted 80–110 mg/dL) does not benefit patients, increases hypoglycemic episodes, and may increase mortality to a slight extent.[52] Target blood glucose levels of 180 mg/dL or less are currently recommended in adult critical care patients. It is unclear what level would be appropriate for pregnant septic patients. Obstetricians are taught to maintain blood glucose levels between 80 and 120 in diabetic patients in labor, so as to reduce the risk of neonatal hypoglycemia: however, antenatal sepsis is a different phenomenon, and maternal benefit is at least as important as neonatal. Ultimately, this decision must be individualized.
- Bicarbonate therapy for sepsis or hyperlactatemia is not recommended.
- Prophylaxis against venous thrombosis: Pharmacoprophylaxis, either with low-molecular-weight heparin (once daily) or unfractionated heparin (2 or 3 times daily), plus pneumatic compression devices. If the patient has a contraindication to anticoagulation (eg, coagulopathy, active bleeding), use compression devices alone. All of these recommendations are valid in pregnancy and the puerperium, although plans for analgesia, anesthesia, and delivery may require modification.
- Stress ulcer prophylaxis: Proton pump inhibitor or H$_2$ blocker if a septic patient has risk factors for upper gastrointestinal bleeding (coagulopathy, prolonged mechanical ventilation). Pregnancy should not alter this recommendation.
- Nutrition: Oral or enteral feeding, rather than parenteral nutrition is recommended. Weak evidence for sepsis, although in general critical care populations there seems to be some benefit from oral or enteral feeding. No data guide a recommendation for nutrition in the septic pregnant patient. Concerns about delayed gastric emptying are valid, but can be vitiated if enteral rather than oral nutrition is delivered. Indwelling central catheters, particularly if used for nutrition, do pose a risk for bacteremia, sepsis, and thrombosis.

DELIVERY CONSIDERATIONS IN MATERNAL SEPSIS

Antepartum sepsis arising from the uterus will require delivery, not just antibiotics, and neonatal survival is strongly correlated with gestational age. Attempts to delay delivery in this setting are fraught with harm for the mother and are likely to fail in any case.

Sepsis arising from a nonuterine source in the antenatal period is trickier. Data are limited here, but preterm labor and birth are common. Acosta and associates[17] found the median gestational age at onset of antenatal sepsis to be 35 weeks, and a median diagnosis-to-delivery interval of 0 days. Eighty percent of antepartum sepsis in this study was nongenital in origin, which suggests that there is little to no latency between any type of maternal sepsis and delivery. It is not possible to distinguish spontaneous preterm birth from medically indicated preterm birth in this paper. However, the maternal inflammatory response in sepsis is systemic, and even distant infection (pyelonephritis, periodontal disease) is associated with spontaneous preterm birth. The role of maternal microbial communities both within and outside of the uterus is not yet understood, but is a focus of research.[53]

Keeping in mind that sepsis is more than infection, it is not necessary to posit direct transplacental spread of pathogens as the proximate cause of preterm birth related to maternal sepsis. A proinflammatory maternal milieu may trigger preterm labor via different mechanisms altogether. In a recent biochemical review, a signature of specifically expressed genes related to infection, immunity, or inflammation was associated with preterm birth, including increased expression of TLR, receptor of advanced glycation end products, and alarmins.[54] Activated TLR or other mediators at the level of the uterus may trigger a cytokine response that induces uterine activity and preterm birth.[55] There is clearly a need for further research in this area. The practicing obstetrician–gynecologist, however, faced with a septic patient who is still pregnant should be prepared for both spontaneous preterm birth and for the potential need for delivery as a component of therapy.

REFERENCES

1. Vincent J-L, Opal SM, Marshall JC, et al. Sepsis definitions: time for change. Lancet 2013;381:774–5.
2. Bone RC, Balk RA, Cerra FR, et al, Members of the American College of Chest Physicians/Society of Critical Care Medicine Consensus Conference Committee. American College of Chest Physicians/Society of Critical Care Medicine Consensus Conference: definitions for sepsis and organ failure and guidelines for the use of innovative therapies in sepsis. Crit Care Med 1992;20:864–74.
3. Levy MM, Fink MP, Marshall JC, et al. 2001 SCCM/ESICM/ACCP/ATS/SIS International Sepsis Definitions Conference. Crit Care Med 2003;31:1250–6.
4. Seymour CW, Liu VX, Iwashyna TJ, et al. Assessment of clinical criteria for sepsis. For the Third International Consensus Definitions for Sepsis and Septic Shock (Sepsis-3). JAMA 2016;315(8):762–74.
5. Shankar-Hari M, Phillips PS, Levy ML, et al, Sepsis Definitions Task Force. Developing a new definition and assessing new clinical criteria for septic shock. For the Third International Consensus Definitions for Sepsis and Septic Shock (Sepsis-3). JAMA 2016;315(8):775–87.
6. Singer M, Deutschman CS, Seymour CW, et al. The Third International Consensus Definitions for Sepsis and Septic Shock (Sepsis-3). JAMA 2016;315(8):801–10.
7. Surgers L, Valin N, Carbonne B, et al. Evolving microbiological epidemiology and high fetal mortality in 135 cases of bacteremia during pregnancy and postpartum. Eur J Clin Microbiol Infect Dis 2013;32:107–13.
8. Deutschman CS, Tracey KJ. Sepsis: current dogma and new perspectives. Immunity 2014;40:463–75.
9. van der Poll T, Opal SM. Host-pathogen interactions in sepsis. Lancet Infect Dis 2008;8:32–43.
10. Wiersinga WJ, Leopold SJ, Cranendonk DR, et al. Host innate immune responses to sepsis. Virulence 2014;5:36–44.
11. Boyd JH, Russell JA, Fjell CD. The meta-genome of sepsis: host genetics, pathogens and the acute immune response. J Innate Immun 2014;6:272–83.

12. Angus CD, van der Poll T. Severe sepsis and septic shock. N Engl J Med 2013; 369:840–51.

13. Bauer ME, Bateman BT, Bauer ST, et al. Maternal sepsis mortality and morbidity during hospitalization for delivery: temporal trends and independent associations for severe sepsis. Anesth Analg 2013;117:944–50.

14. Angus DC, Linde-Zwirble WT, Lidicker J, et al. Epidemiology of severe sepsis in the United States: analysis of incidence, outcome, and associated costs of care. Crit Care Med 2001;29:1303–10.

15. Kumar G, Kumar N, Taneja A, et al, Milwaukee Initiative in Critical Care Outcomes Research (MICCOR) Group of Investigators. Nationwide trends of severe sepsis in the 21st century (2000-2007). Chest 2011;140:1223–31.

16. Kramer HMC, Schutte JM, Zwart JJ, et al. Maternal mortality and severe morbidity from sepsis in the Netherlands. Acta Obstet Gynecol Scand 2009;88:647–53.

17. Acosta CD, Kurinczuk JJ, Lucas DN, et al, United Kingdom Obstetric Surveillance System. Severe maternal sepsis in the UK, 2011-2012: a national case-control study. PLoS Med 2014;11(7):e1001672.

18. Callaghan WM, Creanga AA, Kuklina EV. Identification of severe maternal morbidity during delivery hospitalizations, United States, 1991-2003. Am J Obstet Gynecol 2008;199:133.e1-8.

19. Acosta CD, Knight M, Lee HC, et al. The continuum of maternal sepsis severity: incidence and risk factors in a population-based cohort study. PLoS One 2013; 8(7):e67175.

20. Al-Ostad G, Kezouh A, Spence AR, et al. Incidence and risk factors of sepsis mortality in labor, delivery, and after birth: population-based study in the USA. J Obstet Gynaecol Res 2015;41:1201–6.

21. Oud L, Watkins P. Evolving trends in the epidemiology, resource utilization outcomes of pregnancy-associated severe sepsis: a population-based cohort study. J Clin Med Res 2015;7:400–16.

22. Iwashyna TJ, Ely EW, Smith DM, et al. Long-term cognitive impairment and functional disability among survivors of severe sepsis. JAMA 2010;304:1787–94.

23. Annane D, Sharshar T. Cognitive decline after sepsis. Lancet Respir Med 2015;3: 61–9.

24. Bauer ME, Bauer ST, Rajala B, et al. Maternal physiologic parameters in relationship to systemic inflammatory response syndrome criteria. Obstet Gynecol 2014; 124:535–41.

25. Albright CM, Ali TN, Lopes TN, et al. The Sepsis in Obstetrics Score: a model to identify risk of morbidity from sepsis in pregnancy. Am J Obstet Gynecol 2014; 211:39.e1-8.

26. on behalf of MBRRACE-UK. In: Knight M, Kenyon S, Bricklehurst P, et al, editors. Saving lives, improving mothers' care – lessons learned to inform future maternity care from the UK and Ireland confidential enquiries into maternal deaths and morbidity 2009-12. Oxford: National Perinatal Epidemiology Unit, University of Oxford; 2014.

27. Bauer ME, Lorenz RP, Bauer ST, et al. Maternal deaths due to sepsis in the state of Michigan, 1999-2006. Obstet Gynecol 2015;126:747–52.

28. Dellinger RP, Levy MM, Rhodes A, et al, Surviving Sepsis Campaign Guidelines Committee including the Pediatric Subgroup. Surviving Sepsis Campaign: international guidelines for management of severe sepsis and septic shock: 2012. Crit Care Med 2013;41:580–637.

29. Kumar A, Roberts D, Wood KE, et al. Duration of hypotension before initiation of effective antimicrobial therapy is the critical determinant of survival in human septic shock. Crit Care Med 2006;34:1589–96.

30. Gaieski DF, Mikkelsen ME, Band RA, et al. Impact of time to antibiotics on survival in patients with severe sepsis or septic shock in whom early goal-directed therapy was initiated in the emergency department. Crit Care Med 2010;38:1045–53.

31. Ferrer R, Martin-Loeches I, Phillips G, et al. Empiric antibiotic treatment reduces mortality in severe sepsis and septic shock from the first hour: results from a guideline-based performance improvement program. Crit Care Med 2014;42: 1749–55.

32. Churchill D, Roger A, Clift J, et al, on behalf of the MBRRACE-UK sepsis chapter writing group, on behalf of MBRRACE-UK. Think sepsis. In: Knight M, Kenyon S, Brocklehurst P, et al, editors. Saving lives, improving mothers' care – lessons learned to inform future maternity care from the UK and Ireland confidential enquiries into maternal deaths and morbidity 2009-12. Oxford: National Perinatal Epidemiology Unit, University of Oxford; 2014. p. 27–44.

33. Madsen TE, Napoli AM. The DISPARITY-II Study: delays to antibiotic administration in women with severe sepsis and septic shock. Acad Emerg Med 2014;21: 1499–502.

34. Marshall JC, Maier RV, Jimenez M, et al. Source control in the management of severe sepsis and septic shock: an evidence-based review. Crit Care Med 2004; 32(Suppl):S513–26.

35. Rivers E, Nguyen B, Havstad S, et al, Early Goal-Directed Therapy Collaborative Group. Early goal-directed therapy in the treatment of severe sepsis and septic shock. N Engl J Med 2001;345:1368–77.

36. Guinn DA, Abel DE, Tomlinson MW. Early goal directed therapy for sepsis during pregnancy. Obstet Gynecol Clin North Am 2007;34:459–79.

37. Barton JR, Sibai BM. Severe sepsis and septic shock in pregnancy. Obstet Gynecol 2012;120:689–706.

38. Pacheco LD, Saade GR, Hankins GDV. Severe sepsis during pregnancy. Clin Obstet Gynecol 2014;57:827–34.

39. Yealy DM, Kellum JA, Huang DT, et al, ProCESS Investigators. A randomized trial of protocol-based care for early septic shock. N Engl J Med 2014;370:1683–93.

40. Peake SL, Delaney A, Bailey M, et al, ARISE Investigators, ANZICS Clinical Trials Group. Goal-directed resuscitation for patients with early septic shock. N Engl J Med 2014;371:1496–506.

41. Mouncey PR, Osborn TM, Power S, et al, ProMISe Trial Investigators. Trial of early, goal-directed resuscitation for septic shock. N Engl J Med 2015;372:1301–11.

42. Surviving Sepsis Campaign Bundles. 2015. Available at: http://www.survivingsepsis.org/SiteCollectionDocuments/SSC_Bundle.pdf. Accessed April 24, 2016.

43. Marik PE, Bellomo R. A rational approach to fluid therapy in sepsis. Br J Anaesth 2016;116:339–49.

44. Ragunathan K, Shaw A, Nathanson B, et al. Association between the choice of IV crystalloid and in-hospital mortality among critically ill adults with sepsis. Crit Care Med 2014;42:1585–91.

45. Marik PE. Early management of severe sepsis: concepts and controversies. Chest 2014;145:1407–18.

46. Crozier TM, Wallace EM, Parkin WG. Haemodynamic assessment in pregnancy and pre-eclampsia: a Guytonian approach. Pregnancy Hypertens 2015;5: 177–81.

47. Ngan Kee WD, Lee SWY, Ng FF, et al. Randomized double-blinded comparison of norepinephrine and phenylephrine for maintenance of blood pressure during spinal anesthesia for cesarean delivery. Anesthesiology 2015;122:736–45.
48. Mintzer BH, Johnson RF, Paschall RL, et al. The diverse effects of vasopressors on the fetoplacental circulation of the perfused human placenta. Anesth Analg 2010;110:857–62.
49. Fishburne JI, Meis PJ, Urban RB, et al. Vascular and uterine responses to dobutamine and dopamine in the gravid ewe. Am J Obstet Gynecol 1980;137(8):944–52.
50. Hicks CW, Sweeney DA, Danner RL, et al. Efficacy of selective mineralocorticoid and glucocorticoid agonists in canine septic shock. Crit Care Med 2012;40(1):199–207.
51. Ranieri VM, Thompson BT, Barie PS, et al, PROWESS-SHOCK Study Group. Drotrecogin alfa (activated) in adults with septic shock. N Engl J Med 2012;366:2055–64.
52. The NICE-SUGAR Study Investigators. Intensive versus conventional glucose control in critically ill patients. N Engl J Med 2009;360:1283–97.
53. Vinturache AE, Gyamfi-Bannerman C, Hwang J, et al. Maternal microbiome—a pathway to preterm birth. Semin Fetal Neonatal Med 2016;21:94–9.
54. Noguchi T, Sado T, Naruso K, et al. Evidence for activation of Toll-like receptor and receptor for advanced glycation end products in preterm birth. Mediators Inflamm 2010;2010:490406.
55. Thaxton JE, Nevers TA, Sharma S. TLR-mediated preterm birth in response to pathogenic agents. Infect Dis Obstet Gynecol 2010;2010 [pii:378472].
56. Jai S, Guleria K, Suneja A, et al. Use of the Sequential Organ Failure Assessment Score for evaluating outcome among obstetric patients admitted to the intensive care unit. Int J Gynaecol Obstet 2016;132:332–6.

Immune Regulation in Pregnancy

A Matter of Perspective?

Elizabeth A. Bonney, MD, MPH

KEYWORDS

- Immune regulation • Pregnancy • Maternal tolerance

KEY POINTS

- Elements of host defense, innate immunity, and adaptive immunity alter during pregnancy.
- The maternal immune system meets the needs for both tolerance and protection through complex regulation but not suppression.
- Classic as well as nonclassic models of immune system activation and tolerance can explain elements of maternal tolerance.

WHY IS UNDERSTANDING OF THE IMMUNE SYSTEM IN PREGNANCY CLINICALLY RELEVANT?

The immune system matters. Several areas of clinical relevance should come to mind. First, regulation of the immune system is thought to play a role in both male and female fertility,[1] and dysregulation of the immune system is still thought to play a role in recurrent miscarriage.[2] Women with asthma, autoimmune disease, immune deficiency, and other derangements of the immune system are at risk for poor pregnancy outcomes[3] and it is clear that interactions between pregnancy and the immune system influence women postpartum and beyond.[4] Recent emergence of viruses such as pandemic influenza,[5] Ebola,[6] and Zika[7,8] also underline the utility of focus on the immune system, particularly with regard to vaccine development for pregnant women. In addition, the implications of the interaction between the pregnant mother's immune system and infectious agents extend not only into the health of the woman but also the health of the embryo, fetus, and neonate. Next is a brief overview of the immune system as relates to pregnancy.

Disclosure: The author has nothing to disclose.
Department of Obstetrics, Gynecology and Reproductive Sciences, University of Vermont College of Medicine, Given Building Room C-246, 89 Beaumont Avenue, Burlington, VT 05405, USA
E-mail address: ebonney@uvm.edu

Obstet Gynecol Clin N Am 43 (2016) 679–698
http://dx.doi.org/10.1016/j.ogc.2016.07.004
0889-8545/16/© 2016 Elsevier Inc. All rights reserved.

HOST DEFENSE

The importance of inherent protective mechanisms present in the reproductive tract, including both barrier and antimicrobial actions, has been recognized.[9] Balance within the microbiome of various tissues can mean the difference between health and autoimmune disease.[10] The more than 1 billion organisms living in the vagina are now thought to mediate both immune protective[11] and immune modulatory functions.[12] Moreover, alterations in the vaginal microbiome may be associated with increased risk of preterm birth.[13] Although the association between altered vaginal microbiome and adverse pregnancy has been observed,[14,15] the interaction between pregnancy, the microbiome, and subsequent disease or health has not been formally tested. In addition to bacteria existing in the vagina, there are viruses that interact with bacteria and the local immune system to support health or generate disease.[16] The microorganisms present in the vagina, in addition to other immune factors, are likely influenced by endogenously produced vaginal fluid and agents such as lubricants and foreign objects (eg, pessaries). Although the cyclic nature of vaginal fluid in the nonpregnant state and the overall composition of the vaginal fluid and cervical mucus present during pregnancy has been evaluated, specific antimicrobial and immune modulating mechanisms are still under examination. For example, antimicrobial peptides such as defensins, reviewed elsewhere,[17] are players in the composition of the cervicovaginal fluid and are protectors against ascending infection.

Another important element of host defense during pregnancy is trophoblast. These cells may present a physical barrier to prevent transmission of infection to the fetus.[18,19] In addition, trophoblast expresses molecules that help to limit or prevent persistent infection.[20–23] However, persistent involvement of the placenta may be seen in several viral infections.[24] Fetal cells are thought to be the source of persistent maternal infection with Zika virus.[25]

INNATE IMMUNITY

Inherent immune-protective/modulating properties of cells and products of the vagina and cervix are often spoken of differently from specific cells of the innate immune system. Characteristics attributed to the innate immune system are lack of specificity, rapidity, and lack of memory. However, the last of these 3 characteristics has come into question because it is apparent that some innate immune cells, particularly natural killer (NK) cells are capable of being "educated",[26] possibly by interaction with trophoblast or decidual cells.[27] It is said that a hallmark of pregnancy is increased activation in systemic innate immunity.[28,29] However, local innate immunity is said to be modified during gestation to be functionally active early in pregnancy in order to assist in implantation, downregulated through most of gestation, and then increased with parturition and labor.

Mast cells[30] play a sentinel role in tissues. Stimulation of mast cells by bacteria or other agents via surface-expressed pattern recognition receptors generates mediators that enhance blood flow, smooth muscle contraction, and trafficking of neutrophils, basophils, and eosinophils. Mast cell granules are packed with proteins, including interleukin (IL)6, tumor necrosis factor (TNF), leukotrienes, and histamine.[31] Histamine exerts its actions through 4 G protein–coupled receptors ($H_{1-4}R$). H_1R and H_4R are regulators of inflammatory, allergic, and autoimmune disease,[32–37] and recent evidence suggests that H_2R and H_4R support the generation of regulatory T cells (T_{reg}) that modulate immune responses.[38–40]

Mast cells are present in the uterus and cervix.[41] Interactions between mast cells and other cells at the maternal-fetal interface mediate implantation (H_2R),[42] support angiogenesis,[43,44] and preserve quiescence[45] until term, when histamine from mast cells binds to H_1R and fosters uterine contractions.[46-48] Type I sensitivity induces premature labor in humans[49] and in animals[50] via histamine binding to H_1R in the uterus.[51]

Neutrophils[52] are critical to the innate response through phagocytosis of bacteria and production of reactive oxygen species, lytic enzymes, and peptides that lead to activation of the inflammatory cascade. Activated neutrophils can pass from the blood through endothelial cells by the use of metalloproteinases that disrupt cellular membranes. Some organisms and stimuli induce neutrophils to undergo a unique form of death, Neutrophil Extracellular Traps -osis, which involves extrusion of chromatin and cytoplasmic contents, which in turn can bind and help immobilize bacteria. This process also generates tissue damage and more inflammation.[53] There exist phenotypic subsets of neutrophils, and some of these may have particular relevance to pregnancy. In the first trimester of human pregnancies, a unique subpopulation of neutrophils, so-called N2, becomes prominent.[54] This population may be supported by local expression of transforming growth factor beta (TGF-β) and expresses proteins important to angiogenesis, including vascular endothelial growth factor-A (VEGF-A). At term and in the context of preterm birth, inflammatory, or N1, neutrophils traffic to the uterus in response to molecules such as IL-8, where they may express matrix metalloproteinases that help to dissolve fetal membranes. After delivery, neutrophils traffic to the cervix to participate in tissue repair.[55]

Dendritic cells typically reside in a quiescent state in tissues. When activated, these cells mature and initiate protein antigen processing and traffic to the lymph nodes draining the tissue. Activated dendritic cells are considered to be the most proficient at processing antigenic protein, placing peptides from that protein into the cleft of major histocompatibility molecules, and shunting the major histocompatibility complex (MHC)–plus-peptide complexes to the surface for presentation to T cells. Presentation involves the binding of the MHC-peptide complex to the T cell receptor, binding of other surface molecules on dendritic cells to their receptors on T cells, and elaboration of soluble factors that can modify the T cell response. The result of this interaction can be activation and proliferation of T cells specific for the protein whose peptide is in the MHC molecule. The dendritic cell population is likely to be slightly different depending on the tissue of residence, and this is true with regard to the placenta, uterus, uterine draining node, and spleen.[56] It is possible that tissue-specific differences in the dendritic cell population are developmentally regulated. It has been observed that dendritic cells in the uterus are limited in their ability to traffic to the uterine-draining lymph nodes during pregnancy[57] and that this supports tolerance of the fetus. Other possibilities of control of dendritic cell function may occur at the level of maturation,[58,59] because it has been proposed that immature dendritic cells support immune tolerance of tissue grafts[60] and cancers.[61] However, inflammation can override these mechanisms and produce activation of dendritic cells from the uterus.[56]

Macrophages

Members of the mononuclear phagocyte family include monocytes and macrophages. In general, monocytes are generated in the bone marrow and circulate as diverse populations[31,62,63] until they traffic to tissues in response to specific developmental or environmental signals such as infection or inflammation.[62] Trafficking to tissues induces differentiation to macrophages. Inflammation or infection, including phagocytosis of bacteria and necrotic cells, causes activation and maturation of tissue-resident macrophages to full effector function.[31] Depending on the tissue type and local signals expressed, macrophages may form distinct phenotypes. One, the M1 phenotype, is considered to be the inflammatory phenotype and is marked by expression of inflammatory cytokines such as IL-1β, IL-6, IL-23, and IL-17.[31,62] The development of this phenotypic subset is driven by the local expression of gamma interferon (γIFN) produced by T helper 1 (Th1) T cells and NK cells and also by TNF expressed by activated dendritic cells.[62] Local expression of βIFN by trophoblast can also support generation of this phenotype.[62] A second group of phenotypes, M2, includes M2a, which are generated by interaction with Th2 cell–elaborated cytokines such as IL-4 and IL-13, and primarily participate in wound healing. Another M2 phenotypic subset, sometimes termed regulatory or M2c, can be activated in certain tissues by ligation of their toll-like receptors. Their development can be supported by the action of IL-10 expressed by T_{reg} and can in turn secrete IL-10 themselves and further support T_{reg} development.[62] Another suppressive offshoot of the monocyte lineage is termed the monocytic myeloid-derived suppressor cells, similar to tumor-associated macrophages, which are said to suppress immune response in tumors and other tissues.[64]

During pregnancy, hormonal changes can alter the presence and phenotype of circulating monocytes.[63] In the decidua, macrophages are present and assist with implantation.[65] Through gestation, they are present at fairly constant numbers in the uterus. The presence of macrophages increases in the cervix at term[66] and in preterm labor.[67,68] Macrophage subsets[63] may contribute to the mechanisms leading to disruption of the fetal membranes, because of expression of matrix metalloproteinases,[69] uterine contractions caused by expression of prostaglandins,[70] and softening and dilation of the cervix caused by expression of collagenases.[71] Given the capacity and complexity of macrophage subsets, it is easy to imagine that macrophages also assist with healing and remodeling of the epithelium over the implantation site, and with cervical and uterine remodeling in the postpartum.[72] Further, data suggest that T cells can modify the phenotype of macrophages or monocytes in secondary lymphoid organs draining the uterus.[73] This finding suggests that macrophages may play a part in regulatory circuits that modify inflammation-induced poor pregnancy outcomes.

NK cells are grouped within the innate lymphoid cell (ILC) 1 subset, and represent a population of cells that can augment inflammation in many sites. Although initially thought to be mostly involved in killing of abnormal cells, including virally infected[74] and cancer[75] cells, over time it has been recognized that distinct subpopulations of NK cells exist. These subpopulations express decreased ability to kill but increased ability to provide factors that modify the growth or differentiation of other cells. Adding complexity to the evolving picture of NK cells are the observations that NK cells can "learn" from exposure to cells and factors from their environment. The complexity of NK cells is highlighted by their presence and function at the maternal-fetal interface where they can collaborate with trophoblast and endothelial cells to remodel decidual vessels and increase blood flow through the placenta. In other sites lack of or alteration in MHC tends to cause NK cell killing. However, it seems that, at the maternal-fetal interface, NK cells may learn and retain the ability to limit trophoblast killing despite the limited MHC expression in the placenta. NK cell function is regulated by an array of inhibitory receptors, including killer immunoglobulin (Ig)–like receptors, and activating receptors.[76] Thus relative expression of inhibitory versus activating receptors might regulate the level of cytotoxicity expressed by these cells. The ILC2 innate lymphoid subset expresses cytokines such as IL-4,[77] but little is known about their presence in decidua or placenta.[78] Within the ILC3 group are the lymphoid tissue inducer (LTi), and NK22 cells. In human decidua, LTi produce γIFN and IL-17, both thought to be important in the response to infection, and NK22 cells that are phenotypically similar to NK cells but also secrete the cytokine IL-22, which can be a growth factor for trophoblast.[79]

Natural killer T (NKT) cells have limited specificity but several of the effector functions of classic T cells. NKT cells were originally shown to be inherently capable of producing cytokines such as IL-4.[80] Invariant NKT cells recognize lipid ligands bound to the MHC-like molecule CD1.[81] Within the reproductive tract, activated NKT cells have been shown to mediate pregnancy loss and preterm birth in mouse models.[82] In contrast, the tumor environment can generate NKT cells that downregulate immune responses,[83] which may occur at the maternal-fetal interface.[84]

Gamma Delta T Cells

During development a proportion of T cell–lineage cells generate T cell receptor chains gamma (γ) and delta (δ), instead of alpha (α) and beta (β). These cells develop and populate tissues earlier than their $\alpha\beta$ counterparts, have a limited repertoire, and in addition tend to populate mucosal surfaces.[85] This behavior places them in a unique position to sample the environment in which the animal exists and be a first line of defense. The exact nature of the antigens recognized by $\gamma\delta$ cells is unknown, but it has been suggested that they, like NKT cells, respond to certain lipids in the context of CD1.[85] In addition, this cell type plays a potential regulatory role because they express the capacity to kill activated T cells.[86] These cells are present in the reproductive tract, where they may modify local immunity.[87] Sex steroids influence the development of these cells.[88] They expand during pregnancy and are found in placental villi in humans[89] and in mice.[90] Although genetic deficiency in $\gamma\delta$ T cells does not inhibit successful pregnancy it may be that pregnancies deficient in $\gamma\delta$ T cells are more susceptible to infection.[91]

ADAPTIVE IMMUNITY
T Cells

T cells bearing $\alpha\beta$ T cell receptor chains comprise the primary regulation of the adaptive immune response. T cells express either the CD4 or CD8 coreceptor that restricts its ability to recognize the peptide bound to MHC class II or class I, respectively. Naive T cells of either type leave the thymus to circulate between blood and lymph nodes draining various organs. When a naive T cell interacts productively with an activated dendritic cell that presents the MHC-plus-peptide complex recognized by the T cell's receptor, the T cell begins to change its developmental status. If the correct mix of other signals is also received by the T cell it can begin to divide and produce daughter cells. The other signals include signaling through molecules such as CD28 and T cell–generated cytokines such as IL-2. Further, the cells that present antigen to T cells can produce cytokines and other factors that can modify the T cell subset that is generated by activation. In addition, T cells can directly or indirectly provide signals that support or suppress the kind of effector function in other T cells.

For CD4 T cells, the many possibilities for effector function have not been clearly delineated. Expression of cytokines such as IL-4, IL-5, and IL-13 constitutes a population of CD4 T cells, Th2, that is important in the production of antibody and protection against some parasites. Overactivity of such cells is a hallmark of allergy and asthma. In contrast, expression of cytokines such as interferon gamma and TNF constitutes a population, Th1, that supports cytotoxic immune responses. The Th2-Th1 paradigm has been the focus of interest with regard to maternal tolerance of the fetus, because many observations suggested that pregnancy caused a shift in the maternal immune system toward Th2 versus Th1 responses.[92] However, the idea that pregnancy is critically dependent on this shift waned because deficiency in critical Th2 cytokines results in grossly normal pregnancies in animal models (eg, Ref.[93]).

With regard to the conundrum defined by the competing needs of maternal tolerance of the fetus and maternal and fetal immune protection, a newer paradigm has arisen, focused on the presence and function of 2 other CD4 T cell subsets: T_{reg} and Th17 cells. The hallmark cytokines of the T_{reg} subset are TGF-β and IL-10, both produced by cells of the placenta. It is now thought that T_{reg} are the primary suppressors of immune responses. T_{reg} lineages include those that are thymus derived (tT_{reg}) and developmentally inhabit tissues, in contrast with those that arise after activation by antigen in the periphery (pT_{reg}). This latter group, is thought to prevent overactivation and supports the reestablishment of a quiescent state. In mouse pregnancy, even when mother, father, and offspring are all the same genotype (syngeneic), there is evidence that the hormonal milieu of pregnancy supports the expansion of T_{reg} capable of suppressing local immunity.[94] In addition, exposure to semen can cause the induction of fetal/paternal antigen–specific T_{reg}.[95] Further exposure to fetal antigens during the course of pregnancy expands this population, thus creating a regulatory pool bearing immunologic memory to fetal antigens, which can then support maternal tolerance in subsequent pregnancies. However, exposure of T_{reg} to inflammatory signals, such as ligands for the Toll-like receptor (TLR) and IL-6, can shift T_{reg} to a potent and highly inflammatory subset, Th17, known for its expression of IL-17. Th17 is induced during the inflammatory response to agents such as listeria[96] and influenza,[97] and is a potential mediator of infection-related abortion and premature labor.[98] Other CD4 T cell subsets invoked in regulation of immunity in the maternal-fetal interface include the Th9 subset, which may be important in the local inflammatory response that supports parturition.[99]

CD8 T cells can also express varying classes of responsiveness, depending on innately expressed genes and exposure to particular signals and cytokines from other T cells[100] or antigen-presenting cells.[101] CD8 T cells produce molecules, such as granzyme and perforin, that assist in killing virally infected cells.[102] They also can assist in the disruption of transplanted organs.[103] CD8 T cells are present at the maternal-fetal interface,[104] particularly during viral infection.[24] Although CD8 T cells can be modified by pregnancy, they can still fetal cells in the maternal blood and lymphoid organs.[105,106] In contrast, and adding to the paradigm that T_{reg} support maternal tolerance, is the observation that pregnancy can support the generation of CD8 T_{reg},[99,107] which may modify CD8 T cell cytotoxicity during pregnancy.

Memory

At some point after immune activation in response to antigen, the proliferative response ends, and a significant proportion of the population of antigen-specific effector cells generated die. The result of this process is a pool of memory T cells. On a population level, memory T cells arise from a linearly differentiated subset of antigen-specific T cells.[108] Pregnancy generates a pool of memory T cells that are specific for fetal antigen.[4,105] Moreover, evidence suggests that vaccination or infection during pregnancy does not impair immunologic memory.[24,109]

Recent observations have focused on a new class of tissue-resident T cells that are thought to be critical in the rapid response of mucosal surfaces to viral or other pathogens. Infection in mucosa generates this pool, which can rapidly circulate back to the index tissue with subsequent infections. Both CD4 and CD8 tissue-resident T cells have been observed in the vagina[110,111] and in uterine[112–114] tissues.

B cells give rise to antibody-producing plasma cells. They develop in the bone marrow and circulate to the periphery where they occupy specialized areas within lymph nodes. There, they can be exposed to antigen migrating from tissues into draining lymph nodes or present on lymph node–resident follicular dendritic cells.[115] For a subset of antigens with a particular structure, exposure to B cells may cause direct activation, proliferation, and differentiation. For another set of antigens, binding to antigen-specific B-cell receptors causes antigen uptake, processing, and presentation to T cells. Presentation generates T cell production of soluble and cell-surface molecules that can bind to B cells and mediate immunoglobulin production, class switch, and differentiation to plasma cells.[116] Lineages of B cells include regulatory B cells that express IL-10, downmodulate the B-cell response, and thus repress autoimmune disease.[117] The B-cell compartment undergoes homeostatic changes during pregnancy[118,119] that may increase serum immunoglobulin levels during this time, as well as supporting distribution of immunoglobulins, including immunoglobulin (Ig) A and IgG, through tissues into their respective lumens (eg, Ref.[120]). It also has been observed that pregnancy expands regulatory B cells[121] and the strength and specificity of these B_{reg} may modify both maternal tolerance and protection against infection.

DO GONADAL STEROIDS AFFECT IMMUNE FUNCTION?

Gonadal steroids comprise the environment generated by the X and Y chromosomes by which gene-by-environment interaction produces health or disease.[122] The view that one hormone, estrogen, is proinflammatory and the other, progesterone, is anti-inflammatory is too simplistic. For example, estrogen can support antiviral immunity in the reproductive tract,[123] and this is thought to depend on an inflammatory cytokine. In contrast, estrogen can modulate immunity by supporting the presence of T_{reg},[124] and is used to treat autoimmune disease. For another example, progesterone, long held to be critical to the apparent immune suppression of pregnancy, supports the expression of cytokines, such as IL-15, that enhance the homeostatic proliferation of immune cells.[125–127] The role of gonadal steroids in immune regulation is likely to be complex. The in vitro and in vivo effects of these molecules on immune cells have anchored the experimental evidence used to support the idea that successful pregnancy requires immune modulation. What about the theoretical constructs addressing the immunology of pregnancy?

THEORIES AND MODELS OF IMMUNE TOLERANCE IN THE CONTEXT OF PREGNANCY

Tolerance is an active process by which the immune system does not respond to a given antigen. Despite the differences in placentation among mammalian species, the so-called problem of viviparity is essentially one wherein the developing fetus is in intimate contact with the mother. In humans and rodents, there are at least 4 potential venues for such contact. The hemachorial placenta of these species, as the name implies, is such that blood from the mother directly bathes trophoblast that arises from the fetus and comprise the placenta. In addition, extravillous trophoblast both anchors the placenta and replaces the endothelium of vessels in order to accommodate maternal blood flow into the intervillous space. Fetal cells migrate to the systemic circulation of the mother, and vice versa. This process accounts for long-term microchimerism in both directions and may carry immunologic consequences.

Self-Nonself Models of Immunity

Classically, recognition of what is nonself initiates T cell activation.[128–130] In these models, regulation of the immune response, including tolerance of self-antigens, includes reliance on specific methods of suppression. By these models, another way to generate functional tolerance is to limit the specific class or brand of immune response possible. Thus, a harmful immune response that is mediated by cytotoxic

T cells is suppressed by the shifting of this immune response to one that produces noncytotoxic antibody. Further, classic models of immunity suggest that a final phase of immune tolerance is the limitation of trafficking or function of T cells generated in the course of activation by antigen.

With respect to pregnancy, classic models have, through interpretation of existing data, morphed over time to include highly complex underlying mechanisms. For example, early models suggested that maternal tolerance was simply a matter of failure of maternal T cells to be exposed to fetal antigen.[128] As an extension of this idea, it has been proposed that there is specific limitation of the trafficking of dendritic cells from the uterus to the uterine draining nodes and that this limits presentation of fetal antigens to maternal T cells during pregnancy.[57] However, as previously mentioned, fetal and maternal cells can traffic in both directions,[131,132] and pregnancy produces systemic immunity to fetal antigens.

Many mechanisms have been put forth as preventative of local activation of immunity. The list of molecules thought to provide both global and local suppression of immunity includes molecules such as indolamine 2,3-deoxygenase (IDO).[133,134] These molecules have been used to support the idea that the whole of pregnancy is a state of relative immune suppression, and thus driven to increased susceptibility to infectious disease. Further, the alternatively activated macrophages and NK cells begin the list of cells with immune-suppressive properties that exist within the uterus and placenta during pregnancy. This list of cells recruited into the immune suppression paradigm recent grew to include the regulatory T cell both in its CD4 and possibly CD8 formats.

The Danger Model

This model is the major alternative to classic models of maternal tolerance of the fetus. This model has been discussed in detail in the context of adverse pregnancy outcomes.[135–137] The critical pieces of this model state that T cell, and therefore immune system activation, is not reliant on recognition of nonself but on recognition of 'danger'. Although this may seem a matter of semantics, it does represent a major shift in how clinicians might think about diseases, including infectious diseases, that occur during pregnancy. According to the danger model, the expression of paternal or unique fetal antigens during pregnancy does not necessarily generate T cell activation if danger is not present. Danger is expressed in fetal tissues and in the decidua through dysregulation of critical metabolic processes, necrosis, and similar mechanisms, which produces a signal that activates dendritic cells and possibly alters the processing of locally expressed antigens. Danger is tied to the activation of dendritic cells and their expression of the costimulatory signals needed for T cell activation. According to the model, recognition of fetal antigen in the absence of costimulation leads to T cell death. Even if a population of T cells is generated against fetal antigens, they do not necessarily generate fetal loss and this depends on the structural integrity, growth, and lack of continued expression of danger in fetal tissues. Like the liver, the remaining placenta and related tissues, if healthy, simply outrun or outgrow any insult by potential attacking T cells. In this context, the expansion of antigen-nonspecific or fetal antigen–specific regulatory T cells may represent a bystander effect that supports the placenta's normal growth or the ability to outrun potentially harmful T cells. The fact that disruption of this population of T cells leads to loss of semiallogeneic fetuses neither proves nor disproves the validity of self-nonself recognition as the basis for immune activation. Through this model, the expression of molecules or the expansion of cells with immune-suppressing characteristics is noncritical to successful fetal antigen–specific maternal immune tolerance. What is critical is the metabolic or physiologic health of fetal cells. This model is also consistent with the idea that some diseases of pregnancy carry a maternal component. For example, in pregnancies marked by preeclampsia, if maternal decidual or endothelial cells are rendered dysfunctional by some insult, this may lead to local or systemic maternal dendritic cell activation and processing of local (eg, the source is placental) or systemic (eg, the source is trafficking fetal cells) fetal antigens and presentation of the relevant peptides to maternal T cells. This process may lead to specific antifetal immunity. In other pregnancies, trafficking of T cells into the decidua can occur in the context of infection and not lead to abortion.[24] Regulation of trafficking to this tissue by effector cells is a complex issue, and possibly not a default mechanism of tolerance.

With regard to the relationship between class of immune response and tolerance of the maternal-fetal unit, the danger model suggests that every tissue has a specific tendency toward the type of immune response generated in that tissue.[138] The presence therefore of foreign or, in the case of pregnancy, fetal/paternal antigen, as opposed to self-antigen, does not drive the class of the response. It may be that placental or intrauterine responses are geared toward certain classes as a result of early developmental programming. This possibility may explain the observation of a tendency toward Th2-type immune responses in decidua or the systemic circulation during pregnancy. Moreover, this model supports the idea that the pleotropic nature of cytokines and growth factors is such that pregnancy loss caused by lack of expression of certain Th2 cytokines, such as IL-10, may have more to do with the poor health of trophoblast than the failure of a class switch in maternal immunity. Further, the danger model's likely interpretation of the fact that lack of expression of the proinflammatory cytokine IL-6 leads to increased gestational length[139] is that IL-6 is an important metabolic regulator of the time clocks leading to parturition, not that inherent midgestation suppression of inflammation is the primary goal of pregnancy-associated tissues.

Evolutionary Nonself Model

Although this model does not deal with pregnancy transplantation, or alloimmune recognition in general, it might be useful to speculate, given current data, what evolutionary nonself and related models might say about maternal tolerance of the fetus. In this offshoot of classic immune models, the focus is on activation of the innate immune response as the critical mechanism for overall immune activation.[140]

By this model, T cell receptor recognition of self-peptides in the context of MHC underlines the basis for development in the thymus and survival and initial activation in the periphery. However, full activation is reliant on a costimulatory signal delivered by an activated antigen-presenting cell. The signal for activation of the antigen-presenting cell constitutes the point at which self is discriminated from nonself. Three strategies for immune recognition are envisioned[141]:

- The first is recognition of microbial nonself, which occurs through binding of innate immune cell receptors expressed by dendritic cells or macrophages to pathogen-associated molecular patterns on infecting agents.
- The second is recognition of missing self, which is recognition of molecules that are evolutionarily expressed on cells of the body or immune cells, but not bacteria, for example.
- The third is recognition of altered self, which is said to occur when there is expression of new cellular markers or abnormalities in cellular markers in the wake of viral or other pathologic infection.

Tolerance in this model is an indirect process that occurs because microbial nonself is segregated from cells that could recognize it by inhibitory signals expressed on the tissue of interest, by increased expression of unique self-antigens, and by pathogen-associated mechanisms to decrease expression of altered self after infection. Later versions of this model also rely on the activity of suppressor cells to limit the function of autoreactive T cells.[142] It might be guessed, according to this model, that the presence of fetal antigens at the maternal-fetal interface does not necessarily activate the immune system. However, when infection occurs, the pattern receptor–mediated immune system occurs in order to protect the mother. This thinking supports interpretation obtained through experimental models of infection or inflammation-induced preterm birth.[73,143] The fact that parasitic infection within the placenta leads to dire consequences[144] also fits within this model.

There are observations related to maternal tolerance that are in line with the model's focus on innate immune privilege. For example, the expression on the human zona pellucida of Sialyl-Lewis[x] motifs that bind immune-suppressive ligands such as sieglec-9, expression of the immune-modulating glycoprotein glycodelin-A (reviewed in Ref.[9]) and expression of the mucinous glycoprotein MUC 16 (also known as CA 125) by the endometrium[9] are thought to suppress local activity of immune cells to protect the implanting embryo. For another example, the placenta expresses several small lectin molecules, the galectins, that are thought to be immune modulatory. The roles of other unusual glycoproteins, including their role in immune modulation in the reproductive tract, are being examined.

In the context of this model, the low level of immune cell activation to the organisms present in the reproductive tract and uterus[145,146] might be explained by reproductive tract cell modulation of sialic acid residues,[147] or segregation of these organisms from the immune response by their retention intracellularly.[145,146] Viral infection is common at the maternal-fetal interface, but the loss of pregnancy and other adverse outcomes occurs only in a portion of cases, and this may be related to a so-called second hit that induces innate immune system activation.[148] An explanation consistent with this model is that certain viruses adapt to trophoblast in such a way that viral infection in trophoblast downregulates the expression of altered self and thus prevents immune system activation. Support for the idea of viral adaptation comes from the fact that evolutionary time has produced a placenta whose critical functions depend on genes taken from endogenous retroviruses.[149]

IS THE POSTPARTUM IMMUNE SYSTEM IMPORTANT?

Pregnancy is a time of rapid shifting in physiology. Resolution and new adaptation occur globally during the postpartum state. For example, some degree of pregnancy-induced vascular adaptation continues for weeks to months after delivery.[150–153] Elements of the physiology of pregnancy continue well into women's post-pregnancy lives. Normal pregnancies are generally associated with very low long-term cardiovascular risks, whereas complicated pregnancies, including preeclampsia,[154–156] preterm birth,[157–159] gestational diabetes,[160] and high multiparity,[161] are associated with cardiovascular risk. The postpartum state is likely an important time to ask questions about what happens to the maternal immune system. For example, how can the fetal cell microchimerism after delivery be explained? Classic models suggest that, through microchimerism, the fetus becomes an extension of maternal self[162,163] and that long-lived T_{reg}, impair reactivity to fetal cells. The danger model provides another perspective on these cells. If the trafficking of these cells was not caused by necrosis or dysregulation of tissues within the uterus, and, further, if the trafficking cells settle in their new locations without causing damage or disruption, then no immune response would be expected, and this might lead to the long-term microchimerism that has been reported. Another question is how to explain evidence of new-onset autoimmune disease, such as thyroiditis[164] or peripartum cardiomyopathy,[165] overshoots the baseline in severity of autoimmune disease in the postpartum period? Although classic models suggest that these findings are related to release from immune suppression in the postpartum state, the evolutionary nonself and danger models suggest persistent underlying infection or dysregulation, respectively, of maternal tissues as driving long-term disease risk. However, there may be other models, based on what is known about immune cell homeostasis,[166–170] and these will have to be explored.

REFERENCES

1. Carp HJ, Selmi C, Shoenfeld Y. The autoimmune bases of infertility and pregnancy loss. J Autoimmun 2012;38(2–3):J266–74.
2. Bonney EA, Brown SA. To drive or be driven: the path of a mouse model of recurrent pregnancy loss. Reproduction 2014;147(5):R153–67.
3. Pantham P, Abrahams VM, Chamley LW. The role of anti-phospholipid antibodies in autoimmune reproductive failure. Reproduction 2016;151(5):R79–90.
4. Lissauer D, Piper K, Goodyear O, et al. Fetal-specific CD8+ cytotoxic T cell responses develop during normal human pregnancy and exhibit broad functional capacity. J Immunol 2012;189(2):1072–80.
5. Raj RS, Bonney EA, Phillippe M. Influenza, immune system, and pregnancy. Reprod Sci 2014;21(12):1434–51.
6. Caluwaerts S, Fautsch T, Lagrou D, et al. Dilemmas in managing pregnant women with Ebola: 2 case reports. Clin Infect Dis 2016;62(7):903–5.
7. Duffy MR, Chen T-H, Hancock WT, et al. Zika virus outbreak on Yap Island, Federated States of Micronesia. N Engl J Med 2009;360(24):2536–43.
8. Oliveira Melo AS, Malinger G, Ximenes R, et al. Zika virus intrauterine infection causes fetal brain abnormality and microcephaly: tip of the iceberg? Ultrasound Obstet Gynecol 2016;47(1):6–7.
9. Clark GF, Schust DJ. Manifestations of immune tolerance in the human female reproductive tract. Front Immunol 2013;4:26.
10. Davis-Richardson AG, Triplett EW. A model for the role of gut bacteria in the development of autoimmunity for type 1 diabetes. Diabetologia 2015;58(7): 1386–93.
11. Anahtar MN, Byrne EH, Doherty KE, et al. Cervicovaginal bacteria are a major modulator of host inflammatory responses in the female genital tract. Immunity 2015;42(5):965–76.
12. Rizzo A, Fiorentino M, Buommino E, et al. *Lactobacillus crispatus* mediates anti-inflammatory cytokine interleukin-10 induction in response to *Chlamydia trachomatis* infection in vitro. Int J Med Microbiol 2015;305(8):815–27.
13. Nelson DB, Shin H, Wu J, et al. The gestational vaginal microbiome and spontaneous preterm birth among nulliparous African American women. Am J Perinatol 2016;33(9):887–93.
14. Baldwin EA, Walther-Antonio M, MacLean AM, et al. Persistent microbial dysbiosis in preterm premature rupture of membranes from onset until delivery. PeerJ 2015;3:e1398.
15. Jacob JA. Another frontier in microbiome research: Preterm birth. JAMA 2015; 314(15):1550–1.
16. Wylie KM, Mihindukulasuriya KA, Zhou Y, et al. Metagenomic analysis of double-stranded DNA viruses in healthy adults. BMC Biol 2014;12:71.

17. Yarbrough VL, Winkle S, Herbst-Kralovetz MM. Antimicrobial peptides in the female reproductive tract: a critical component of the mucosal immune barrier with physiological and clinical implications. Hum Reprod Update 2015;21(3):353–77.

18. McConkey CA, Delorme-Axford E, Nickerson CA, et al. A three-dimensional culture system recapitulates placental syncytiotrophoblast development and microbial resistance. Sci Adv 2016;2(3):e1501462.

19. Zeldovich VB, Clausen CH, Bradford E, et al. Placental syncytium forms a biophysical barrier against pathogen invasion. PLoS Pathog 2013;9(12):e1003821.

20. Penkala I, Wang J, Syrett CM, et al. LNCRHOXF1: a long noncoding RNA from the X-chromosome that suppresses viral response genes during development of the early human placenta. Mol Cell Biol 2016;36(12):1764–75.

21. Racicot K, Kwon JY, Aldo P, et al. Type I interferon regulates the placental inflammatory response to bacteria and is targeted by virus: mechanism of polymicrobial infection-induced preterm birth. Am J Reprod Immunol 2016;75(4):451–60.

22. Aldo PB, Mulla MJ, Romero R, et al. Viral ssRNA induces first trimester trophoblast apoptosis through an inflammatory mechanism. Am J Reprod Immunol 2010;64(1):27–37.

23. Zdravkovic M, Knudsen HJ, Liu X, et al. High interferon alpha levels in placenta, maternal, and cord blood suggest a protective effect against intrauterine herpes simplex virus infection. J Med Virol 1997;51(3):210–3.

24. Constantin CM, Masopust D, Gourley T, et al. Normal establishment of virus-specific memory CD8 T cell pool following primary infection during pregnancy. J Immunol 2007;179(7):4383–9.

25. Driggers RW, Ho C-Y, Korhonen EM, et al. Zika virus infection with prolonged maternal viremia and fetal brain abnormalities. N Engl J Med 2016;374(22):2142–51.

26. Cooper MA, Yokoyama WM. Memory-like responses of natural killer cells. Immunol Rev 2010;235(1):297–305.

27. Sharkey AM, Xiong S, Kennedy PR, et al. Tissue-specific education of decidual NK cells. J Immunol 2015;195(7):3026–32.

28. Sacks GP, Studena K, Sargent K, et al. Normal pregnancy and preeclampsia both produce inflammatory changes in peripheral blood leukocytes akin to those of sepsis. Am J Obstet Gynecol 1998;179(1):80–6.

29. Southcombe JH, Redman CW, Sargent IL, et al. Interleukin-1 family cytokines and their regulatory proteins in normal pregnancy and pre-eclampsia. Clin Exp Immunol 2015;181(3):480–90.

30. St John AL, Abraham SN. Innate immunity and its regulation by mast cells. J Immunol 2013;190(9):4458–63.

31. Galli SJ, Borregaard N, Wynn TA. Phenotypic and functional plasticity of cells of innate immunity: macrophages, mast cells and neutrophils. Nat Immunol 2011;12(11):1035–44.

32. Simon T, Gogolak P, Kis-Toth K, et al. Histamine modulates multiple functional activities of monocyte-derived dendritic cell subsets via histamine receptor 2. Int Immunol 2012;24(2):107–16.

33. Case LK, Moussawi M, Roberts B, et al. Histamine H1 receptor signaling regulates effector T cell responses and susceptibility to coxsackievirus B3-induced myocarditis. Cell Immunol 2012;272(2):269–74.

34. Sirois J, Menard G, Moses AS, et al. Importance of histamine in the cytokine network in the lung through H2 and H3 receptors: stimulation of IL-10 production. J Immunol 2000;164(6):2964–70.

35. Botturi K, Lacoeuille Y, Vervloet D, et al. Histamine induces Th2 activation through the histamine receptor 1 in house dust mite rhinitic but not asthmatic patients. Clin Exp Allergy 2010;40(5):755–62.

36. Meretey K, Fekete MI, Bohm U, et al. Effect of H1 and H2 agonists on the chemiluminescence of human blood mononuclear cells induced by phytohaemagglutinin. Immunopharmacology 1985;9(3):175–80.

37. Teuscher C, Subramanian M, Noubade R, et al. Central histamine H_3 receptor signaling negatively regulates susceptibility to autoimmune inflammatory disease of the CNS. Proc Natl Acad Sci U S A 2007;104(24):10146–51.

38. del Rio R, Noubade R, Saligrama N, et al. Histamine H4 receptor optimizes T regulatory cell frequency and facilitates anti-inflammatory responses within the central nervous system. J Immunol 2012;188(2):541–7.

39. Dijkstra D, Leurs R, Chazot P, et al. Histamine downregulates monocyte CCL2 production through the histamine H4 receptor. J Allergy Clin Immunol 2007; 120(2):300–7.

40. Emerson MR, Orentas DM, Lynch SG, et al. Activation of histamine H2 receptors ameliorates experimental allergic encephalomyelitis. Neuroreport 2002;13(11): 1407–10.

41. Menzies FM, Higgins CA, Shepherd MC, et al. Mast cells reside in myometrium and cervix, but are dispensable in mice for successful pregnancy and labor. Immunol Cell Biol 2012;90(3):321–9.

42. Zhao X, Ma W, Das SK, et al. Blastocyst H(2) receptor is the target for uterine histamine in implantation in the mouse. Development 2000;127(12):2643–51.

43. Bosquiazzo VL, Ramos JG, Varayoud J, et al. Mast cell degranulation in rat uterine cervix during pregnancy correlates with expression of vascular endothelial growth factor mRNA and angiogenesis. Reproduction 2007;133(5):1045–55.

44. Woidacki K, Meyer N, Schumacher A, et al. Transfer of regulatory T cells into abortion-prone mice promotes the expansion of uterine mast cells and normalizes early pregnancy angiogenesis. Sci Rep 2015;5:13938.

45. McNeill JH, Verma SC. Histamine2 receptors in rat uterus. Res Commun Chem Pathol Pharmacol 1975;11(4):639–44.

46. Castelli MC, Vadora E, Bacchi Modena A, et al. In vitro effects of histamine on human pregnant myometrium contractility. Boll Soc Ital Biol Sper 1993;69(12): 783–9.

47. Willets JM, Taylor AH, Shaw H, et al. Selective regulation of H1 histamine receptor signaling by G protein-coupled receptor kinase 2 in uterine smooth muscle cells. Mol Endocrinol 2008;22(8):1893–907.

48. Bytautiene E, Vedernikov YP, Saade GR, et al. IgE-independent mast cell activation augments contractility of nonpregnant and pregnant guinea pig myometrium. Int Arch Allergy Immunol 2008;147(2):140–6.

49. Romero R, Kusanovic JP, Gomez R, et al. The clinical significance of eosinophils in the amniotic fluid in preterm labor. J Matern Fetal Neonatal Med 2010;23(4): 320–9.

50. Bytautiene E, Vedernikov YP, Maner WL, et al. Challenge with ovalbumin antigen increases uterine and cervical contractile activity in sensitized guinea pigs. Am J Obstet Gynecol 2008;199(6):658.e1-6.

51. Bytautiene E, Vedernikov YP, Saade GR, et al. Degranulation of uterine mast cell modifies contractility of isolated myometrium from pregnant women. Am J Obstet Gynecol 2004;191(5):1705–10.

52. Giaglis S, Stoikou M, Grimolizzi F, et al. Neutrophil migration into the placenta: good, bad or deadly? Cell Adh Migr 2016;10(1–2):208–25.

53. Brinkmann V, Zychlinsky A. Neutrophil extracellular traps: is immunity the second function of chromatin? J Cell Biol 2012;198(5):773–83.
54. Amsalem H, Kwan M, Hazan A, et al. Identification of a novel neutrophil population: proangiogenic granulocytes in second-trimester human decidua. J Immunol 2014;193(6):3070–9.
55. Mahendroo M. Cervical remodeling in term and preterm birth: insights from an animal model. Reproduction 2012;143(4):429–38.
56. Bizargity P, Bonney EA. Dendritic cells: a family portrait at mid-gestation. Immunology 2009;126(4):565–78.
57. Collins MK, Tay C-S, Erlebacher A. Dendritic cell entrapment within the pregnant uterus inhibits immune surveillance of the maternal/fetal interface in mice. J Clin Invest 2009;119(7):2062–73.
58. Kwan M, Hazan A, Zhang J, et al. Dynamic changes in maternal decidual leukocyte populations from first to second trimester gestation. Placenta 2014;35(12): 1027–34.
59. Pomeroy B, Sipka A, Klaessig S, et al. Monocyte-derived dendritic cells from late gestation cows have an impaired ability to mature in response to *E. coli* stimulation in a receptor and cytokine-mediated fashion. Vet Immunol immunopathol 2015;167(1–2):22–9.
60. Gao XW, Fu Y, Li WJ, et al. Mechanism of immune tolerance induced by donor derived immature dendritic cells in rat high-risk corneal transplantation. Int J Ophthalmol 2013;6(3):269–75.
61. Scholz C, Rampf E, Toth B, et al. Ovarian cancer-derived glycodelin impairs in vitro dendritic cell maturation. J Immunother 2009;32(5):492–7.
62. Mosser DM, Edwards JP. Exploring the full spectrum of macrophage activation. Nat Rev Immunol 2008;12:958–69.
63. Ning F, Liu H, Lash GE. The role of decidual macrophages during normal and pathological pregnancy. Am J Reprod Immunol 2016;75(3):298–309.
64. Kumar V, Patel S, Tcyganov E, et al. The nature of myeloid-derived suppressor cells in the tumor microenvironment. Symp Soc Exp Biol 2016;37(3):208–20.
65. Jasper MJ, Care AS, Sullivan B, et al. Macrophage-derived LIF and IL1B regulate alpha(1,2)fucosyltransferase 2 (Fut2) expression in mouse uterine epithelial cells during early pregnancy. Biol Reprod 2011;84(1):179–88.
66. Payne KJ, Clyde LA, Weldon AJ, et al. Residency and activation of myeloid cells during remodeling of the prepartum murine cervix. Biol Reprod 2012;87(5):106.
67. Gomez-Lopez N, StLouis D, Lehr MA, et al. Immune cells in term and preterm labor. Cell Mol Immunol 2014;11(6):571–81.
68. Yellon SM, Dobyns AE, Beck HL, et al. Loss of progesterone receptor-mediated actions induce preterm cellular and structural remodeling of the cervix and premature birth. PLoS One 2013;8(12):e81340.
69. Newby AC. Metalloproteinase production from macrophages - a perfect storm leading to atherosclerotic plaque rupture and myocardial infarction. Exp Physiol 2016. [Epub ahead of print].
70. Norwitz ER, Lopez Bernal A, Starkey PM. Tumor necrosis factor-alpha selectively stimulates prostaglandin F2 alpha production by macrophages in human term decidua. Am J Obstet Gynecol 1992;167(3):815–20.
71. Ogawa K, Funaba M, Tsujimoto M. The effects of TGF-beta1 on the expression of type IV collagenases in mouse peritoneal macrophages. Mol Biol Rep 2011; 38(2):1451–6.
72. Timmons BC, Fairhurst AM, Mahendroo MS. Temporal changes in myeloid cells in the cervix during pregnancy and parturition. J Immunol 2009;182(5):2700–7.

73. Bizargity P, Del Rio R, Phillippe M, et al. Resistance to lipopolysaccharide-induced preterm delivery mediated by regulatory T cell function in mice. Biol Reprod 2009;80(5):874–81.

74. Orange JS. Natural killer cell deficiency. J Allergy Clin Immunol 2013;132(3):515–25 [quiz: 526].

75. Eguizabal C, Zenarruzabeitia O, Monge J, et al. Natural killer cells for cancer immunotherapy: pluripotent stem cells-derived NK cells as an immunotherapeutic perspective. Front Immunol 2014;5:439.

76. Vacca P, Montaldo E, Croxatto D, et al. Identification of diverse innate lymphoid cells in human decidua. Mucosal Immunol 2015;8(2):254–64.

77. Shih HY, Sciume G, Mikami Y, et al. Developmental acquisition of regulomes underlies innate lymphoid cell functionality. Cell 2016;165(5):1120–33.

78. Furcron AE, Romero R, Plazyo O, et al. Vaginal progesterone, but not 17alpha-hydroxyprogesterone caproate, has antiinflammatory effects at the murine maternal-fetal interface. Am J Obstet Gynecol 2015;213(6):846.e1-e19.

79. Wang Y, Xu B, Li MQ, et al. IL-22 secreted by decidual stromal cells and NK cells promotes the survival of human trophoblasts. Int J Clin Exp Pathol 2013;6(9):1781–90.

80. Bendelac A, Hunziker RD, Lantz O. Increased interleukin 4 and immunoglobulin E production in transgenic mice overexpressing NK1 T cells. J Exp Med 1996;184(4):1285–93.

81. Lawson V. Turned on by danger: activation of CD1d-restricted invariant natural killer T cells. Immunology 2012;137(1):20–7.

82. Boyson JE, Nagarkatti N, Nizam L, et al. Gestation stage-dependent mechanisms of invariant natural killer T cell-mediated pregnancy loss. Proc Natl Acad Sci U S A 2006;103(12):4580–5.

83. Huijts CM, Schneiders FL, Garcia-Vallejo JJ, et al. mTOR inhibition per se induces nuclear localization of FOXP3 and conversion of invariant NKT (iNKT) cells into immunosuppressive regulatory iNKT cells. J Immunol 2015;195(5):2038–45.

84. Uemura Y, Suzuki M, Liu TY, et al. Role of human non-invariant NKT lymphocytes in the maintenance of type 2 T helper environment during pregnancy. Int Immunol 2008;20(3):405–12.

85. Adams EJ, Gu S, Luoma AM. Human gamma delta T cells: evolution and ligand recognition. Cell Immunol 2015;296(1):31–40.

86. Roessner K, Wolfe J, Shi C, et al. High expression of Fas ligand by synovial fluid-derived gamma delta T cells in Lyme arthritis. J Immunol 2003;170(5):2702–10.

87. Alcaide ML, Strbo N, Romero L, et al. Bacterial vaginosis is associated with loss of gamma delta T Cells in the female reproductive tract in women in the Miami Women Interagency HIV Study (WIHS): a cross sectional study. PLoS One 2016;11(4):e0153045.

88. Chapman JC, Chapman FM, Michael SD. The production of alpha/beta and gamma/delta double negative (DN) T-cells and their role in the maintenance of pregnancy. Reprod Biol Endocrinol 2015;13:73.

89. Bonney EA, Pudney J, Anderson DJ, et al. Gamma-delta T cells in midgestation human placental villi. Gynecol Obstet Invest 2000;50(3):153–7.

90. Heyborne KD, Cranfill RL, Carding SR, et al. Characterization of gamma delta T lymphocytes at the maternal-fetal interface. J Immunol 1992;149(9):2872–8.

91. Fujihashi K, McGhee JR, Kweon MN, et al. gamma/delta T cell-deficient mice have impaired mucosal immunoglobulin A responses. J Exp Med 1996;183(4):1929–35.

92. Krishnan L, Guilbert LJ, Russell AS, et al. Pregnancy impairs resistance of C57BL/6 mice to *Leishmania major* infection and causes decreased antigen-specific IFN-gamma response and increased production of T helper 2 cytokines. J Immunol 1996;156(2):644–52.
93. Bonney EA, Onyekwuluje J. Maternal tolerance to H-Y is independent of IL-10. Immunol Invest 2004;33(4):385–95.
94. Aluvihare VR, Kallikourdis M, Betz AG. Regulatory T cells mediate maternal tolerance to the fetus. Nat Immunol 2004;5(3):266–71.
95. Moldenhauer LM, Diener KR, Thring DM, et al. Cross-presentation of male seminal fluid antigens elicits T cell activation to initiate the female immune response to pregnancy. J Immunol 2009;182(12):8080–93.
96. Curtis MM, Way SS. Interleukin-17 in host defence against bacterial, mycobacterial and fungal pathogens. Immunology 2009;126(2):177–85.
97. Gopal R, Rangel-Moreno J, Fallert Junecko BA, et al. Mucosal pre-exposure to Th17-inducing adjuvants exacerbates pathology after influenza infection. Am J Pathol 2014;184(1):55–63.
98. Ito M, Nakashima A, Hidaka T, et al. A role for IL-17 in induction of an inflammation at the fetomaternal interface in preterm labour. J Reprod Immunol 2010; 84(1):75–85.
99. Gomez-Lopez N, Olson DM, Robertson SA. Interleukin-6 controls uterine Th9 cells and CD8+ T regulatory cells to accelerate parturition in mice. Immunol Cell Biol 2016;94(1):79–89.
100. Guerder S, Matzinger P. A fail-safe mechanism for maintaining self-tolerance. J Exp Med 1992;176(2):553–64.
101. Ridge JP, Di Rosa F, Matzinger P. A conditioned dendritic cell can be a temporal bridge between a CD4+ T-helper and a T-killer cell. Nature 1998;393(6684): 474–8.
102. Nguyen ML, Hatton L, Li J, et al. Dynamic regulation of permissive histone modifications and GATA3 binding underpin acquisition of granzyme A expression by virus-specific CD8(+) T cells. Eur J Immunol 2016;46(2):307–18.
103. Valujskikh A, Lantz O, Celli S, et al. Cross-primed CD8(+) T cells mediate graft rejection via a distinct effector pathway. Nat Immunol 2002;3(9):844–51.
104. Tilburgs T, Strominger JL. CD8+ effector T cells at the fetal-maternal interface, balancing fetal tolerance and antiviral immunity. Am J Reprod Immunol 2013; 69(4):395–407.
105. Bonney EA, Onyekwuluje J. The H-Y response in mid-gestation and long after delivery in mice primed before pregnancy. Immunol Invest 2003;32(1–2):71–81.
106. Norton MT, Fortner KA, Oppenheimer KH, et al. Evidence that CD8 T-cell homeostasis and function remain intact during murine pregnancy. Immunology 2010; 131(3):426–37.
107. Wang SC, Li YH, Piao HL, et al. PD-1 and Tim-3 pathways are associated with regulatory CD8+ T-cell function in decidua and maintenance of normal pregnancy. Cell Death Dis 2015;6:e1738.
108. Jelley-Gibbs DM, Strutt TM, McKinstry KK, et al. Influencing the fates of CD4 T cells on the path to memory: lessons from influenza. Immunol Cell Biol 2008; 86(4):343–52.
109. Kay AW, Blish CA. Immunogenicity and clinical efficacy of influenza vaccination in pregnancy. Front Immunol 2015;6:289.
110. Iijima N, Iwasaki A. T cell memory. A local macrophage chemokine network sustains protective tissue-resident memory CD4 T cells. Science 2014;346(6205): 93–8.

111. Cuburu N, Graham BS, Buck CB, et al. Intravaginal immunization with HPV vectors induces tissue-resident CD8+ T cell responses. J Clin Invest 2012;122(12): 4606–20.

112. Yeaman GR, Collins JE, Fanger MW, et al. CD8+ T cells in human uterine endometrial lymphoid aggregates: evidence for accumulation of cells by trafficking. Immunology 2001;102(4):434–40.

113. Tabanelli V, Valli R, Righi S, et al. A unique case of an indolent myometrial T-cell lymphoproliferative disorder with phenotypic features resembling uterine CD8+ resident memory T cells. Pathobiology 2014;81(4):176–82.

114. van Egmond A, van der Keur C, Swings GM, et al. The possible role of virus-specific CD8(+) memory T cells in decidual tissue. J Reprod Immunol 2016; 113:1–8.

115. Heesters BA, Myers RC, Carroll MC. Follicular dendritic cells: dynamic antigen libraries. Nat Rev Immunol 2014;14(7):495–504.

116. Dienz O, Eaton SM, Bond JP, et al. The induction of antibody production by IL-6 is indirectly mediated by IL-21 produced by CD4+ T cells. J Exp Med 2009; 206(1):69–78.

117. Menon M, Blair PA, Isenberg DA, et al. A regulatory feedback between plasmacytoid dendritic cells and regulatory B Cells is aberrant in systemic lupus erythematosus. Immunity 2016;4(3):683–97.

118. Muzzio DO, Soldati R, Ehrhardt J, et al. B cell development undergoes profound modifications and adaptations during pregnancy in mice. Biol Reprod 2014; 91(5):115.

119. Norton MT, Fortner KA, Bizargity P, et al. Pregnancy alters the proliferation and apoptosis of mouse splenic erythroid lineage cells and leukocytes. Biol Reprod 2009;81(3):457–64.

120. Schaefer K, Brown N, Kaye PM, et al. Cervico-vaginal immunoglobulin G levels increase post-ovulation independently of neutrophils. PLoS One 2014;9(12): e114824.

121. Rolle L, Memarzadeh Tehran M, Morell-Garcia A, et al. Cutting edge: IL-10-producing regulatory B cells in early human pregnancy. Am J Reprod Immunol 2013;70(6):448–53.

122. Ober C, Loisel DA, Gilad Y. Sex-specific genetic architecture of human disease. Nat Rev Genet 2008;9(12):911–22.

123. Anipindi VC, Bagri P, Roth K, et al. Estradiol enhances CD4+ T-cell anti-viral immunity by priming vaginal DCs to Induce Th17 responses via an IL-1-dependent pathway. PLoS Pathog 2016;12(5):e1005589.

124. Spanier JA, Nashold FE, Mayne CG, et al. Vitamin D and estrogen synergy in Vdr-expressing CD4(+) T cells is essential to induce Helios(+)FoxP3(+) T cells and prevent autoimmune demyelinating disease. J Neuroimmunol 2015;286:48–58.

125. Okada H, Nakajima T, Sanezumi M, et al. Progesterone enhances interleukin-15 production in human endometrial stromal cells in vitro. J Clin Endocrinol Metab 2000;85(12):4765–70.

126. Gattinoni L, Finkelstein SE, Klebanoff CA, et al. Removal of homeostatic cytokine sinks by lymphodepletion enhances the efficacy of adoptively transferred tumor-specific CD8+ T cells. J Exp Med 2005;202(7):907–12.

127. Oelert T, Papatriantafyllou M, Pougialis G, et al. Irradiation and IL-15 promote loss of CD8 T-cell tolerance in response to lymphopenia. Blood 2010;115(11): 2196–202.

128. Medawar PB. Some immunological and endocrinological problems raised by the evolution of viviparity in vertebrates. Symp Soc Exp Biol 1954;7:320–8.
129. Burnet FM. The immunological significance of the thymus: an extension of the clonal selection theory of immunity. Australas Ann Med 1962;1:79–91.
130. Bretscher P, Cohn M. A theory of self-nonself discrimination. Science 1970; 169(3950):1042–9.
131. Bonney EA, Matzinger P. The maternal immune system's interaction with circulating fetal cells. J Immunol 1997;158(1):40–7.
132. Mold JE, Michaelsson J, Burt TD, et al. Maternal alloantigens promote the development of tolerogenic fetal regulatory T cells in utero. Science 2008;322(5907): 1562–5.
133. Bonney EA, Matzinger P. Much IDO about pregnancy. Nat Med 1998;4(10): 1128–9.
134. Munn DH, Zhou M, Attwood JT, et al. Prevention of allogeneic fetal rejection by tryptophan catabolism. Science 1998;281(5380):1191–3.
135. Matzinger P. Tolerance, danger, and the extended family. Annu Rev Immunol 1994;12:991–1045.
136. Anderson CC, Matzinger P. Danger: the view from the bottom of the cliff. Semin Immunol 2000;12(3):231–8 [discussion: 257–344].
137. Bonney EA. Preeclampsia: a view through the danger model. J Reprod Immunol 2007;76(1–2):68–74.
138. Matzinger P, Kamala T. Tissue-based class control: the other side of tolerance. Nat Rev Immunol 2011;11(3):221–30.
139. Robertson SA, Christiaens I, Dorian CL, et al. Interleukin-6 is an essential determinant of on-time parturition in the mouse. Endocrinology 2010;151(8): 3996–4006.
140. Janeway CA Jr. The immune system evolved to discriminate infectious nonself from noninfectious self. Immunol Today 1992;13(1):11–6.
141. Medzhitov R, Janeway CA Jr. Decoding the patterns of self and nonself by the innate immune system. Science 2002;296(5566):298–300.
142. Medzhitov R. Approaching the asymptote: 20 years later. Immunity 2009;30(6): 766–75.
143. Elovitz MA, Wang Z, Chien EK, et al. A new model for inflammation-induced preterm birth: the role of platelet-activating factor and Toll-like receptor-4. Am J Pathol 2003;163(5):2103–11.
144. Kabyemela E, Goncalves BP, Prevots DR, et al. Cytokine profiles at birth predict malaria severity during infancy. PLoS One 2013;8(10):e77214.
145. Stout MJ, Conlon B, Landeau M, et al. Identification of intracellular bacteria in the basal plate of the human placenta in term and preterm gestations. Am J Obstet Gynecol 2013;208(3):226.e1-7.
146. Cao B, Mysorekar IU. Intracellular bacteria in placental basal plate localize to extravillous trophoblasts. Placenta 2014;35(2):139–42.
147. Kline KA, Schwartz DJ, Gilbert NM, et al. Immune modulation by group B Streptococcus influences host susceptibility to urinary tract infection by uropathogenic Escherichia coli. Infect Immun 2012;80(12):4186–94.
148. Cardenas I, Means RE, Aldo P, et al. Viral infection of the placenta leads to fetal inflammation and sensitization to bacterial products predisposing to preterm labor. J Immunol 2010;185(2):1248–57.
149. Sugimoto J, Schust DJ. Review: human endogenous retroviruses and the placenta. Reprod Sci 2009;16(11):1023–33.

150. Morris EA, Hale SA, Badger GJ, et al. Pregnancy induces persistent changes in vascular compliance in primiparous women. Am J Obstet Gynecol 2015;212(5): 633.e1-6.

151. Hilgers RH, Bergaya S, Schiffers PM, et al. Uterine artery structural and functional changes during pregnancy in tissue kallikrein-deficient mice. Arterioscler Thromb Vasc Biol 2003;23(10):1826–32.

152. Clapp JF 3rd, Capeless E. Cardiovascular function before, during, and after the first and subsequent pregnancies. Am J Cardiol 1997;80(11):1469–73.

153. Euser AG, Cipolla MJ. Resistance artery vasodilation to magnesium sulfate during pregnancy and the postpartum state. Am J Physiol Heart Circ Physiol 2005; 288(4):H1521–5.

154. Bruckmann A, Seeliger C, Lehmann T, et al. Altered retinal flicker response indicates microvascular dysfunction in women with preeclampsia. Hypertension 2015;66(4):900–5.

155. Pruthi D, Khankin EV, Blanton RM, et al. Exposure to experimental preeclampsia in mice enhances the vascular response to future injury. Hypertension 2015; 65(4):863–70.

156. Garovic VD, Bailey KR, Boerwinkle E, et al. Hypertension in pregnancy as a risk factor for cardiovascular disease later in life. J Hypertens 2010;28(4):826–33.

157. Ngo A, Chen J, Figtree G, et al. Preterm birth and future risk of maternal cardiovascular disease – is the association independent of smoking during pregnancy? BMC Pregnancy Childbirth 2015;15(1):1–11.

158. Robbins CL, Hutchings Y, Dietz PM, et al. History of preterm birth and subsequent cardiovascular disease: a systematic review. Am J Obstet Gynecol 2014;210(4):285–97.

159. Bonamy A-KE, Parikh NI, Cnattingius S, et al. Birth characteristics and subsequent risks of maternal cardiovascular disease: effects of gestational age and fetal growth. Circulation 2011;124(25):2839–46.

160. Gunderson EP, Chiang V, Pletcher MJ, et al. History of gestational diabetes mellitus and future risk of atherosclerosis in mid-life: the Coronary Artery Risk Development in Young Adults study. J Am Heart Assoc 2014;3(2):e000490.

161. Ness RB, Harris T, Cobb J, et al. Number of pregnancies and the subsequent risk of cardiovascular disease. N Engl J Med 1993;328(21):1528–33.

162. Adams KM, Yan Z, Stevens AM, et al. The changing maternal "self" hypothesis: a mechanism for maternal tolerance of the fetus. Placenta 2007;28(5–6): 378–82.

163. Adams KM, Nelson JL. Microchimerism: an investigative frontier in autoimmunity and transplantation. JAMA 2004;291(9):1127–31.

164. Lazarus JH, Parkes AB, Premawardhana LD. Postpartum thyroiditis [Review] [55 refs]. Autoimmunity 2002;35(3):169–73.

165. Ansari AA, Fett JD, Carraway RE, et al. Autoimmune mechanisms as the basis for human peripartum cardiomyopathy. Clin Rev Allergy Immunol 2002;23(3): 301–24.

166. Smith KA, Popmihajlov Z. The quantal theory of immunity and the interleukin-2-dependent negative feedback regulation of the immune response. Immunol Rev 2008;224:124–40.

167. Schluns KS, Kieper WC, Jameson SC, et al. Interleukin-7 mediates the homeostasis of naive and memory CD8 T cells in vivo. Nat Immunol 2000; 1(5):426–32.

168. Sprent J, Surh CD. T cell memory. Annu Rev Immunol 2002;20:551–79.

169. Mueller SN, Ahmed R. High antigen levels are the cause of T cell exhaustion during chronic viral infection. Proc Natl Acad Sci U S A 2009;106(21):8623–8.
170. Gupta PK, Godec J, Wolski D, et al. CD39 expression identifies terminally exhausted CD8+ T cells. PLoS Pathog 2015;11(10):e1005177.

Respiratory Considerations Including Airway and Ventilation Issues in Critical Care Obstetric Patients

Holly Ende, MD*, Dirk Varelmann, MD

KEYWORDS

- Airway changes of pregnancy • Acute respiratory distress syndrome
- Lung protective ventilation
- Extracorporeal membrane oxygenation during pregnancy
- Reactive airway disease in pregnancy

KEY POINTS

- Physiologic changes of pregnancy predispose to difficulty with mask ventilation and intubation, rapid desaturation during periods and apnea, and high airway pressures during mechanical ventilation.
- Hypoxic respiratory failure in the parturient can be due to a multitude of causes, both related and unrelated to pregnancy. Acute respiratory distress syndrome is a common final pathway by which many of these etiologies lead to arterial hypoxemia.
- Treatment of hypoxic respiratory failure should focus on lung-protective ventilation with low tidal volumes and moderate levels of positive end–expiratory pressure as well as careful fluid management. For refractory cases, neuromuscular blockade, prone positioning, and extracorporeal membrane oxygenation may be considered.
- Reactive airway disease in pregnancy is common, and consideration should be given to administration of inhaled corticosteroids to improve outcomes.

INTRODUCTION

Critical care management of the obstetric patient can present unique challenges to obstetricians, intensivists, anesthesiologists, and consultants. Parturients who present with respiratory distress can suffer from a multitude of etiologies (**Table 1**), both related and unrelated to their gravid state, and each diagnosis must be pursued as appropriate to the clinical picture. Normal physiologic changes of pregnancy may

Disclosure Statement: Authors have no disclosures.
Department of Anesthesiology, Perioperative and Pain Medicine, Brigham and Women's Hospital, 75 Francis Street, CWN L1, Boston, MA 02115, USA
* Corresponding author.
E-mail address: holly.b.ende@gmail.com

Table 1 Etiologies of respiratory failure in pregnancy	
Hypoxic respiratory failure: pregnancy specific	AFE Pulmonary edema secondary to tocolytics Pulmonary edema secondary to preeclampsia/eclampsia Cardiogenic pulmonary edema secondary to peripartum cardiomyopathy ARDS secondary to placental abruption, obstetric hemorrhage, chorioamnionitis, or endometritis
Hypoxic respiratory failure: nonpregnancy Specific	Aspiration pneumonia/pneumonitis Viral/bacterial pneumonia Pulmonary embolism Venous air embolism Cardiogenic pulmonary edema secondary to heart failure unrelated to pregnancy Atelectasis Pneumothorax ARDS secondary to transfusion-associated acute lung injury, pulmonary contusion, sepsis, trauma, burns.
Hypercarbic respiratory failure	Reactive airway disease/asthma Drug overdose Neuromuscular disorders Myasthenia gravis Guillain-Barre

Data from Mighty HE. Acute respiratory failure in pregnancy. Clin Obstet Gynecol 2010;53(2): 360–8.

obscure the presentation and diagnosis, and irrelevant of the cause, pregnancy may complicate the management of both hypoxic and hypercarbic respiratory failure in this patient population. In addition to these concerns, both anticipated and unanticipated difficult airway management, including difficulty ventilating and intubating, are more common during pregnancy and may be encountered during endotracheal tube placement.

PHYSIOLOGIC CHANGES OF PREGNANCY

During pregnancy, many normal alterations occur within the pulmonary system, both as the result of hormonal changes and mechanical compression by the gravid uterus. Changes in respiratory mechanics and lung volumes are summarized in **Table 2**. Increased minute ventilation during pregnancy occurs as early as 12 weeks gestational age and is attributable to stimulation of respiratory centers by progesterone. This increase leads to a decline in the $Paco_2$ to 30 mm Hg. The resulting metabolic compensation for this respiratory alkalosis leads to a decreased serum bicarbonate concentration to approximately 20 mEq/L, which decreases the buffering capacity of the blood in the pregnant population. The normal $Paco_2$ to end–tidal CO_2 gradient is also decreased during pregnancy as a result of increased cardiac output, which decreases the proportion of alveolar dead space ventilation.[1]

AIRWAY MANAGEMENT OF THE PREGNANT PATIENT

If during the course of respiratory failure, a pregnant patient requires intubation, the likelihood of difficult mask ventilation and subsequent intubation attempts is

Table 2
Physiologic changes of pregnancy

	Description	Cause	Result
Anatomy	Increased subcostal angle Increased antero-posterior and transverse chest wall diameter	Enlarging gravid uterus	Decreased chest wall compliance; increased inspiratory pressures may be required during mechanical ventilation
	Elevation of diaphragm	Enlarging gravid uterus	Inspiration at term mostly attributable to diaphragm excursion
	Decreased lower esophageal sphincter tone Increased intra-abdominal pressure	Enlarging gravid uterus; elevated serum progesterone	Increased risk of aspiration
Lung volumes/ capacities	Increased tidal volume (TV)	Increased respiratory drive due to progesterone	Largest contributor to increased minute ventilation
	Decreased functional residual capacity (FRC)	Decreased total lung capacity with increased inspiratory capacity	Alveolar collapse during tidal volume breathing if closing capacity exceeds FRC
Ventilation	Increased minute ventilation	Increased TV and respiratory rate	Increased oxygen delivery to fetus; respiratory alkalosis

Data from Mighty HE. Acute respiratory failure in pregnancy. Clin Obstet Gynecol 2010;53(2): 360–8.

significantly increased compared with the general population. This occurs as a result of anatomic airway changes that occur during gestation. The proportion of women with Mallampati class IV airway examination, indicating potential difficulty with endotracheal tube insertion, has been shown to increase by 34% between 12 and 38 weeks gestational age (**Fig. 1**).[2] In addition, during labor and delivery, airway classification can increase further. Kodali and colleagues[3] showed that 33% of women demonstrate a worsened airway classification by at least 1 class from the start to end of labor. Airway edema as a result of preeclampsia, respiratory infections, or prolonged second stage of labor can further exacerbate these baseline changes. Furthermore, physiologic changes that occur during pregnancy, including decreased functional residual capacity and increased oxygen consumption, decrease the amount of time from onset of apnea to significant oxygen desaturation.[1] As a result, prolonged periods of apnea as can occur with difficult intubation are less tolerated in pregnancy and can lead to clinically significant hypoxia and even cardiac arrest. These factors influence the risk/benefit analysis when deciding when and how to intubate a pregnant patient with respiratory failure, and consideration should be given for the most experienced operator to perform laryngoscopy.

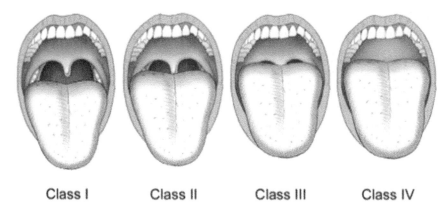

Class I   Class II   Class III   Class IV

Fig. 1. Mallampati airway classification—Mallampati classification of airways involves visual inspection of the oropharynx for visibility of the uvula and palate. (*From* Nuckton TJ, Glidden DV, Browner WS, et al. Physical examination: Mallampati score as an independent predictor of obstructive sleep apnea. Sleep 2006;29(7):904; with permission.)

HYPOXIC RESPIRATORY FAILURE

There are many potential etiologies of hypoxic respiratory failure in pregnancy and the postpartum period (see **Table 1**). Some, such as amniotic fluid embolism (AFE) and pulmonary edema resulting from preeclampsia or tocolytics, are specific to parturients. Many others, however, can occur outside of the obstetric population but may have particularly devastating complications when encountered during pregnancy. Acute respiratory distress syndrome (ARDS), while not an etiology in itself, represents a final common pathway by which many of these disorders lead to arterial hypoxemia.

Acute Respiratory Distress Syndrome

ARDS represents a shared pathophysiologic process within the lungs that can be initiated by a variety of insults, both intrapulmonary and extrapulmonary. These insults lead to neutrophil activation and damage of the pulmonary endothelium, ultimately resulting in pulmonary edema, increased shunt fraction, and decreased lung compliance.[4] Patients typically present with nonspecific symptoms including dyspnea and tachypnea, and examination may reveal pulmonary rales or cyanosis. The diagnosis of ARDS is based on The Berlin Criteria published by the ARDS Definition Task Force in 2012 and summarized in **Table 3**.[5] These criteria represent an improvement over previously utilized criteria, because they offer an estimation of mortality based on the severity of hypoxemia. These mortality predictions, however, have not been validated in pregnant patients, and thus extrapolation should be made with care. Potential etiologies of ARDS in general include sepsis (most common cause of ARDS in both the obstetric and nonobstetric populations), transfusion-related acute lung injury (TRALI), lung contusion, trauma, aspiration, and venous air embolism. Additional etiologies unique to pregnancy consist of preeclampsia, amniotic fluid embolism, and infections of pregnancy such as chorioamnionitis and endometritis. Many of these etiologies will be discussed in detail. Maternal and neonatal outcomes with ARDS are mainly derived from case series, which indicate that maternal mortality may be as high as 35% to 60% and most often results from multiple organ dysfunction syndrome.[6] Management of ARDS in the general population concentrates on elucidating the etiology, minimizing ongoing injury, supportive therapy, and utilization of low-tidal volume ventilatory

Table 3	
The Berlin definition of acute respiratory distress syndrome	
Timing	Within 1 week of a known clinical insult or new or worsening respiratory symptoms
Chest imaging	Bilateral opacities not fully explained by effusions, lobar/lung collapse, or nodules
Origin of edema	Respiratory failure not fully explained by cardiac failure or fluid overload
Oxygenation	Mild – 200 mm Hg < Pao_2/Fio_2 $\leq$ 300 mm Hg with PEEP or CPAP $\geq$ 5 cm H_2O Moderate – 100 mm Hg < Pao_2/Fio_2 $\leq$ 200 mm Hg with PEEP $\geq$ 5 cm H_2O Severe – Pao_2/Fio_2 $\leq$ 100 mm Hg with PEEP $\geq$ 5 cm H_2O

Abbreviations: CPAP, continuous positive airway pressure; Fio_2, fraction of inspired oxygen; Pao_2, partial pressure of arterial oxygen; PEEP, positive end–expiratory pressure.

From ARDS Definition Task Force, Ranieri VM, Rubenfeld GD, et al. Acute respiratory distress syndrome: the Berlin Definition. JAMA 2012;307(23):2530.

strategies to minimize barotrauma. In the obstetric population, evaluation and management should further include an assessment of fetal wellbeing and development of a plan for delivery if applicable.

Amniotic Fluid Embolus

AFE is a rare and serious obstetric complication caused by entry of fetal debris or amniotic fluid into the circulation of the mother during the peripartum period. Although the clinical picture of AFE can be dominated by cardiovascular collapse, respiratory manifestations are also common. Evidence from case series indicates that 48% to 72% of women experience dyspnea at the time of AFE, and hypoxia is thought to be an important premonitory symptom to the development of the subsequent cardiovascular and coagulation changes.[7] This hypoxemia is initially caused by extreme ventilation-to-perfusion mismatch as a result of the embolus. Cardiogenic pulmonary edema may subsequently arise as a result of left ventricular failure. Finally, capillary leak may develop, leading to noncardiogenic exudative edema.[8] The progression of these initial respiratory symptoms to ARDS is one of the major causes of mortality in this patient population.[7] Chest radiograph typically shows bilateral opacities, which are indistinguishable from many other pulmonary pathologies.[7] Treatment of AFE is supportive, and maintaining oxygenation usually requires early intubation and controlled ventilation with titration of positive end–expiratory pressure (PEEP) and inspired oxygen concentration. Cardiopulmonary bypass and extracorporeal membrane oxygenation are additional modalities that have been successfully used when mechanical ventilation is insufficient to provide adequate oxygenation.[9] A complete discussion of AFE (see Amir A. Shamshirsaz, Steven L. Clark's article, "Amniotic Fluid Embolism," in this issue).

Aspiration

Parturients are at elevated risk of aspiration as a result of the physiologic and anatomic changes of pregnancy. Compression from the gravid uterus increases intragastric pressure; progesterone effects lead to a decreased lower esophageal sphincter tone, and during labor gastric emptying is also delayed.[10] Should aspiration occur, the subsequent clinical course can range from mild and clinically insignificant alveolar infiltrates to respiratory failure requiring mechanical ventilation. Immediate treatment includes suctioning of the upper airway and intubation and suctioning of primary bronchi as indicated. Lung lavage, empiric antibiotic administration, and corticosteroids are not recommended in the routine care following aspiration.[11] Additional supportive measures may include oxygen supplementation and PEEP as needed.

Pulmonary Embolism

Thromboembolism represents one of the greatest causes of mortality in the obstetric population, although the incidence appears to be decreasing. Risk factors for thrombosis are many and include[12] obesity, increased age, ethnicity, family history, previous history, and immobility.

The clinical diagnosis of pulmonary embolism (PE) in the nonobstetric population includes symptoms such as leg swelling, dyspnea, tachypnea, tachycardia, and palpitations, all of which are common in pregnancy. Because of this, objective testing in the form of lung imaging must be utilized for diagnosis of PE in the pregnant patient.[13]

Summary of Management of Hypoxic Respiratory Failure

Although the etiologies of hypoxic respiratory failure are many, the mainstay of treatment for all focuses on provision of supplemental oxygen, which can be provided in increasingly invasive forms. Patients often require endotracheal intubation and mechanical ventilation in order to achieve adequate arterial oxygenation. The fraction of inspired oxygen can be titrated from a room air concentration of 21% to 100% of inspired gases. PEEP can also be utilized to sustain alveolar inflation throughout the respiratory cycle, which improves the delivery of oxygen from the alveolus to the pulmonary venous blood.

Lung-Protective Ventilation

Within the subset of patients with hypoxic respiratory failure who suffer from ARDS, pulmonary consolidations lead to decreased static lung compliance. Because of this decreased compliance, higher inspiratory pressures are required to maintain adequate tidal volumes, subsequently leading to barotrauma and volutrauma. Understanding these mechanisms for lung injury, much research has focused on the effect of limiting tidal volumes during ventilation of patients with ARDS. This requires accepting higher levels of arterial carbon dioxide and the associated effects of respiratory acidosis. Conventional ventilation typically employs tidal volumes of 10 to 15 mL/kg of body weight while low tidal volume ventilation is defined as 5 to 7 mL/kg. Combined with moderate PEEP, this low-volume strategy has been termed lung-protective ventilation and has been shown to decrease overall mortality and increase ventilator-free days in ARDS within the general nonpregnant population.[14,15] No studies have been performed evaluating the effects of these strategies in parturients.

Positive End–Expiratory Pressure

Additionally, moderate-to-high levels of PEEP can aid oxygenation in ARDS by maintaining open alveoli throughout the entire cycle of ventilation. This prevents trauma to the lung parenchyma caused by repetitive opening and closing of alveolar units. Alveolar-to-arterial oxygen transfer is also enhanced, leading to improvement in arterial hypoxemia.[16] Recommended Fio_2 and PEEP setting combinations are shown in **Table 4**.[14]

Mode of Ventilation

Regarding specific modes of ventilation, current data are inconclusive, and no mode has been shown to confer benefit when utilized for respiratory failure in the intensive care unit (ICU) setting. A full summary of modes of ventilation is shown in **Table 5**. Controlled, assist-controlled, and intermittent mandatory modes can all utilize volume- or pressure-limited breath strategies, neither of which has been shown to be superior.[17]

Table 4
Fraction of inspired oxygen and positive end–expository pressure settings recommended by the Acute Respiratory Distress Syndrome Network

Lower PEEP/higher Fio_2

Fio_2	0.3	0.4	0.4	0.5	0.5	0.6	0.7	0.7	0.7	0.8	0.9	0.9	0.9	1.0
PEEP	5	5	8	8	10	10	10	12	14	14	14	16	18	18–24

Higher PEEP/lower Fio_2

Fio_2	0.3	0.3	0.3	0.3	0.3	0.4	0.4	0.5	0.5	0.5–0.8	0.8	0.9	1.0	1.0
PEEP	5	8	10	12	14	14	16	16	18	20	22	22	22	24

Adapted from The Acute Respiratory Distress Syndrome Network. Ventilation with lower tidal volumes as compared with traditional tidal volumes for acute lung injury and the acute respiratory distress syndrome. N Engl J Med 2000;342(18):1303.

Neuromuscular Blockade

The use of neuromuscular blockade (NMB) in the critical care setting to improve ventilation to perfusion matching and oxygenation in patients with ARDS remains controversial. However, many recent studies have shown lower hospital mortality and lower risk of barotrauma when NMB is utilized in the early phase of ARDS.[18–20] Potential complications of this therapy may include weakness or critical illness myopathy, but current data do not suggest that short-term infusions (<48 hours) increase the incidence of this complication.[18]

Table 5
Modes of ventilation

Mode	Definition	Details/Uses
Controlled mode	All breaths are initiated by the ventilator and the ventilator performs entire work of inspiration during each breath	Set minute ventilation Utilized with general anesthesia and/or paralysis
Assist control mode	Breaths can be initiated by either the ventilator or the patient, but the ventilator assists every breath	Set minimum minute ventilation, can be increased by patient effort Commonly used in ICU setting
Intermittent mandatory mode (IMV)	Breaths can be initiated by either the ventilator or the patient, and patient initiated breaths can be assisted or not depending on ventilator settings	Set minimum minute ventilation, can be increased by patient effort
Synchronized intermittent mandatory ventilation (SIMV)	IMV in which ventilator triggered breaths are synchronized to patient's inspiratory efforts	Set minimum minute ventilation, can be increased by patient effort Commonly used in ICU setting
Pressure support ventilation (PSV)	All breaths are patient triggered	Used to assist spontaneously ventilating patient

Data from Mighty HE. Acute respiratory failure in pregnancy. Clin Obstet Gynecol 2010;53(2): 360–8.

Prone Positioning

In addition, some have advocated the use of prone positioning (PP) in the most refractory cases of hypoxic respiratory failure in order to improve lung mechanics and gas exchange. Mortality following this intervention may be improved, although a recent review failed to show a statistically significant difference in the treated group. Three subsets of patients were, however, shown to benefit from the PP:

1. Recruited within 48 hours of meeting entry criteria
2. Treated with PP for at least 16 hours per day
3. More severe arterial hypoxemia upon initiation of PP

On the other hand, the use of PP can confer additional risk to patients and has been specifically shown to increase the risk of pressure sores and tracheal tube obstructions in a recent review.[21]

Fluid Management

ARDS is characterized by increased capillary permeability and subsequent pulmonary edema, which can increase intrapulmonary shunt and lead to hypoxia. Management of ARDS includes maneuvers aimed at decreasing the formation and increasing the resorption of this fluid. This is generally accomplished by

1. Maintaining net zero fluid balance through the use of fluid restriction and diuretics (this has been shown to increase the number of ventilator-free days in ARDS patients without shock or renal failure)[22]
2. Providing fluid resuscitation when ARDS is accompanied by hemodynamic compromise
3. Pulmonary vasodilation via inhaled agents (the theoretic benefit of vasodilation includes a decreased filtration pressure, which decreases fluid migration out of the pulmonary vasculature and into the lungs)
4. Colloids including albumin have not been shown to be beneficial in improving outcomes in ARDS despite the theoretic advantage of improving intravascular oncotic pressure[23]

Use of Extracorporeal Respiratory Support During Pregnancy

Extracorporeal membrane oxygenation (ECMO) is a treatment modality consisting of an extracorporeal pump and oxygenator used to improve hypoxemia in patients with refractory respiratory failure. Veno-arterial ECMO (VA-ECMO) augments both gas exchange and hemodynamics as blood is pumped out of the venous system and returned, oxygenated, to the arterial circulation. Veno-venous ECMO (VV-ECMO), conversely, facilitates only gas exchange, as blood is both pumped out of and returned to the venous system. The type of ECMO chosen depends on the patient's underlying condition, with VA-ECMO required for cases of hypoxic respiratory failure accompanied by ventricular dysfunction, such as may be the case with AFE. Successful use of both VV- and VA-ECMO has been described in pregnancy for ARDS associated with H1N1 influenza and AFE.[9,24,25] VA-ECMO for AFE poses significant bleeding risk as a result of necessary anticoagulation in the setting of potential underlying DIC, and was not recommended by a recent guideline published by the Society for Maternal–Fetal Medicine.[26]

HYPERCARBIC RESPIRATORY FAILURE

In contrast to hypoxic respiratory failure, the causes of hypercarbic respiratory failure are much fewer, and treatment is somewhat more straightforward. In general, hypercarbia is caused by decreased minute ventilation, which can result from obstruction to airflow within the airways themselves or inability to produce sufficient respiratory effort secondary to muscle weakness. The latter may be attributable to drug overdose, primary neurologic or muscle disorders, and other more rare causes. The treatment of this subset of cases is mainly supportive, aimed at addressing the underlying cause, and overall beyond the scope of this article. Hypercarbic respiratory failure as the result of airflow obstruction, however, is commonly encountered during pregnancy and will be addressed in detail.

Reactive Airway Disease/Status Asthmaticus

Asthma is a common respiratory comorbidity encountered in pregnant patients, and about one-third of parturients with a history of asthma will experience an exacerbation during pregnancy.[27] Most are mild and will not require ICU admission or intubation. Initial management includes administration of supplemental oxygen and inhaled beta-agonists to relieve bronchospasm. Multiple prospective studies have evaluated the use of inhaled corticosteroids in this patient population and found a statistically significant decrease in acute asthma attacks and readmission rates in pregnant asthmatic patients prescribed steroids.[27,28] Although some concern over potential teratogenic effects of these medications has been raised in the past, no data currently suggest adverse fetal effects. In severe cases, intravenous epinephrine may be required to treat refractory bronchospasm. Ongoing evaluation of the patient for response to treatment should include peak flow and arterial blood gas measurements when clinically indicated. Assisted ventilation may be provided in the form of noninvasive positive pressure ventilation or endotracheal intubation and mechanical ventilation as necessary.

REFERENCES

1. Hegewald MJ, Crapo RO. Respiratory physiology in pregnancy. Clin Chest Med 2011;32(1):1–13, vii.
2. Pilkington S, Carli F, Dakin MJ, et al. Increase in Mallampati score during pregnancy. Br J Anaesth 1995;74(6):638–42.
3. Kodali BS, Chandrasekhar S, Bulich LN, et al. Airway changes during labor and delivery. Anesthesiology 2008;108(3):357–62.
4. Collop NA, Sahn SA. Critical illness in pregnancy. An analysis of 20 patients admitted to a medical intensive care unit. Chest 1993;103(5):1548–52.
5. ARDS Definition Task Force, Ranieri VM, Rubenfeld GD, et al. Acute respiratory distress syndrome: the Berlin Definition. JAMA 2012;307(23):2526–33.
6. Cole DE, Taylor TL, McCullough DM, et al. Acute respiratory distress syndrome in pregnancy. Crit Care Med 2005;33(10 Suppl):S269–78.
7. Conde-Agudelo A, Romero R. Amniotic fluid embolism: an evidence-based review. Am J Obstet Gynecol 2009;201(5):445.e1-3.
8. O'Shea A, Eappen S. Amniotic fluid embolism. Int Anesthesiol Clin 2007;45(1):17–28.
9. Hsieh YY, Chang CC, Li PC, et al. Successful application of extracorporeal membrane oxygenation and intra-aortic balloon counterpulsation as lifesaving therapy for a patient with amniotic fluid embolism. Am J Obstet Gynecol 2000;183(2):496–7.
10. Macfie A, Magides A, Richmond M, et al. Gastric emptying in pregnancy. Br J Anaesth 1991;67:54–7.
11. Mighty HE. Acute resp failure pregnancy. Clin Obstet Gynecol 2010;53(2):360–8.

12. Cantwell R, Clutton-Brock T, Cooper G, et al. Saving mothers' lives: reviewing maternal deaths to make motherhood safer: 2006-2008. The eighth report of the confidential enquiries into maternal deaths in the United Kingdom. BJOG 2011;118(Suppl 1):1–203.

13. Stone SE, Morris TA. Pulmonary embolism during and after pregnancy. Crit Care Med 2005;33(10 Suppl):S294–300.

14. Ventilation with lower tidal volumes as compared with traditional tidal volumes for acute lung injury and the acute respiratory distress syndrome. The Acute Respiratory Distress Syndrome Network. N Engl J Med 2000;342(18):1301–8.

15. Petrucci N, De Feo C. Lung protective ventilation strategy for the acute respiratory distress syndrome. Cochrane Database Syst Rev 2013;(2):CD003844.

16. Santa Cruz R, Rojas JI, Nervi R, et al. High versus low positive end-expiratory pressure (PEEP) levels for mechanically ventilated adult patients with acute lung injury and acute respiratory distress syndrome. Cochrane Database Syst Rev 2013;(6):CD009098.

17. Chacko B, Peter J, Tharyan P, et al. Pressure-controlled versus volume-controlled ventilation for acute respiratory failure due to acute lung injury (ALI) or acute respiratory distress syndrome (ARDS). Cochrane Database Syst Rev 2015;(1):CD008807.

18. Alhazzani W, Alshahrani M, Jaeschke R, et al. Neuromuscular blocking agents in acute respiratory distress syndrome: a systematic review and meta-analysis of randomized controlled trials. Crit Care 2013;17(2):R43.

19. Gainnier M, Roch A, Forel JM, et al. Effect of neuromuscular blocking agents on gas exchange in patients presenting with acute respiratory distress syndrome. Crit Care Med 2004;32(1):113–9.

20. Papazian L, Forel J-M, Gacouin A, et al. Neuromuscular blockers in early acute respiratory distress syndrome. N Engl J Med 2010;363(12):1107–16.

21. Bloomfield R, Noble DW, Sudlow A. Prone position for acute respiratory failure in adults. Cochrane Database Syst Rev 2015;11:CD008095.

22. National Heart, Lung, and Blood Institute Acute Respiratory Distress Syndrome (ARDS) Clinical Trials Network, Wiedemann HP, Wheeler AP, Bernard GR. Comparison of two fluid-management strategies in acute lung injury. N Engl J Med 2006;354(24):2564–75.

23. Roch A, Guervilly C, Papazian L. Fluid management in acute lung injury and ards. Ann Intensive Care 2011;1(1):16.

24. Grasselli G, Bombino M, Patroniti N, et al. Use of extracorporeal respiratory support during pregnancy: a case report and literature review. ASAIO J 2012;58: 281–4.

25. Saad AF, Rahman M, Maybauer DM, et al. Extracorporeal membrane oxygenation in pregnant and postpartum women with H1N1-related acute respiratory distress syndrome: a systematic review and meta-analysis. Obstet Gynecol 2016;127(2): 241–7.

26. Hankins GD, Clark SL. Society for Maternal-Fetal Medicine (SMFM) with the assistance of. Electronic address: pubs@smfm.org, Pacheco LD, Saade G. SMFM Clinical guidelines No. 9: Amniotic fluid embolism: diagnosis and management. Am J Obstet Gynecol 2016. http://dx.doi.org/10.1016/j.ajog.2016.03.012.

27. Stenius-Aarniala BS, Hedman J, Teramo KA. Acute asthma during pregnancy. Thorax 1996;51(4):411–4.

28. Wendel P, Ramin S, Barnett-Hamm C, et al. Asthma treatment in pregnnacy: a randomized controlled study. Am J Obstet Gynecol 1996;175(1):150–4.

Cardiac Lesions in the Critical Care Setting

Manisha Gandhi, MD, Amir A. Shamshirsaz, MD*

KEYWORDS

- Maternal cardiac disease • Congenital heart disease • Pregnancy
- Valvular heart disease

KEY POINTS

- Physiologic changes in pregnancy can place extra demands on cardiac function.
- Preconception counseling is key to improving pregnancy outcomes.
- The most commonly encountered cardiac events are pulmonary edema and dysrhythmias.
- A team approach to antepartum care is recommended and should include maternal-fetal medicine, cardiology, and anesthesia as indicated, particularly for patients with congenital cardiac disease.

INTRODUCTION

Although cardiac disease complicates only 1% to 4% of all pregnancies in the United States, such conditions continue to account for up to 10% to 25% of maternal mortality.[1–3] Intensive care unit (ICU) admissions owing to cardiac disease make up 15% of obstetrics ICU admissions.[4–8] Rheumatic fever and its valvular sequelae of heart failure is no longer the most common cause of maternal mortality. Both maternal congenital heart disease and acquired heart disease, such as myocardial infarction and cardiomyopathy, now are the predominant causes of maternal death. With advances in the diagnosis and treatment of congenital heart disease in newborns and children, more young women with these conditions are reaching reproductive age and attempting pregnancy. Also, the incidence of an acute coronary event is increasing during pregnancy because of older maternal age at child bearing and higher rates of hypertension and obesity in women.[9]

The long-held belief that pregnancy is absolutely contraindicated in maternal cardiovascular disease is no longer justifiable using evidence-base medicine. There are some conditions in which pregnancy is contraindicated, and high maternal risk and poor fetal outcome can be predicted. However, in many women with heart disease,

Division of Maternal-Fetal Medicine, Department of Obstetrics & Gynecology, Baylor College of Medicine, Texas Children's Pavilion for Women, 6651 Main Street, Houston, TX 77030, USA
* Corresponding author.
E-mail address: ashamshi@bcm.edu

Obstet Gynecol Clin N Am 43 (2016) 709–728
http://dx.doi.org/10.1016/j.ogc.2016.07.003
0889-8545/16/© 2016 Elsevier Inc. All rights reserved.

obgyn.theclinics.com

a more favorable maternal and fetal outcome is expected. This article focusses on the cardiac conditions that require more attention and have the potential to require observation in the ICU setting.

PHYSIOLOGIC CHANGES IN PREGNANCY

Cardiovascular adaptations to pregnancy are well tolerated by healthy young women. However, these adaptations are of such magnitude that they can significantly compromise women with abnormal or damaged hearts. Comprehensive understanding of the normal physiologic adaptations to pregnancy is essential to successful treatment of patients with cardiac disease. Conditions that may be asymptomatic when the patient is not pregnant can deteriorate in the pregnant state. **Box 1** outlines key physiologic changes in a normal singleton gestation. **Table 1** provides an overview of changes in cardiovascular test during pregnancy.

Physiologic Consideration in Patients with Cardiac Disease

The unique problems encountered by the pregnant woman with cardiac disease are secondary to 4 principle physiologic changes:

1. A 50% increase in intravascular volume is seen in normal pregnancy. In patients whose cardiac output is limited by intrinsic myocardial dysfunction, valvular lesions, or ischemic cardiac disease, volume overload is poorly tolerated and may lead to congestive heart failure or worsening ischemia. In patients with an anatomic predisposition, such volume expansion may result in aneurysm formation or dissection (eg, Marfan syndrome).[10]
2. Decreased systemic vascular resistance (SVR) becomes especially important in patients with the potential for a right-to-left shunt, which will be invariably increased by a decreasing SVR during pregnancy. Such alterations in cardiac afterload also complicate adaptation to pregnancy in patients with certain types of valvular disease such as mitral stenosis.[10]
3. Marked fluctuations in cardiac output normally occur during pregnancy, particularly during labor and delivery.[11] Such changes increase progressively from the first stage of labor, reaching in some cases an additional 50% by the late second stage.[12] The potential for further dramatic volume shifts occurs around the time of delivery, both secondary to postpartum hemorrhage and as the results of autotransfusion, which occurs with the release of vena caval obstruction and sustained uterine contraction. Such volume shifts may be poorly tolerated by women whose cardiac output is highly dependent on adequate preload (pulmonary hypertension) or in those with fixed cardiac output (mitral stenosis).[12]
4. The hypercoagulability associated with pregnancy increases the need for adequate anticoagulation in patients at risk for arterial thrombosis (artificial valves and some subsets of atrial fibrillation) at a time when optimum anticoagulation with coumarin derivatives may have adverse fetal consequence. For women receiving any type of therapeutic anticoagulation, the risk of serious postpartum hemorrhage is also increased.[10]

COUNSELING THE PREGNANT PATIENT

Maternal and fetal outcome in the cardiac patients depends on the type of cardiac disease, myocardial function, maternal function status, presence and severity of

---

Box 1

Expected physiologic changes occurring in the antepartum, intrapartum, and postpartum periods

Antepartum

- Blood volume increases by 20% to 50%

- Systemic vascular resistance decreased by 20%

- Blood pressure (BP) (taken in sitting position)
  - BP ≥140/90 abnormal at any time in gestation
  - BP decreases to lowest point at 28 weeks
  - After 28 weeks, BP increases to nonpregnant level by term

- Mean arterial pressure unchanged

- Heart rate increased by 10 to 15 beats/min

- Stroke volume increased by 30%

- Cardiac output increases by 30% to 50%

- Pulmonary capillary wedge pressure unchanged

- Central venous pressure (preload to right heart) unchanged

- Pulmonary vascular resistance decreased by 30%

- Increase hypercoagulable state

Intrapartum

- During a contraction
  - 300 to 500 mL of blood enters circulation
  - Heart rate increases
  - Cardiac output increased by 30%
  - Blood pressure increased by 10 to 20 mm Hg

- Supine position may decrease cardiac output by 20%

Postpartum

- Cardiac output increased by 50% in immediate postpartum period

- Stroke volume increases 60% in the immediate postpartum period

- Reflex bradycardia occurs (15%)

- These changed persist for 2 weeks after delivery

Modified from Gandhi M, Martin SR. Cardiac disease in pregnancy. In: Foley MR, Strong TH, Garite TJ, editors. Obstetric intensive care manual. 4th edition. McGraw-Hill; 2014. p. 103–22; with permission.

---

cyanosis, pulmonary vascular pressure, and prior surgical procedures along with any uncorrected lesions and residua and sequelae of repair.

Maternal Risk

Risk stratification of the mother based on her cardiac diagnosis can be helpful in the preconception evaluation and counseling. Functional status for patients with cardiac disease is commonly classified according to the New York Heart Association (NYHA) classification system as outlined in **Box 2**.[13] Siu and Colleagues,[14] as part of the Cardiac Disease in Pregnancy (CARPREG) investigators found that, in their cohort of 599 women with heart disease, there was a 13% incidence of a cardiac event, notably pulmonary edema, arrhythmia, stroke, or cardiac death. The authors developed a score

Table 1 Changes in cardiovascular tests during pregnancy	
Cardiovascular Examination	**Findings in Pregnancy**
Chest radiograph	Apparent cardiomegaly Enlarged left atrium Increased vascular markings
Electrocardiography	Right axis deviation Right bundle branch block ST-segment depression of 1 mm on left precordial leads Q waves in lead III T-wave inversion in leads III, V2, and V3
Echocardiography	Trivial tricuspid regurgitation Pulmonary regurgitation Increased left atrial size Increased left ventricular end- diastolic dimensions by 6% to 10% Mitral regurgitation Pericardial effusion

From Gandhi M, Martin SR. Cardiac disease in pregnancy. In: Foley MR, Strong TH, Garite TJ, editors. Obstetric intensive care manual. 4th edition. McGraw-Hill; 2014. p. 103–22; with permission.

to predict adverse maternal outcomes, which is outlined in **Table 2**.[14] **Box 3** classifies various cardiac abnormalities according to maternal death risk estimates; however, the patient's particular history is not included in these estimates.[10]

Fetal Risk

Maternal heart disease is associated with fetal and neonatal complications, such as fetal growth restriction, fetal loss, and prematurity.[15] These complications are more common in cases of maternal cyanosis, anticoagulation, NYHA class III and IV, left heart obstruction lesions, maternal smoking, or multifetal gestation.[16] These complications include small for gestational age infants, delivery before 34 weeks of gestation, and neonatal death.[17] In women who have congenital heart disease (CHD), the risk of CHD in the offspring is 7% to 8%, for conditions with no chromosomal abnormality or family history.[18] When the father has CHD, the risk of CHD in the fetus is roughly

---

Box 2
New York Heart Association functional classification system

Class I
  No limitation of physical activity. Ordinary physical activity does not precipitates cardiovascular symptoms such as dyspnea, angina, fatigue, or palpitations.

Class II
  Slight limitation of physical activity. Ordinary physical activity will precipitates cardiovascular symptoms. Patients are comfortable at rest.

Class III
  Less than ordinary physical activity precipitates symptoms that markedly limit activity. Patients are comfortable at rest.

Class IV
  Patients have discomfort with any physical activity. Symptoms are present at rest.

Table 2
Cardiac Disease in Pregnancy (CARPREG) Risk Score: predictors of maternal cardiovascular events

New York Heart Association (NYHA) functional class > II
Cyanosis (room air saturation <90%)
Prior cardiovascular event
Systemic ventricular ejection fraction <40%
Left heart obstruction (eg, Mitral valve area <2 cm^2 or aortic valve area <1.5 cm^2, or left ventricular outflow gradient of >30 mm Hg)

Risk Estimation of Maternal Cardiovascular Complications	
No. of Predictors	*Risk of Cardiac Events in Pregnancy (%)*
0	5
1	27
>1	75

Adapted from Franklin WJ, Gandhi M. Congenital heart disease in pregnancy. Cardiol Clin 2012;30(3):383–94; with permission.

3% to 4%.[19] Nonetheless, CHD in the fetus approaches 50% in single gene disorders such as Marfan syndrome. Genetic counseling is recommended if there is a dysmorphism or a chromosomal abnormality suggested.[20] **Table 3** demonstrates the risk of fetal cardiac abnormality by maternal lesion.

GENERAL PRINCIPLES IN MANAGEMENT
Preconception Care

Box 4 shows the principles of preconception care in patients with cardiac disease. Medical and surgical intervention may be necessary before conception to optimize cardiac function and to minimize the risks of pregnancy. All cardiac medications should be reviewed, with cessation of any contraindicated drugs and substitution of suitable alternatives (**Box 5**). Comorbidities should also be well controlled, including hypertension, diabetes, and obesity.

Possible Contraindications to Pregnancy

Box 6 outlines the possible contraindications to pregnancy. Patients with such conditions should be strongly recommended against pregnancy.[14,19]

Antepartum Considerations

A multidisciplinary approach including specialists in cardiology, maternal fetal medicine, and obstetrics anesthesiology is recommended. In some cases, an adult intensivist should be consulted if the mother is high risk, and a neonatologist should be consulted if the baby is considered at risk. Patients should be evaluated regularly for signs and symptoms of cardiac decompensation. Fetal echocardiogram between 20 and 24 weeks is indicated because of increased risk of fetal CHD. Periodic ultrasound scans should be started from 24 weeks to assess fetal growth (especially in complex cardiac diseases). At 28 to 30 weeks of gestation (when maternal plasma volume is highest), the delivery plan, including hospital location, mode of delivery, anesthesia type, and bacterial endocarditis prophylaxis plan, should be confirmed.[15] Antepartum fetal surveillance can be considered starting at 32 to 34 weeks if there is any concern for fetal growth restriction or maternal complications such as preeclampsia or hypoxia.

Box 3
Maternal mortality associated with pregnancy

Group 1: Mortality rate less than 1%

ASD

VSD

Patent ductus arteriosus

Mitral stenosis: NYHA class I and II

Pulmonic/tricuspid valve disease

Corrected tetralogy of Fallot

Bioprosthetic valve

Group 2: Mortality rate 5%–15%

Mitral stenosis: NYHA class III and IV

Aortic stenosis

Coarctation of aorta without valvular involvement

Uncorrected tetralogy of Fallot

Previous myocardial infarction

Marfan syndrome with normal aorta

Mitral stenosis with atrial fibrillation

Artificial valve

Group 3: Mortality rate 25%–50%

Pulmonary hypertension
    Primary
    Eisenmenger syndrome

Coarctation of aorta with valvular involvement

Marfan syndrome with aortic involvement

Peripartum cardiomyopathy with persistent left ventricular dysfunction

Modified from Gandhi M, Martin SR. Cardiac disease in pregnancy. In: Foley MR, Strong TH, Garite TJ, editors. Obstetric intensive care manual. 4th edition. McGraw-Hill; 2014. p. 103–22; with permission.

Interventional Considerations

Percutaneous cardiovascular intervention

If percutaneous cardiac catheterization and intervention are necessary, the preferred time is after the fourth month in the second trimester, as by this gestational age, organogenesis is complete; the fetal thyroid is small and there is greater distance between the fetus and mother's chest than in later weeks. The gravid uterus should be double shielded from direct radiation, and unfractionated heparin should be used (generally 40–70 U/kg), with an activated clotting time of at least 200 seconds but not exceeding 300 seconds.[15]

Cardiac surgery and cardiopulmonary bypass

Cardiac surgery is recommended only when medical or interventional procedures fail, and the mother's life is threatened. The maternal mortality is now similar to that of nonpregnant women. However, there is significant morbidity including late neurologic

Table 3
Risk of fetal cardiac abnormality by maternal lesion

Maternal Lesion	Risk if Mother is Affected (%)
Tetralogy of Fallot	2–4.5
Aortic coarctation	4–14.1
ASD	4.6–11
VSD	6–15.6
Pulmonary stenosis	5.3–6.5
Aortic stenosis	8–17.9
PDA	4.1
Marfan syndrome	50
22q11 deletion syndromes	50

Modified from Gandhi M, Martin SR. Cardiac disease in pregnancy. In: Foley MR, Strong TH, Garite TJ, editors. Obstetric intensive care manual. 4th edition. McGraw-Hill; 2014. p. 103–22; with permission.

impairment in 3% to 6% of neonates, and fetal mortality remains high.[21] During cardiopulmonary bypass, fetal heart rate should be followed closely (if fetus is viable) in addition to standard monitoring. Pump flow greater than 2.5 L/min/m^2 and perfusion pressure greater than 70 mm Hg are necessary to attain adequate uteroplacental perfusion.[22] Maintenance of the maternal hematocrit greater than 28% is recommended to optimize oxygen delivery.[15] If possible, normothermic perfusion is best, and careful management of pH is recommended to avoid hypocapnia, which can lead to uteroplacental vasoconstriction and fetal hypoxia. In general, neonatal survival at 26 weeks is approximately 80%, with 20% of newborns having a significant neurologic abnormality. Thus, cesarean section may be considered before cardiopulmonary bypass if gestational age is beyond 26 weeks.[20,23]

Delivery and postpartum care
The mode of delivery is usually determined by obstetric instead of cardiac condition. Most patients can safely undergo a trial of labor and experience a vaginal birth. In certain circumstances, an operative vaginal delivery in second stage should be considered to limit the stress associated with pushing, such as cases of severe maternal aortic stenosis.[15] In general, cesarean delivery is reserved for normal obstetric indications.[24] Despite the increased risks of hemorrhage, infection, and large fluid shifts, there are a few conditions in which labor is ill advised and cesarean delivery is recommended (**Box 7**).

Box 4
Preconception care in patients with cardiac disease

- Baseline evaluation of cardiac function
- Counseling regarding pregnancy risk for mother and fetus
- Consultation with cardiologist, maternal fetal medicine specialist, if possible obstetrics anesthesiologist
- Review current medication to determine appropriateness of their use in pregnancy
- Routine preconception care as for all patients: assessment of immunization status, screening for genetic diseases as indicated, supplemental folic acid

Box 5
Cardiac drugs to avoid/use with caution

Angiotensin-converting enzyme inhibitors

Angiotensin-II receptor blockers

Amiodarone

Warfarin[a]

Spironolactone

[a] Use during first trimester is contraindicated unless less than 5 mg or in extremely high-risk lesions. Warfarin may be used from weeks 13 to 35, and then heparin may be used until delivery.
From Franklin WJ, Gandhi M. Congenital heart disease in pregnancy. Cardiol Clin 2012;30(3):383–94; with permission.

Attention should be to strict fluid intake and output. All intravenous fluids should be maintained on an infusion pump. There is lack of consensus regarding the use of invasive monitoring during labor and delivery. Although many centers have decreased the use of pulmonary artery catheter, peripheral arterial lines and central venous lines can be used to assess a patient's cardiovascular status during the peripartum period. The supine position should be avoided to maintain adequate preload. Supplemental oxygen should be administered to maintain the oxygen saturation greater than 95%. Early epidural placement can decrease the sympathetic stimulation and myocardial oxygen consumption associated with labor and is recommended for most women with heart disease.[25] **Table 4** summarizes anesthesia recommendations depending on each cardiac lesion. In patients with fixed cardiac output, the initiation of epidural analgesia must be performed slowly with careful attention to fluid balance and clinical status.

Endocarditis prophylaxis
Infective endocarditis prophylaxis is no longer recommended for vaginal or cesarean deliveries in the absence of infection irrespective of the type of maternal heart disease. The current recommendation from the American Heart Association is that only when

Box 6
Possible contraindication to pregnancy

- Pulmonary arterial hypertension of any cause
- Marfan syndrome, with dilated aortic root greater than 40 mm
- Aortic dilation greater than 50 mm in aortic disease associated with bicuspid aortic valve
- Severe left heart obstructive lesions (severe mitral stenosis, severe symptomatic aortic stenosis, or severe coarctation)
- Severe systemic left ventricular (LV) dysfunction with LV ejection fraction less than 30%, NYHA III/IV
- Previous peripartum cardiomyopathy particularly with any residual impairment of LV function

From Franklin WJ, Gandhi M. Congenital heart disease in pregnancy. Cardiol Clin 2012;30(3):383–94; with permission.

> **Box 7**
> **Contraindication to vaginal delivery in patients with cardiac disease**
>
> - Dilated aortic root (more than 4 cm) or aortic aneurysm
> - Acute severe congestive heart failure
> - History of recent myocardial infarction
> - Severe symptomatic aortic stenosis
> - Warfarin administration within 2 weeks of delivery
> - Need for emergency valve replacement immediately after delivery

deliveries are associated with infection should patients with high-risk cardiac lesions receive intrapartum prophylaxis (**Box 8**).[26]

Management of Specific Cardiac Lesions

Valvular cardiac disease

Most valvular lesions, which may be congenital or acquired, occur secondary to rheumatic fever, which accounts for 90% of cardiac disorders in pregnancy worldwide. Heart

Table 4
Anesthesia and maternal cardiac lesion

Maternal Lesion	Anesthesia Recommendations
Pulmonic and tricuspid lesions	Epidural acceptable
Mitral stenosis	Epidural acceptable. May help control tachycardia in labor. Avoid abrupt sympathetic blockage owing to potential decrease in preload.
Mitral insufficiency	Epidural acceptable
Aortic stenosis/idiopathic hypertrophic subaortic stenosis	Cautious use of epidural to avoid hypotension. May consider narcotic epidural.
Aortic insufficiency	Epidural acceptable
Mechanical heart valves	Epidural acceptable but requires coordination with last dose of anticoagulation to minimize epidural hematoma risk. High-dose LMWH should be discontinued at least 24 h before epidural placement. For those on high doses of UFH, normal aPTT should be documented before epidural placement.
ASD, VSD, PDA	Epidural acceptable in absence of pulmonary hypertension or known Eisenmenger syndrome.
Severe pulmonary hypertension and Eisenmenger syndrome	Epidural is contraindicated, although narcotic-only epidural may be acceptable.
Coarctation of the aorta	Epidural acceptable
Marfan syndrome	Epidural acceptable. May help in control of tachycardia associated with pain and avoid urge to Valsalva.
Peripartum cardiomyopathy	Epidural acceptable and decreases preload and afterload and minimizes tachycardia associated with pain.

Abbreviations: aPTT, activated partial thromboplastin time; LMWH, low-molecular-weight heparin; UFH, unfractionated heparin.

Box 8
Indications for intrapartum endocarditis prophylaxis

1. Prosthetic cardiac valve or prosthetic material used for cardiac valve repair

2. Previous infective endocarditis

3. Congenital heart disease that meets one of the following conditions:
   a. Unrepaired cyanotic defect including palliative shunts and conduits
   b. Completely repaired defects with prosthetic material or device whether placed by surgery of catheter intervention during the first 6 months after the procedure
   c. Repaired defect with residual defects at the site or adjacent to the site of a prosthetic patch or prosthetic device

Adapted from Wilson W, Taubert KA, Gewitz M, et al. Prevention of infective endocarditis: guidelines from the American Heart Association. Circulation 2007;116(15):1736–54.

---

failure is the most common complication, and patients with acquired valvular heart disease have a higher mortality rate than those with congenital heart disease.[27] The specific valve lesion, number of valves involved, and the degree of valvular obstruction, particularly of the mitral and aortic valves, determines the degree of risk for development of complications such as dysrhythmias and pulmonary edema. **Table 5** summarizes the recommendations for management for the lesions discussed in this section.

Pulmonary/Tricuspid Stenosis and Regurgitation

Pulmonic stenosis/regurgitation and tricuspid stenosis/regurgitation are both typically well tolerated in pregnancy with minimal risk of right heart failure and are rarely of any consequence in pregnancy. Echocardiogram is recommended to evaluate severity of right outflow obstruction (>60 mm Hg consistent with severe obstruction). Medical therapy is generally not indicated.

Mitral Stenosis

Mitral stenosis is the most common valvular lesion in pregnancy. Stenosis of the mitral valve impedes flow of blood from left atrium to the left ventricle, and elevated left atrial pressures are necessary to maintain adequate left ventricular filling through restricted opening. Patients with moderate or severe stenosis are most likely to have cardiac complications. Patients may be asymptomatic until physiologic changes of pregnancy unmask the disease. Symptomatic patients may undergo balloon valvulotomy during pregnancy.

Recommended workup and clinical findings

- Echocardiogram to establish severity of stenosis and size of left atrium
- Symptoms unusual until valve area less than 2 cm^2
- Moderate mitral stenosis: 1 to 1.5 cm^2 valve area
- Severe mitral stenosis: less than 1 cm^2 valve area
- Electrocardiogram (ECG) to exclude atrial fibrillation from enlarged left atrium may show left atrial enlargement, right ventricular hypertrophy, and right atrial enlargement in cases of pulmonary hypertension
- Auscultation: loud first heart sound, an opening snap and rumbling diastolic murmur

Potential complications

- Pulmonary edema, atrial fibrillation, and supraventricular tachycardia are the most common maternal complications.

- Sixty percent have the initial episode of pulmonary edema antepartum, at a mean gestational age of 30 weeks.
- Thromboembolism can develop as a result of left atrial dilation. This condition may present as a stroke.

MITRAL AND AORTIC INSUFFICIENCY

Mitral and aortic insufficiencies are well tolerated in pregnancy. Longstanding regurgitation may lead to ventricular dysfunction or left atrial enlargement.

Recommended Workup and Clinical Findings

Echocardiogram to assess severity of regurgitation and evaluate left atrial enlargement and ventricular function.

Potential Complications

- Complications are unlikely. Risk related to underlying left ventricular dysfunction.
- Rarely may be associated with pulmonary edema and dysrhythmias.

AORTIC STENOSIS/IDIOPATHIC HYPERTROPHIC SUBAORTIC STENOSIS

Idiopathic hypertrophic subaortic stenosis is autosomal dominant in inheritance with similar risks and management to aortic stenosis. The condition is characterized by hypertrophy of the ventricular septum, which can obstruct left ventricular outflow. When isolated, stenosis is often caused by bicuspid aortic valve. If multiple valves are involved, it is usually rheumatic in origin.

- Valve diameter normally 3 to 4 cm^2
- Mild disease (valve area >1.5 cm^2, peak gradient <50 mm Hg), tolerated well in pregnancy
- Severe disease (valve area <1 cm^2, peak gradient >75 mm Hg, or an ejection fraction <55%), at significant risk, preconception correction recommended.

Stenotic Valve Leads to Fixed Cardiac Output

The presence of symptoms worsens outcomes. Patients with severe disease should limit activity. Complications may develop from underperfusion or excessive flow. Consequences of underperfusion typically are more life threatening than pulmonary edema from fluid overload. Goal pulmonary artery wedge pressures (if measured) are 15 to 17 mm Hg. Diuretics should be used cautiously to avoid underperfusion.

Recommended workup and clinical findings

- Echocardiogram to evaluate size of aortic valve opening, gradient of flow across the valve, and ejection fraction
- ECG to show left ventricular hypertrophy and left atrial enlargement; arrhythmias possible if significant left atrial enlargement
- Harsh systolic ejection murmur

Potential complications

If unable to overcome obstruction and maintain adequate cardiac output:

- Angina: caused by decreased coronary perfusion
- Syncope: caused by poor cerebral perfusion
- Sudden death: caused by arrhythmias
- Hypervolemia: may lead to pulmonary edema

Table 5
Management of maternal cardiac lesions in pregnancy

Maternal Cardiac Lesion	Therapy	Key Avoids	Anticoagulation	Labor and Delivery
Pulmonary/tricuspid stenosis and insufficiency	None	None	None	Cesarean for obstetric indications
Mitral stenosis	Beta blockers for HR control. Diuretics if pulmonary edema and digoxin if atrial fibrillation.	Avoid tachycardia, fluid overload, decrease in SVR or PVR	If left atrium dilation or chronic atrial fibrillation	Avoid terbutaline. Hemodynamic monitoring if severe disease. Cesarean for obstetric indications although assisted 2nd stage if severe disease.
Mitral and aortic insufficiency	Only if dysrhythmia	Avoid arrhythmia, bradycardia, increase in SVR, myocardial-depressant drugs	If left atrium dilation or chronic atrial fibrillation	Cesarean for obstetric indications
Aortic stenosis	Only if dysrhythmia. Diuretics if pulmonary edema.	Avoid hypotension, decreased venous return, bradycardia, hypervolemia.	None	Cesarean for obstetric indications. Assisted 2nd stage if severe disease.
Mechanical heart valves	Anticoagulation as addressed	Avoid warfarin beyond 6 wk, insufficient anticoagulation, waiting too long postpartum to resume anticoagulation.	Start LMWH or UFH 4–6 h postpartum. Start warfarin same day. Continue UFH or LMWH until warfarin therapeutic.	Cesarean for obstetric indications. Assisted 2nd stage if severe disease. Operative vaginal delivery may have increased risk of bleeding related to anticoagulation. Operative delivery poses increased risk of bleeding related to need for anticoagulation.

ASD, VSD, PDA	Only if dysrhythmia.	Avoid hypertension, decrease in PVR, tachycardia and supraventricular arrhythmias.	None	Cesarean for obstetric indications. Consider air filters to all venous lines.
Eisenmenger syndrome	Pulmonary artery vasodilators	Avoid hypotension, excessive blood loss, increases in PVR.	Prophylactic anticoagulation	Outcomes similar with vaginal and cesarean delivery with high mortality rates. Continuous pulse oximetry and keep oxygen >90%. Avoid air embolism.
Coarctation of the aorta	Antihypertensives	Avoid excessive blood loss, myocardial depressant drugs, bradycardia, and Valsalva efforts	None	Cesarean delivery rates higher owing to perceived risk of intracranial hemorrhage or aortic dissection. Vaginal delivery may occur with strict pain and blood pressure control, maintaining adequate cardiac preload, and minimizing Valsalva.
The Marfan syndrome	Beta blockers to avoid tachycardia	Avoid hypertension, tachycardia, and Valsalva	None	Avoid tachycardia. Consider assisted 2nd stage to avoid Valsalva. Consider cesarean delivery in those with aortic root >4 cm^2 or aortic dissection or heart failure.
Peripartum cardiomyopathy	Diuretics, vasodilators, digoxin, beta blockers	Avoid hypertension, excessive fluid, and increasing cardiac demand	Consider if significant ventricular dilation or atrial arrhythmia	Cesarean for obstetric indications. Assisted 2nd stage if severe disease.

Abbreviations: HR, heart rate; LMWH, low molecular weight heparin; PVR, pulmonary vascular resistance; UFH, unfractionated heparin.

MITRAL VALVE PROLAPSE

Mitral valve prolapse is one of the most common cardiac lesions during pregnancy. Most women are asymptomatic but may have palpitations. Pregnancy is typically tolerated well, and no changes in antenatal or intrapartum management are recommended.

MECHANICAL HEART VALVES

The primary management challenge in pregnancy is the prevention of valve thrombosis in those with mechanical valves, and patients with mechanical valve prostheses require lifelong anticoagulation. Warfarin is the recommended anticoagulant in the nonpregnant population. Nonmechanical tissue valves do not significantly increase risk for thromboembolism and do not require anticoagulation unless other risk factors such as atrial fibrillation are present.

Patients with any of the following are considered at high risk for thrombosis[28]:

- Any mechanical mitral valve
- A mechanical aortic valve with any of the following risk factors: atrial fibrillation, previous thromboembolism, ejection fraction less than 30%, a hypercoagulable state, older generation thrombogenic valves, or multiple valves
- Older more thrombogenic valves, including aortic caged-ball or tilting disc valves (ie, Lillehei-Kaster, Omniscience, Starr-Edwards)

The 10-year survival for patients with mechanical valves is 70% although pregnancy does not appear to shorten expected survival.[29]

Recommended Workup and Clinical Findings

- Echocardiogram should be done to establish location and type of valve and exclude thrombosis. Evaluation of left ventricular dysfunction is also important.
- ECG should be done to establish baseline and exclude atrial fibrillation. Findings are variable like aortic caged-ball or tilting disc valves (eg, Lillehei-Kaster, Omniscience, Starr-Edwards).
- Auscultation can reveal a variety of findings based on the type and location of the valve. Clicking of the valve may be audible.

Potential Complications

- Maternal mortality risk is approximately 3%.[30]
- Valve failure may occur independent of pregnancy.
- Thrombosis of the valve is primary concern.
- Over- and underanticoagulation can pose risks for maternal and fetal complications.
- Rates of pregnancy loss are increased, particularly with warfarin use.

Anticoagulation

- Anticoagulation decisions are tailored to patient's risk factors and preference as well as compliance.
- The 2008 Eighth American College of Chest Physicians guidelines for anticoagulation are summarized in **Box 9**.[31]
- Daily low-dose aspirin may be added to patients at significant increased risk for thrombosis.

Box 9
The 2008 Eighth American College of Chest Physicians guidelines for anticoagulation

Option 1: High-dose low-molecular-weight heparin (LMWH) therapy throughout gestation. Start enoxaparin, 1 mg/kg q 12 h. Goal anti-Xa level 4 h postinjection is ~1 (0.7–1.2) U/mL.

Option 2: High-dose unfractionated heparin (UFH) throughout gestation. UFH subcutaneously q 12 h. Goal anti-Xa level mid interval is 0.35 to 0.7 U/mL or goal mid interval aPTT ≥2 times control.

Option 3: Either of the above regimens through completed week 12, then change to warfarin until ~36 wk or close to delivery. Goal international normalized ratio ~3 (2.5–3.5). UFH or LMWH can then be resumed until delivery.

Option 4: Coumadin throughout gestation until close to delivery. Given increase in fetal complications, this regimen should be considered only for patients at highest risk (prior thromboembolism, older generation prosthesis at mitral location).

Data from Bates SM, Greer IA, Pabinger I, et al. Venous thromboembolism, thrombophilia, antithrombotic therapy, and pregnancy: American College of Chest Physicians Evidence-Based Clinical Practice Guidelines (8th Edition). Chest 2008;133(6 Suppl):844S–86S.

CONGENITAL CARDIAC LESIONS
Atrial Septal Defect, Ventricular Septal Defect, and Patent Ductus Arteriosus

Pregnancy is generally well tolerated with these lesions if they are small or have been corrected. Most of these defects are diagnosed and corrected in childhood. Larger lesions allow for more equal flow between the left and right heart and are more likely associated with increased pulmonary pressures and Eisenmenger syndrome in the adult.

Recommended workup and clinical findings

- Echocardiogram to evaluate size of defect, severity of shunting, and measure pulmonary artery pressures
- ECG
  ○ Atrial septal defect (ASD): partial right bundle branch block, right axis deviation, and sometimes right ventricular hypertrophy
  ○ Ventral septal defect (VSD)/patent ductus arteriosus (PDA): usually normal, may show left or right ventricular hypertrophy
- Auscultation
  ○ ASD: systolic ejection murmur at left sternal border and wide fixed split second heart sound
  ○ VSD: holosystolic thrill and murmur at left sternal border
  ○ PDA: grade 3/6 continuous systolic and diastolic murmur in infraclavicular region (Gibson murmur)

Potential complications

- Patients with a large defect and significant left-to-right shunt may develop atrial arrhythmias (atrial fibrillation) and congestive heart failure in pregnancy.
- Pulmonary hypertension may be present and may lead to Eisenmenger syndrome.
- Paradoxic emboli: emboli originating in lower extremities and pelvis or from the defect may travel across defect to brain, causing stroke.

SECONDARY PULMONARY HYPERTENSION AND EISENMENGER SYNDROME

Secondary pulmonary hypertension results from excess flow into the pulmonary circulation from chronic left-to-right (systemic-to-pulmonary) shunting across an intracardiac communication (most commonly ASD, VSD, and PDA). When pulmonary pressures exceed systemic pressures, flow across the shunt reverses to right to left. The result is decreased pulmonary perfusion, hypoxemia, and worsening pulmonary hypertension as a result of hypoxemia. This reversal defines Eisenmenger syndrome.

The maternal-fetal mortality rate is nearly 50% and occurs most often in the peripartum or recent postpartum period.[32] Pregnancy termination should be discussed with the patient.

Recommended Workup and Clinical Findings

In patients with suspected secondary pulmonary hypertension, the following evaluation is recommended:

- Pulse oximetry, including finger and toe oximetry, with and without administration of supplemental oxygen
- ECG to show ventricular hypertrophy with associated ST-T wave changes or a right atrial abnormality
- Chest radiograph abnormalities—dilatation of the central pulmonary arteries, abrupt termination of peripheral pulmonary artery branches (pruning), and right heart enlargement
- Complete blood count and nuclear lung scintigraphy
- Transthoracic and transesophageal echocardiography, cardiovascular magnetic resonance imaging, or computed tomography
- Cyanosis and clubbing as well as poor exercise tolerance
- Polycythemia

Potential Complications

- Decreased systemic vascular resistance of pregnancy leads to worsening of the right-to-left shunt, worsening hypoxemia, and death in 30% to 50% of patients.
- Death usually occurs in the first week postpartum.
- Most common causes of death are worsening and intractable hypoxemia, volume depletion, preeclampsia, and thromboembolism.

Avoid the Following

- Hypotension: can lead to a decrease in systemic vascular resistance and causes massive right-to-left shunting, bypassing the pulmonary circulation, and worsening pulmonary hypertension
- Excessive blood loss and volume depletion: causes hypotension by decreasing venous return
- Increases in pulmonary vascular resistance (ie, hypoxemia, hypercarbia, metabolic acidosis, excess catecholamines)
- Myocardial-depressant drugs, iron deficiency, high altitude, and exercise

COARCTATION OF AORTA

Coarctation of the aorta is typically corrected during childhood, and the classic presentation in adults is hypertension. The most common site of coarctation is distal to the left subclavian artery, so hypertension will be measured equally in both arms. The femoral pulse is delayed compared with the brachial pulse, and the lower extremity pressures are low. Surgical repair is recommended for adults with a peak-to-peak gradient greater than 20 mm Hg (the difference between the peak pressure distal and proximal to the narrowing).[33] After repair, patients remain at risk for complications including recoarctation, aortic aneurysm and dissection, and hypertension.

Thirty percent to 40% of patients will also have a bicuspid aortic valve. Ten percent of patients will also have intracranial aneurysms (vs 2% in the general population). All patients should have magnetic resonance angiography of the thoracic aorta and intracranial vessels performed at least once.[33]

Recommended Workup and Clinical Findings

- Echocardiogram to identify severity of the narrowing, evaluate left ventricular function, and exclude additional cardiac defects
- ECG: usually normal, may show left ventricular hypertrophy
- Auscultation: may be normal; various murmurs possible based on presence of associated anomalies and size of collateral vessel development

Potential Complications

Adults with uncorrected coarctation (native) are likely to have hypertension and coronary artery disease and are at risk for dissection and heart failure. This may be exacerbated by pregnancy.

THE MARFAN SYNDROME

The Marfan syndrome is an autosomal dominant condition, and most will have cardiac effects of the disease. Aneurysmal dilation and dissection of the aorta account for most of the morbidity and mortality with the Marfan syndrome. Sixty percent to 80% of adults with the Marfan syndrome will have aortic root dilation with or without aortic regurgitation. Risk of aortic rupture or dissection during pregnancy is approximately 10% if aortic root diameter is greater than 4 cm.[34] Rupture and dissection can occur even with normal aortic dimension (<1%). An aortic root diameter greater than 4.5 cm is an indication for preconception repair if patient desires pregnancy. The risk for dissection is decreased but not eliminated after surgical correction.

Recommended Workup and Clinical Findings

- Echocardiogram should be performed to establish size of aortic root. This should be followed serially even if the baseline diameter is normal.
- The Marfan syndrome is associated with other clinical abnormalities including joint hypermobility, ectopia lentis, pectus excavatum, arm span exceeding height, scoliosis, and arachnodactyly.

Potential Complications

Aortic root dissection and rupture are the most significant risks in pregnancy.

PERIPARTUM CARDIOMYOPATHY

Peripartum cardiomyopathy is classically defined by the following:

- Development of cardiac failure in last month or within 5 months postpartum
- Absence of an identifiable cause for cardiac failure
- Absence of recognizable heart disease before last month of pregnancy

- Left ventricular systolic dysfunction: ejection fraction less than 45%, shortening fraction less than 30%, and left ventricular end-diastolic dimension greater than 2.7 cm/m^2 body surface area[35]

Ninety percent of cases occur in the first 2 months postpartum, and half of deaths occur in the first 6 weeks postpartum. There is a high rate of recurrence in subsequent pregnancies even with apparent recovery of cardiac function. Patients with incomplete recovery (ejection fraction <50%) have a high rate of decompensation and should be counseled against future pregnancies.

Recommended Workup and Clinical Findings

- Echocardiogram: establish baseline and repeat every trimester or with worsening symptoms
- If electrocardiogram is nonspecific, possibly atrial fibrillation
- Chest radiograph to show cardiomegaly and pulmonary edema
- Shortness of breath, orthopnea, fatigue, and leg edema
- Markedly elevated B-type natriuretic peptide

Potential Complications

- Worsening cardiac failure and pulmonary edema. Patients with an initial ejection fraction of less than 25% are at greatest risk for subsequent cardiac transplantation.
- Failure to normalize cardiac function within 6 months postpartum carries mortality rate of 85% by 5 years.
- Cause of death commonly dysrhythmias, progressive cardiac failure, or thromboembolic phenomena. Atrial fibrillation is the most common dysrhythmia in patients with peripartum cardiomyopathy.[36]

REFERENCES

1. Koonin LM, Atrash HK, Rochat RW, et al. Maternal mortality surveillance, United States, 1980-1985. MMWR CDC Surveill Summ 1988;37(5):19–29.
2. Koonin LM, Atrash HK, Lawson HW, et al. Maternal mortality surveillance, United States, 1979-1986. MMWR CDC Surveill Summ 1991;40(2):1–13.
3. Berg CJ, Atrash HK, Koonin LM, et al. Pregnancy-related mortality in the United States, 1987-1990. Obstet Gynecol 1996;88(2):161–7.
4. el-Solh AA, Grant BJ. A comparison of severity of illness scoring systems for critically ill obstetric patients. Chest 1996;110(5):1299–304.
5. Mabie WC, Sibai BM. Treatment in an obstetric intensive care unit. Am J Obstet Gynecol 1990;162(1):1–4.
6. Mahutte NG, Murphy-Kaulbeck L, Le Q, et al. Obstetric admissions to the intensive care unit. Obstet Gynecol 1999;94(2):263–6.
7. Naylor DF, Olson MM. Critical care obstetrics and gynecology. Crit Care Clin 2003;19(1):127–49.
8. Zeeman GG, Wendel GD, Cunningham FG. A blueprint for obstetric critical care. Am J Obstet Gynecol 2003;188(2):532–6.
9. Roos-Hesselink JW, Duvekot JJ, Thorne SA. Pregnancy in high risk cardiac conditions. Heart 2009;95(8):680–6.
10. Foley M, Rokey R, Belfort M. Cardiac disease. In: Belfort MA, Saade G, Foley M, et al, editors. Critical care obstetrics. 5th edition. New Jersey: Wiley-Blackwell; 2010. p. 256–82.

11. van Oppen AC, Stigter RH, Bruinse HW. Cardiac output in normal pregnancy: a critical review. Obstet Gynecol 1996;87(2):310–8.
12. Clark SL, Cotton DB, Lee W, et al. Central hemodynamic assessment of normal term pregnancy. Am J Obstet Gynecol 1989;161(6 Pt 1):1439–42.
13. Hsieh TT, Chen KC, Soong JH. Outcome of pregnancy in patients with organic heart disease in Taiwan. Asia Oceania J Obstet Gynaecol 1993;19(1):21–7.
14. Siu SC, Sermer M, Colman JM, et al. Prospective multicenter study of pregnancy outcomes in women with heart disease. Circulation 2001;104(5):515–21.
15. Franklin WJ, Gandhi M. Congenital heart disease in pregnancy. Cardiol Clin 2012; 30(3):383–94.
16. Khairy P, Ouyang DW, Fernandes SM, et al. Pregnancy outcomes in women with congenital heart disease. Circulation 2006;113(4):517–24.
17. Siu SC, Colman JM, Sorensen S, et al. Adverse neonatal and cardiac outcomes are more common in pregnant women with cardiac disease. Circulation 2002; 105(18):2179–84.
18. Drenthen W, Pieper PG, Roos-Hesselink JW, et al. Outcome of pregnancy in women with congenital heart disease: a literature review. J Am Coll Cardiol 2007;49(24):2303–11.
19. Thorne SA. Pregnancy in heart disease. Heart 2004;90(4):450–6.
20. Regitz-Zagrosek V, Blomstrom Lundqvist C, Borghi C, et al. ESC Guidelines on the management of cardiovascular diseases during pregnancy: the Task Force on the Management of Cardiovascular Diseases during Pregnancy of the European Society of Cardiology (ESC). Eur Heart J 2011;32(24):3147–97.
21. Chambers CE, Clark SL. Cardiac surgery during pregnancy. Clin Obstet Gynecol 1994;37(2):316–23.
22. Chandrasekhar S, Cook CR, Collard CD. Cardiac surgery in the parturient. Anesth Analg 2009;108(3):777–85.
23. Parry AJ, Westaby S. Cardiopulmonary bypass during pregnancy. Ann Thorac Surg 1996;61(6):1865–9.
24. Fernandes SM, Arendt KW, Landzberg MJ, et al. Pregnant women with congenital heart disease: cardiac, anesthetic and obstetrical implications. Expert Rev Cardiovasc Ther 2010;8(3):439–48.
25. Kuczkowski KM. Labor pain and labor analgesia. J Gynecol Obstet Biol Reprod (Paris) 2004;33(5):450.
26. Wilson W, Taubert KA, Gewitz M, et al. Prevention of infective endocarditis: guidelines from the American Heart Association: a guideline from the American Heart Association Rheumatic Fever, Endocarditis, and Kawasaki Disease Committee, Council on Cardiovascular Disease in the Young, and the Co. Circulation 2007; 116(15):1736–54.
27. Roos-Hesselink JW, Ruys TPE, Stein JI, et al. Outcome of pregnancy in patients with structural or ischaemic heart disease: results of a registry of the European Society of Cardiology. Eur Heart J 2013;34(9):657–65.
28. Douketis JD, Berger PB, Dunn AS, et al. The perioperative management of antithrombotic therapy: American College of Chest Physicians Evidence-Based Clinical Practice Guidelines (8th Edition). Chest 2008;133(6 Suppl):299S–339S.
29. North RA, Sadler L, Stewart AW, et al. Long-term survival and valve-related complications in young women with cardiac valve replacements. Circulation 1999; 99(20):2669–76.
30. Chan WS, Anand S, Ginsberg JS. Anticoagulation of pregnant women with mechanical heart valves: a systematic review of the literature. Arch Intern Med 2000;160(2):191–6.

31. Bates SM, Greer IA, Pabinger I, et al. Venous thromboembolism, thrombophilia, antithrombotic therapy, and pregnancy: American College of Chest Physicians Evidence-Based Clinical Practice Guidelines (8th Edition). Chest 2008;133(6 Suppl):844S–86S.

32. Presbitero P, Somerville J, Stone S, et al. Pregnancy in cyanotic congenital heart disease. Outcome of mother and fetus. Circulation 1994;89(6):2673–6.

33. Warnes CA, Williams RG, Bashore TM, et al. ACC/AHA 2008 Guidelines for the Management of Adults With Congenital Heart Disease. J Am Coll Cardiol 2008; 52(23):e143–263.

34. Expert consensus document on management of cardiovascular diseases during pregnancy. Eur Heart J 2003;24(8):761–81.

35. Pearson GD, Veille JC, Rahimtoola S, et al. Peripartum cardiomyopathy: National Heart, Lung, and Blood Institute and Office of Rare Diseases (National Institutes of Health) workshop recommendations and review. JAMA 2000;283(9):1183–8.

36. Habli M, O'Brien T, Nowack E, et al. Peripartum cardiomyopathy: prognostic factors for long-term maternal outcome. Am J Obstet Gynecol 2008;199(4):415.e1-5.

Evaluation and Management of Maternal Cardiac Arrhythmias

 CrossMark

Torri D. Metz, MD, MS[a,b,]*, Amber Khanna, MD[c]

KEYWORDS

- Arrhythmia • Cardiac • Maternal • Pregnancy • Treatment

KEY POINTS

- Cardiac arrhythmias are common in pregnancy.
- A majority of women presenting with palpitations have a benign finding on clinical work-up and assessment for arrhythmia.
- Pregnant women with arrhythmias other than sinus tachycardia should be evaluated and comanaged with a cardiologist.
- For most cardiac arrhythmias, treatment is the same in the pregnant and nonpregnant populations. Special considerations for pregnancy predominantly include avoidance of certain medications and appropriate planning for the intrapartum and postpartum period.

INTRODUCTION

Palpitations, or the unpleasant awareness of an abnormally beating heart, are common symptoms during pregnancy.[1,2] These symptoms can represent the full spectrum from normal physiology to life-threatening arrhythmias. Arrhythmias in pregnancy can occur in isolation or with structural heart disease. Heart disease can be known prior to pregnancy or diagnosed during the pregnancy and can be congenital or acquired. Optimal management of maternal cardiac arrhythmia includes identification of the specific arrhythmia, diagnosis of comorbid conditions, and appropriate intervention. In general, management of maternal cardiac arrhythmias is similar to that of the general population. Special consideration must be given, however, as to the effects of medications and procedures on both the mother and fetus.

The authors have no conflicts of interest related to the material presented in this article. There was no funding source for this work.

[a] Department of Obstetrics and Gynecology, University of Colorado School of Medicine, 12631 East 17th Avenue, Aurora, CO 80045, USA; [b] Department of Obstetrics and Gynecology, Denver Health Medical Center, 777 Bannock Street, MC 0660, Denver, CO 80204, USA; [c] Division of Cardiology, Department of Medicine, University of Colorado School of Medicine, 12401 East 17th Avenue, Aurora, CO 80045, USA
* Corresponding author. Department of Obstetrics and Gynecology, Denver Health Medical Center, 777 Bannock Street, MC 0660, Denver, CO 80204.
E-mail address: torri.metz@dhha.org

Obstet Gynecol Clin N Am 43 (2016) 729–745
http://dx.doi.org/10.1016/j.ogc.2016.07.014
0889-8545/16/© 2016 Elsevier Inc. All rights reserved.

NORMAL CARDIOVASCULAR CHANGES OF PREGNANCY

During pregnancy, maternal blood volume increases by approximately 50%. This is accompanied by an increase in cardiac output, which is mediated by an increase in stroke volume and a slight increase in heart rate.[3] The mechanism by which pregnancy predisposes women to arrhythmias has not been fully elucidated. As blood volume and cardiac work increase, there is thought to be atrial stretch that may result an increased predisposition to arrhythmia.[4,5] In addition, the higher resting heart rate in pregnancy may increase the risk of arrhythmia. Soliman and colleagues[6] found an elevated resting heart rate to be associated with triggers for ventricular arrhythmia in an unselected group of patients (N = 867) referred for Holter monitoring at a single center. In pregnancy, heart rate typically increases 10 beats per minutes (bpm) to 15 bpm above baseline.[5] Hormonal changes in pregnancy may also increase the risk of arrhythmia and promote the unmasking of new foci that result in arrhythmias.[7]

EPIDEMIOLOGY OF ARRHYTHMIAS IN PREGNANCY

Overall the incidence of arrhythmia in reproductive age women is increased during pregnancy.[8] In a large cohort of admitted pregnant women (N = 136,422), sinus tachycardia and sinus bradycardia were the most common rhythm disturbances, with a frequency of 104 per 100,000 pregnancies based on diagnostic codes.[9] Supraventricular tachycardia (SVT) was noted at a frequency of 24 per 100,000 pregnancies, with other arrhythmias potentially requiring treatment occurring at a much lower frequency. SVT accounted for approximately 14% of the women with documented arrhythmias in pregnancy. Atrial fibrillation, atrial flutter, and ventricular tachycardia (VT) each accounted for approximately 1% of admissions for maternal cardiac arrhythmia. The overall rate of pregnancy admission, however, for any maternal arrhythmia in the cohort was only 0.17%, indicating that admission for a cardiac arrhythmia in pregnancy is rare.[9]

RISK FACTORS FOR CARDIAC ARRHYTHMIAS
History of Arrhythmia

There are many risk factors for arrhythmias during pregnancy. A major risk factor is a history of arrhythmia prior to pregnancy. The risk of recurrence is highest for women who had paroxysmal atrial fibrillation or atrial flutter (52%) and SVT (50%).[10] It is lower for ventricular arrhythmias (27%).

Congenital Heart Disease

Structural heart disease is associated with arrhythmias in both pregnant and nonpregnant patients. Patients with congenital heart disease have a lifetime risk of atrial arrhythmias of approximately 50%.[11] The highest risk patients are those with Ebstein malformation of the tricuspid valve, transposition of the great arteries, univentricular hearts, atrial septal defects, and tetralogy of Fallot. Up to 35% of patients with Ebstein anomaly have greater than or equal to 1 accessory pathway.[12] The etiology of atrial arrhythmias in the other forms of congenital heart disease is likely scar-mediated and/or pressure and volume loading of the atria.[13] Patients with congenital heart disease are also at risk of ventricular arrhythmias, particularly if they have undergone a ventriculotomy as part of their repair or if they have ventricular dysfunction. In patients with tetralogy of Fallot, a population where both prior ventriculotomy and ventricular dysfunction is common, the prevalence of VT is 3% to 14%.[13]

Other forms of structural heart disease that are not traditionally classified as congenital, such as hypertrophic cardiomyopathy and arrhythmogenic right ventricular cardiomyopathy, are associated with atrial and ventricular arrhythmias. In a case series of 100 women with hypertrophic cardiomyopathy who had 199 live births, there were 2 cases of sudden cardiac death, both in women with high-risk features.[14] One had severe left ventricular hypertrophy and a high resting outflow tract gradient; the other had a strong family history of sudden death.

The largest case series of pregnancy in women with arrhythmogenic right ventricular cardiomyopathy included 26 women during 39 pregnancies.[15] In 5 pregnancies (13%), a single ventricular arrhythmia occurred. The cardiac event rate was not different in pregnant versus nonpregnant women with this cardiomyopathy.

Acquired Heart Disease

Acquired heart disease is also associated with arrhythmias. Rheumatic heart disease affects 16 to 20 million people worldwide.[16] Approximately 39% of patients with rheumatic heart disease have atrial fibrillation.[17] Of those, the risk of thromboembolism is 17% to 18% per year, making anticoagulation imperative.[16] Other forms of acquired heart disease, such as endocarditis or degenerative valve disease, can also have associated arrhythmias.

Genetic Predisposition to Arrhythmia

There are genetically mediated arrhythmias in structurally normal hearts, including long QT syndrome, Brugada syndrome, progressive cardiac conduction defect, catecholaminergic polymorphic VT, and others. Women with long QT syndrome are at reduced risk of a cardiac event (syncope, aborted cardiac arrest, and sudden death) during pregnancy (hazard ratio 0.28; 95% CI, 0.10–0.76; $P = .01$) but increased risk in the 9 months postpartum (hazard ratio 2.7; 95% CI, 1.8–4.3; $P<.001$).[18] Treatment with β-blockers minimizes the risk.

NEW-ONSET ARRHYTHMIA IN PREGNANCY
Typical Presentation

The 2 major symptoms suggestive of an arrhythmia are palpitations and syncope. The most important aspect of arrhythmia evaluation is a detailed history. Patients should be asked to describe the rhythm disturbance because this can help with narrowing the differential diagnosis. For example, patients may notice skipped beats that are often premature atrial or ventricular contractions. A symptom of a racing heart is more concerning for arrhythmia. In these cases, tapping out the rate and rhythm by hand can be helpful. The heart rate during SVT is often too fast to count. An irregular heart rate can still have a pattern, such as trigeminy, or it may have no pattern as in atrial fibrillation.

Other important features of the history include onset and offset. Sudden onset and offset are more concerning for arrhythmia than a gradual speeding up and slowing down of the heart rate. Associated symptoms can be helpful in delineating the likelihood of a concerning arrhythmia (**Table 1**). Identifying triggers can be useful, particularly if they can be modified, such as caffeine intake. If a patient can do something, such as Valsalva maneuver or drinking ice water, to relieve the symptoms, then SVT is more likely.

Obtaining a history for syncope focuses on activities at the time of onset. The most common types of syncope are vasovagal, orthostatic, and cardiovascular. Vasovagal typically has an identified trigger, such as pain, anxiety, or blood. Patients generally describe a prodrome of lightheadedness, nausea, feeling too hot or too cold, weakness, and changes in vision. They often appear pale. If they remain standing, they lose

Table 1
Classification of symptoms of arrhythmia

	Symptom	More Likely Benign	Concerning for Arrhythmia
Palpitations	Heart pounding at normal rate	X	—
	Heart rate >180 bpm at rest	—	X
	Skipped beats	X	—
	Only occurs when laying on left side	X	—
Syncope	Sustains an injury	—	X
	Identifiable trigger, such as sight of blood	X	—
Palpitations or syncope	Structurally abnormal heart	—	X
	Family history of sudden death	—	X
	Exertional symptoms	—	X

consciousness. Muscle twitching/jerking may occur. When they are lying down, they quickly regain consciousness but full recovery may take an extended period of time. Because of the prodrome, even patients who lose consciousness are typically able to break their fall and protect themselves from injury.

Orthostatic syncope is common during pregnancy due to peripheral vasodilation and lower baseline blood pressure. Patients may notice lightheadedness when they move from lying or sitting to standing or when doing something that causes more peripheral vasodilation, such as taking a hot shower.

Cardiogenic syncope can be structural or related to heart rhythm. Hypertrophic cardiomyopathy and aortic stenosis can both cause exertional syncope due to inability to augment cardiac output. Patients with structurally normal hearts may tolerate significant bradycardia or tachycardia, including VT, with lightheadedness but not loss of consciousness so lack of overt syncope is not completely reassuring.

Evaluation of New-Onset Arrhythmia

Electrocardiogram
Initial evaluation of any arrhythmia is a 12-lead ECG. The computer interpretation has variable accuracy, so physician analysis remains vital. It is important to have a systematic approach to interpretation, including rate, rhythm, intervals, QRS axis, evidence of chamber enlargement or hypertrophy, Q waves, ST changes, and any other pertinent findings.

Labs
Laboratory testing for arrhythmias is focused on ruling out underlying etiologies (discussed later). Abnormal potassium and magnesium can contribute to arrhythmias and should be corrected if abnormal.

Cardiac monitors
There are many different types of heart rhythm monitors. Selection depends on the description and frequency of symptoms as well as monitor availability and insurance coverage (**Table 2**). All the monitors have a way for a patient to mark a specific time when she feels symptomatic.

MANAGEMENT OF COMMON ARRHYTHMIAS
Sinus Tachycardia

Sinus tachycardia is common during pregnancy and can be a result of a broad range of diagnoses. The work-up for sinus tachycardia includes consideration of infectious

Table 2
Types of cardiac monitors

Monitor Type	Duration	Continuous or Intermittent Recording	Physician Notification	Common Indication
Continuous ambulatory ECG (Holter)	24 h or 48 h	Continuous	Readily available and covered by most insurances	Multiple episodes per day Quantifying heart rate, PVC rate, asymptomatic arrhythmias
Long term continuous (Zio patch [iRhythm, San Francisco, CA])	7–14 d	Continuous	One large sticker placed on the chest After 2 wk sticker is removed and sent to company for analysis	Episodes every few days Unlikely to find arrhythmia that necessitates urgent intervention
Event recorder	24 h or 48 h	Intermittent	Multiple stickers on the chest Many options to transmit events immediately to device company Some devices have autodetect features for arrhythmias	Episodes once a week Multiple different types of episodes, potential need for urgent intervention
Implantable loop recorders	3 y	Intermittent	Placed under skin of chest as outpatient procedure Can transmit to physician or have device interrogated at physician's office	Infrequent episodes (<1/mo) that are potentially serious

causes, anemia, thyroid dysfunction, pain, anxiety, stimulant or drug use, and more morbid and potentially life-threatening conditions, such as a pulmonary embolus. Often, the history and physical can help guide the clinician as to the etiology of the sinus tachycardia. Treatment of sinus tachycardia is most often targeted at the underlying etiology of the arrhythmia.

Supraventricular Tachycardia

SVT, a tachyarrhythmia originating above the level of the ventricles, is the most common sustained arrhythmia in pregnancy. Rates are regular and typically 150 bpm to 250 bpm. In some cases, SVT can be terminated with Valsalva or carotid sinus massage. If conservative measures are unsuccessful, acute treatment of SVT in pregnancy is best achieved with adenosine.[19] The starting dose of adenosine is 6 mg as an IV push with immediate flush. If conversion is not successful with 6 mg, then 12 mg can be used. After successful conversion to sinus rhythm, maintenance medications (typically β-blockers) can be initiated to prevent recurrence (**Table 3**). Despite some literature demonstrating an association between β-blockers and fetal growth restriction,[20] more recent literature indicates that this association is more likely related to

Table 3
Medications for treating arrhythmias in pregnancy

Medication	Mechanism of Action	Type of Arrhythmia Prevented	Safety in Pregnancy	Safety in Lactation	Other Considerations
Propranolol	β-Blocker	SVT, VT, atrial fibrillation rate control	Possible fetal growth restriction	No known adverse effects	
Metoprolol	β-Blocker	SVT, VT, atrial fibrillation rate control	Possible fetal growth restriction	No known adverse effects	
Atenolol	β-Blocker	SVT, VT, atrial fibrillation rate control	Possible fetal growth restriction Possible association with hypospadias	Concentrates in breast milk	Generally avoided in favor of propranolol or metoprolol
Verapamil	Calcium channel blocker	SVT, VT, atrial fibrillation rate control	No known adverse effects	No known adverse effects	Can cause reflex tachycardia Headache is a common side effect
Diltiazem	Calcium channel blocker	SVT, atrial fibrillation rate control	No known adverse effects	No known adverse effects (although experience limited when compared with verapamil)	Can cause reflex tachycardia Headache is a common side effect
Sotalol	Potassium channel blocker	SVT (including atrial fibrillation and flutter), AV nodal reentrant tachycardia, VT	No known adverse effects	No known adverse effects	Also used for treatment of fetal arrhythmias
Amiodarone	Potassium channel blocker	Recurrent VT	Rare reports of fetal goiter and hypothyroidism Possible fetal growth restriction Possible birth defects	Concentrates in breast milk, long half-life, avoid in lactation	Generally avoided except in cases of life-threatening arrhythmias given reported adverse fetal effects

Drug	Class	Indication			Comments
Procainamide	Sodium channel blocker	Recurrent VT, atrial fibrillation, acute treatment wide complex tachycardia	No known adverse effects	No known adverse effects	Can cause lupus-like syndrome with prolonged use
Quinidine	Sodium channel blocker	Recurrent VT, atrial fibrillation	No known adverse effects	No known adverse effects; Can concentrate in the liver	Serum levels must be monitored
Lidocaine	Sodium channel blocker	Unstable VT	No known adverse effects	No known adverse effects	Often used in conjunction with emergent cardioversion
Flecainide	Sodium channel blocker	Recurrent VT, SVT	No known adverse effects	No known adverse effects	Also used for treatment of fetal arrhythmias; Contraindicated in patients with prior infarction or underlying structural heart disease
Digoxin		SVT (including atrial fibrillation and flutter)	Possible association with growth restriction	No known adverse effects	Monitor carefully given potential toxicity; Also used for treatment of fetal arrhythmias
Adenosine	Endogenous nucleoside	Acute treatment of SVT	No known adverse effects	No known adverse effects, none suspected with short half life	Very short half-life, <10 s; Give medication in 1 push followed by IV flush

the severity of the underlying cardiac condition that necessitates the β-blocker therapy rather than the β-blocker itself.[21] Consideration can be given to assessing fetal growth by ultrasound in the third trimester for women requiring β-blocker therapy.

In cases of recurrent SVT, ablation of the aberrant pathway can be considered. Data regarding ablation in pregnancy is limited, with a recent review identifying only 16 published studies with 27 patients who underwent ablation during pregnancy.[22] Many of these cases were performed for recurrent arrhythmias refractory to medical therapy. There were not evident complications related to the ablations, and all ablations were successful.

If a decision is made to pursue ablation in pregnancy, radiation should be minimized as much as possible (including shielding of the maternal abdomen), and general guidelines for optimizing perfusion to the fetus during the procedure can be used, including positioning the patient with a leftward tilt to avoid compression of the inferior vena cava. If a recent report of successful ablation with less than 2 minutes of fluoroscopy time is reproducible, it may result in a lower threshold for ablation in pregnancy.[23] Continuous fetal monitoring should also be considered in the setting of a viable fetus. Ablation during organogenesis (first trimester) should be avoided if possible given the associated radiation.

Atrial Fibrillation/Flutter

Atrial fibrillation and flutter are rare in pregnancy outside of known underlying structural heart disease.[24] Atrial rates of flutter are typically 240 bpm to 340 bpm with ventricular rates of 75 bpm to 150 bpm (**Fig. 1**). An echocardiogram is indicated for women with new-onset atrial fibrillation or flutter during pregnancy to assess for underlying structural abnormalities and/or thrombus. If there is no underlying structural disease, a diagnosis of pulmonary embolus can also be considered and evaluated for with standard diagnostic testing.[25] Drug testing should also be pursued if there is clinical suspicion of stimulant use.

Initial treatment of atrial fibrillation or flutter in a stable patient is rate control. This is typically accomplished with intravenous (IV) β-blockers or calcium channel blockers (see **Table 3**).[25] Atrial fibrillation or flutter causing hemodynamic compromise should

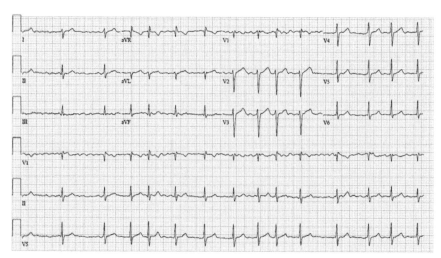

Fig. 1. ECG demonstrating atrial fibrillation. There are not identifiable P waves. The ventricular rate is irregular.

be treated with immediate cardioversion. The need for anticoagulation in women with atrial fibrillation is discussed later.

Bradyarrhythmias and Heart Block

Bradycardia, defined as a heart rate less than 60 bpm, is unusual during pregnancy. Even among women who exercise regularly, mean heart rate is 85 bpm $\pm$ 11 bpm in the third trimester.[26] Bradycardia can be due to either slow heart rate generation at the sinus node or impaired conduction through the atrioventricular (AV) node. In the absence of structural heart disease, sinus bradycardia is unusual but well tolerated. If it is due to an athletic heart, the heart rate responds to activity. Medications, such as β-blockers and calcium channel blockers contribute to sinus bradycardia. There are some situations where a slower heart rate improves cardiac output, including mitral stenosis and hypertrophic cardiomyopathy with left ventricular outflow tract obstruction. Sometimes bradycardia is a side effect of what the medication is prescribed for, such as aortic root dilation in Marfan syndrome or left ventricular dysfunction. Risk/benefit analysis of the medication may favor continuing it.

In the presence of structural heart disease, sinus bradycardia may be due to sinus node dysfunction and can be associated with decreased cardiac output, exercise intolerance, dizziness, and syncope. Treatment of sinus node dysfunction requires a pacemaker (unless an offending medication can be reduced or stopped). Ideally pacemakers are implanted prior to conception so the fetus is not exposed to radiation, but radiation exposure can be minimized (discussed later).

Pacemakers implanted for sinus node dysfunction usually have a rate response algorithm set. The purpose of rate responsiveness is to simulate the typical increase in heart rate during activity that patients with normal sinus nodes experience. There are different mechanisms to detect physical activity, including vibration, minute ventilation, or change in right ventricular impedance. Different aspects of responsiveness are programmable, including range of heart rate, pace of increase and decrease in rate, and degree of activity required to initiate a response. **Fig. 2** for an example of a paced rhythm.

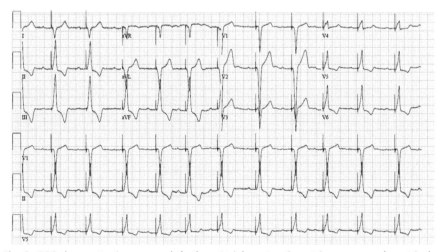

Fig. 2. ECG demonstrating a paced rhythm. Atrial contractions trigger a paced ventricular response. The vertical lines indicate that the pacemaker fired.

Because a vast majority of pacemakers are implanted in older patients, the manufacturer default settings are often not appropriate for pregnant women. It generally takes a period of trial and error to find the settings that feel most comfortable. There are no guidelines for changing the paced heart rate during pregnancy, but in patients who are atrially paced, the authors' practice has had good results with increasing the lower rate to 80 bpm in the second trimester and 100 bpm at the time of delivery. The rate is lowered to 80 after delivery and back down to prior settings at 6 weeks postpartum. These values can be further adjusted based on specific maternal conditions (twin gestation, poor cardiac function, and symptoms).

Rate response during delivery depends on the particular pacemaker. If it uses minute ventilation, it should respond appropriately. If it uses vibration it may not, but physically tapping on the device, or having the patient move her arms, may help. Placing a magnet on a pacing device has variable effect depending on the device and may or may not be helpful. This is usually noted in the interrogation report. Consultation with an electrophysiologist familiar with pregnancy-related changes is invaluable.

Complete heart block, or interruption in the connection between the atria and ventricles, is either congenital or acquired (**Fig. 3**). Congenital heart block is usually autoimmune related to maternal lupus erythematosus and transplacental transfer of anti-Ro/SSA or anti-La/SSB antibodies. Although not all patients with congenital heart block require a pacemaker in infancy, 75% have one by the age of 10.[27] The issue of pacemaker implantation should be readdressed preconception in patients with heart block without a pacemaker. Acquired complete heart block can be due to degeneration of the conduction tissue, a common occurrence in levo-transposition of the great arteries, or surgical, particularly in valve replacement and ventricular septal defect closure.[28,29]

Given that heart block may be intermittent and patients may have an adequate escape rhythm, not all patients are pacemaker dependent. Management during pregnancy is more straightforward when the sinus node functions normally because rates do not need to be manually adjusted. Women with high rates of right ventricular pacing are at risk of left ventricular dysfunction so should have periodic echocardiograms to

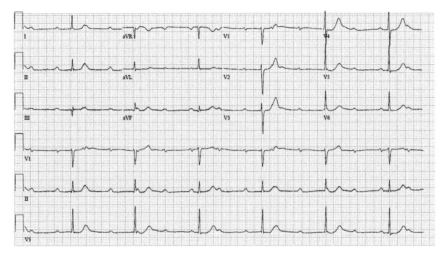

Fig. 3. ECG demonstrating complete heart block. Both the P waves and the QRS complexes are regular. There is not an association between the 2, however, and there are P waves that are not conducted to the ventricle.

monitor ejection fraction. Patients with symptomatic left ventricular systolic dysfunction and either a left bundle branch block or high rate of right ventricular pacing should be considered for a coronary sinus lead to improve synchronization. Ideally this should be considered preconception because implantation requires a significant amount of fluoroscopy time.[30]

Ventricular Arrhythmias

Ventricular arrhythmias span the spectrum of benign premature ventricular contractions (PVCs) to life-threatening VT and ventricular fibrillation (VF). The prevalence of PVCs is high during pregnancy, at 40% to 50%.[31] Although some women may feel the PVCs, they do not have clinical significance in isolation. Sometimes PVCs have identifiable triggers, such as caffeine, which can be avoided. If PVCs are symptomatic and bothersome, they may be suppressed with β-blockers. Because they are benign, the risk/benefit analysis generally favors avoiding medications during pregnancy and most women are happy with reassurance.

Ventricular tachyarrhythmias, including VT (**Fig. 4**) and VF, are much less common and can be much more serious. Management is complex and must be tailored to the individual patient. The most serious situation is aborted sudden cardiac death and/or unstable VT (See Bennett and colleagues article, Cardiac Arrest and Resuscitation Unique to Pregnancy, in this issue for further details regarding appropriate management).

Some patients with ventricular arrhythmias are hemodynamically stable. The arrhythmia may be remote from the time of presentation (seen on remote monitoring or on interrogation of implantable device) or ongoing at the time of evaluation. Initial management is focused on assessing the hemodynamic stability of the patient, reversing any aggravating factors (eg, hypokalemia), and preparing for another episode with medication and/or defibrillation. The diagnostic work-up consists of an ECG, telemetry monitoring to capture onset, offset, and morphology of arrhythmia, and an echocardiogram to evaluate for underlying heart disease. Medical management depends on the severity of the arrhythmia, with the least toxic medications (ie, β-blockers) preferred over more toxic medications, such as amiodarone

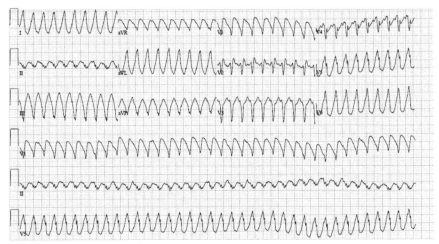

Fig. 4. ECG demonstrating VT. The pattern of wide QRS complex tachycardia is strongly suggestive of VT.

(see **Table 3**). Cardioversion is indicated for ventricular arrhythmia associated with hemodynamic compromise and can be considered for arrhythmias refractory to medical management (discussed later).[32]

ANTIARRHYTHMIC MEDICATIONS

A majority of antiarrhythmics are considered safe for use in pregnancy (see **Table 3**). Many of these medications cross the placenta, however, so fetal exposure is anticipated when using these therapies for maternal indications. Attention to side-effect profiles, known teratogenesis, and concentration in breast milk during lactation is imperative. One medication that deserves special attention is amiodarone. In a small case series, neonates exposed to amiodarone were found to have adverse fetal effects, including thyroid dysfunction, fetal growth restriction, and possibly neurologic abnormalities.[33] In another series of 3 cases of exposure, 1 neonate was born with a ventricular septal defect.[34] Amiodarone is also thought to concentrate in the breastmilk, and close monitoring of the neonate is advised if the mother is continued on amiodarone and elects to breastfeed.

When initiating or continuing an antiarrhythmic or any medication during pregnancy and lactation, the risks of the medication are weighed against the benefits while remembering that optimization of maternal status also optimizes fetal status. During pregnancy, there is an increase in glomerular filtration rate, and an increase in blood volume that may result in decreased levels of cardiac medications.[35] These changes may result in the need for frequent monitoring of levels and dose adjustment throughout the pregnancy as needed to achieve therapeutic benefit.[35]

CARDIOVERSION

Cardioversion can be performed in pregnancy. There are numerous case reports of cardioversion in pregnancy without any evident adverse effects.[36] Cardioversion can be used liberally in the setting of unstable maternal arrhythmia. Specifically, cardioversion can be considered in SVT that is refractory to medical therapy with adenosine, or with any arrhythmia, resulting in an unstable patient. Fetal monitoring during cardioversion is recommended in women with a pregnancy at a viable gestational age, because there are reports of fetal compromise after cardioversion, resulting in fetal death and/or the need for emergent cesarean delivery.[36] Despite these cases of rare complication, cardioversion should be used when indicated for hemodynamic instability because the decreased uterine perfusion associated with hypotension and hypoperfusion of the uterus are not tolerated by the fetus over time.

OTHER MANAGEMENT CONSIDERATIONS
Electrophysiology Procedures

Electrophysiology procedures are diagnostic, therapeutic, or both. The risks of these procedures to all patients include vascular complication, tricuspid valve damage, pulmonary embolism, hemorrhage, tamponade, infection, stroke, and death.[37] In pregnancy, there is added risk of altered hemodynamics that affect how well a woman can tolerate the complication. There are also fetal risks, including radiation and hypoperfusion. The risks and benefits need to be carefully weighed for both mother and fetus. The amount of radiation varies greatly depending on the specific type of procedures and can range from minimal exposure to more than an hour of fluoroscopy time.[38] There are multiple techniques that can reduce the amount of radiation, including minimizing overall fluoroscopy time, using narrower angulation, and adjustments to the protocol settings.[39] Abdominal shielding can further reduce the radiation exposure to the fetus.[40,41] Some electrophysiology procedures can be done without any radiation.[42–45]

High doses of radiation are associated with an increased risk of childhood cancer but it is not clear if there is a safe dose.[46,47] In addition, although the overall risk of childhood leukemia increases with 1 rad to 2 rad of radiation, the absolute risk remains low, with an increase from 1 in 3000 to 1 in 2000.[48] Radiation should be avoided in the first trimester if possible and minimized throughout the pregnancy when feasible. Consultation with an expert experienced in reproductive and developmental radiation risks may be helpful in pregnant women requiring multiple studies or procedures.

Anticoagulation

Anticoagulation is typically recommended before and after cardioversion for atrial fibrillation. In a woman with symptoms for less than 48 hours prior to cardioversion, anticoagulation is controversial but recommended in patients at high risk of thromboembolic events. It is not known if pregnancy should be considered a high-risk state.[49] In women with a longer duration of symptoms, anticoagulation is initiated prior to cardioversion and continued for 3 to 4 weeks.[49] In some cases of a prolonged period of suspected rhythm abnormality, a transesophageal echocardiogram is performed to rule out thrombus prior to proceeding with cardioversion.

In patients with chronic atrial fibrillation, anticoagulation can be considered with either low-molecular-weight heparin or unfractionated heparin. Warfarin should not be used in pregnancy outside of the setting of a mechanical valve, which has a high thrombotic risk. Even in the setting of a mechanical valve, the use of warfarin during pregnancy requires extensive counseling regarding the known teratogenicity and the subsequent risk of fetal intracranial hemorrhage. Warfarin should not be used for anticoagulation for maternal arrhythmia, either low-molecular-weight heparin or unfractionated heparin can be used. Newer anticoagulants have limited safety data in pregnancy and should not be used.

GENERAL PRINCIPLES FOR OBSTETRIC MANAGEMENT

Women with arrhythmias requiring ongoing maintenance medical therapy or women with underlying structural heart disease are candidates for assessments of fetal growth by ultrasound and antenatal fetal surveillance with nonstress tests.

In addition, women with a known arrhythmia typically require telemetry monitoring intrapartum. Ideally this is provided on labor and delivery to maximize obstetric care and outcomes with the cardiac team consulting and being alerted to any telemetry events remotely. Fluid shifts at the time of delivery and in the postpartum period can result in maternal cardiac compromise. Women at risk for arrhythmias, especially women with known congenital heart defects predisposing them to arrhythmias, often have telemetry monitoring through the first 24 hours postpartum.

Maternal anxiety and pain result in an increase in heart rate that can increase the risk of arrhythmia in women who are predisposed. Adequate pain control intrapartum is important in women with recurrent arrhythmias.

A side effect of some tocolytics (terbutaline and nifedipine) is maternal tachycardia. Given that maternal tachycardia can predispose women to arrhythmias, the risks and benefits of administration of tocolytics should be weighed prior to administering them to women with known arrhythmias or an underlying predisposition to arrhythmias. Alternate tocolytics can be considered if indicated for obstetric care.

Timing and Mode of Delivery

Women with stable arrhythmias do not require early induction of labor outside of standard obstetric indications. In contrast, women with recurrent, symptomatic arrhythmias may require earlier delivery dependent on the degree of symptomatology and overall cardiac status. There are no specific cardiac arrhythmias that alone would warrant delivery by cesarean. Some women, however, may have underlying structural heart disease that may prompt a cesarean delivery and this decision should be made on a case-by-case basis in consultation with cardiology. Further discussion of mode of delivery in women with structural heart disease is outside the scope of this article.

Women who require anticoagulation during the pregnancy also require more intensive peripartum planning. Further discussion of the peripartum management of anticoagulation is outside the scope of this article.

PRIMARY PREVENTION OF ARRHYTHMIAS IN WOMEN AT RISK

There are many indications for primary prevention implantable cardioverter-defibrillator (ICD) therapy, which are outlined in American Heart Association task force guidelines.[50,51] The most well-defined indication for ICD therapy is cardiomyopathy with a reduced ejection fraction.

In general, contraindications to ICD implant include incessant VT or VF, arrhythmias due to reversible causes, or a life expectancy less than 1 year.

Defibrillation threshold testing is common in current practice.[52] It involves inducing VF and ensuring the ICD can defibrillate the patient back into a normal rhythm.[53] There are hemodynamic consequences of this testing so the risk/benefit ratio must be considered in pregnant women.

IMPORTANCE OF A MULTIDISCIPLINARY APPROACH

Most women with a new-onset arrhythmia in pregnancy have a benign arrhythmia, such as isolated premature atrial contractions, or sinus tachycardia of a noncardiac etiology. When pregnant women are found to have a nonbenign or potentially treatable arrhythmia, however, the importance of multidisciplinary care is emphasized. For some women, this may be a general adult cardiologist or an electrophysiologist alone. For other women with congenital heart disease, the team may include an adult congenital cardiologist. Regardless, the obstetrician should take a leading role in the coordination of cardiology, anesthesia, nursing, and pediatrics to ensure comprehensive antepartum, intrapartum, and ongoing postpartum care for pregnant women with cardiac arrhythmias.

REFERENCES

1. Choi HS, Han SS, Choi HA, et al. Dyspnea and palpitation during pregnancy. Korean J Intern Med 2001;16(4):247–9.
2. van Mook WN, Peeters L. Severe cardiac disease in pregnancy, part I: hemodynamic changes and complaints during pregnancy, and general management of cardiac disease in pregnancy. Curr Opin Crit Care 2005;11(5):430–4.
3. Ouzounian JG, Elkayam U. Physiologic changes during normal pregnancy and delivery. Cardiol Clin 2012;30(3):317–29.
4. Franz MR, Cima R, Wang D, et al. Electrophysiological effects of myocardial stretch and mechanical determinants of stretch-activated arrhythmias. Circulation 1992;86(3):968–78.

5. Hunter S, Robson SC. Adaptation of the maternal heart in pregnancy. Br Heart J 1992;68(6):540–3.
6. Soliman EZ, Elsalam MA, Li Y. The relationship between high resting heart rate and ventricular arrhythmogenesis in patients referred to ambulatory 24 h electro-cardiographic recording. Europace 2010;12(2):261–5.
7. Nakagawa M, Katou S, Ichinose M, et al. Characteristics of new-onset ventricular arrhythmias in pregnancy. J Electrocardiol 2004;37(1):47–53.
8. Widerhorn J, Widerhorn AL, Rahimtoola SH, et al. WPW syndrome during pregnancy: increased incidence of supraventricular arrhythmias. Am Heart J 1992;123(3):796–8.
9. Li JM, Nguyen C, Joglar JA, et al. Frequency and outcome of arrhythmias complicating admission during pregnancy: experience from a high-volume and ethnically-diverse obstetric service. Clin Cardiol 2008;31(11):538–41.
10. Silversides CK, Harris L, Haberer K, et al. Recurrence rates of arrhythmias during pregnancy in women with previous tachyarrhythmia and impact on fetal and neonatal outcomes. Am J Cardiol 2006;97(8):1206–12.
11. Bouchardy J, Therrien J, Pilote L, et al. Atrial arrhythmias in adults with congenital heart disease. Circulation 2009;120(17):1679–86.
12. Attenhofer Jost CH, Connolly HM, Dearani JA, et al. Ebstein's anomaly. Circulation 2007;115(2):277–85.
13. Kumar S, Tedrow UB, Triedman JK. Arrhythmias in adult congenital heart disease: diagnosis and management. Cardiol Clin 2015;33(4):571–88, viii.
14. Autore C, Conte MR, Piccininno M, et al. Risk associated with pregnancy in hypertrophic cardiomyopathy. J Am Coll Cardiol 2002;40(10):1864–9.
15. Hodes AR, Tichnell C, Te Riele AS, et al. Pregnancy course and outcomes in women with arrhythmogenic right ventricular cardiomyopathy. Heart 2016;102:303–12.
16. Marijon E, Mirabel M, Celermajer DS, et al. Rheumatic heart disease. Lancet 2012;379(9819):953–64.
17. Diker E, Aydogdu S, Ozdemir M, et al. Prevalence and predictors of atrial fibrillation in rheumatic valvular heart disease. Am J Cardiol 1996;77(1):96–8.
18. Seth R, Moss AJ, McNitt S, et al. Long QT syndrome and pregnancy. J Am Coll Cardiol 2007;49(10):1092–8.
19. Joglar JA, Page RL. Management of arrhythmia syndromes during pregnancy. Curr Opin Cardiol 2014;29(1):36–44.
20. Ersboll AS, Hedegaard M, Sondergaard L, et al. Treatment with oral beta-blockers during pregnancy complicated by maternal heart disease increases the risk of fetal growth restriction. BJOG 2014;121(5):618–26.
21. Ruys TP, Maggioni A, Johnson MR, et al. Cardiac medication during pregnancy, data from the ROPAC. Int J Cardiol 2014;177(1):124–8.
22. Driver K, Chisholm CA, Darby AE, et al. Catheter ablation of arrhythmia during pregnancy. J Cardiovasc Electrophysiol 2015;26(6):698–702.
23. Raman AS, Sharma S, Hariharan R. Minimal use of fluoroscopy to reduce fetal radiation exposure during radiofrequency catheter ablation of maternal supraventricular tachycardia. Tex Heart Inst J 2015;42(2):152–4.
24. Knotts RJ, Garan H. Cardiac arrhythmias in pregnancy. Semin Perinatol 2014;38(5):285–8.
25. DiCarlo-Meacham A, Dahlke J. Atrial fibrillation in pregnancy. Obstet Gynecol 2011;117(2 Pt 2):489–92.
26. May LE, Knowlton J, Hanson J, et al. Effects of exercise during pregnancy on maternal heart rate and heart rate variability. PM R 2016;8(7):611–7.

27. Izmirly PM, Saxena A, Kim MY, et al. Maternal and fetal factors associated with mortality and morbidity in a multi-racial/ethnic registry of anti-SSA/Ro-associated cardiac neonatal lupus. Circulation 2011;124(18):1927–35.

28. Ferrari AD, Sussenbach CP, Guaragna JC, et al. Atrioventricular block in the post-operative period of heart valve surgery: incidence, risk factors and hospital evolution. Rev Bras Cir Cardiovasc 2011;26(3):364–72.

29. Lin A, Mahle WT, Frias PA, et al. Early and delayed atrioventricular conduction block after routine surgery for congenital heart disease. J Thorac Cardiovasc Surg 2010;140(1):158–60.

30. Morris GM, Salih Z, Wynn GJ, et al. Patient radiation dose during fluoroscopically guided biventricular device implantation. Acta Cardiol 2014;69(5):491–5.

31. Shotan A, Ostrzega E, Mehra A, et al. Incidence of arrhythmias in normal pregnancy and relation to palpitations, dizziness, and syncope. Am J Cardiol 1997; 79(8):1061–4.

32. Jeejeebhoy FM, Zelop CM, Lipman S, et al. Cardiac arrest in pregnancy: a scientific statement from the American Heart Association. Circulation 2015;132(18): 1747–73.

33. Magee LA, Downar E, Sermer M, et al. Pregnancy outcome after gestational exposure to amiodarone in Canada. Am J Obstet Gynecol 1995;172(4 Pt 1): 1307–11.

34. Ovadia M, Brito M, Hoyer GL, et al. Human experience with amiodarone in the embryonic period. Am J Cardiol 1994;73(4):316–7.

35. Joglar JA, Page RL. Treatment of cardiac arrhythmias during pregnancy: safety considerations. Drug Saf 1999;20(1):85–94.

36. Barnes EJ, Eben F, Patterson D. Direct current cardioversion during pregnancy should be performed with facilities available for fetal monitoring and emergency caesarean section. BJOG 2002;109(12):1406–7.

37. Horowitz LN, Kay HR, Kutalek SP, et al. Risks and complications of clinical cardiac electrophysiologic studies: a prospective analysis of 1,000 consecutive patients. J Am Coll Cardiol 1987;9(6):1261–8.

38. Rogers DP, England F, Lozhkin K, et al. Improving safety in the electrophysiology laboratory using a simple radiation dose reduction strategy: a study of 1007 radiofrequency ablation procedures. Heart 2011;97(5):366–70.

39. Nof E, Lane C, Cazalas M, et al. Reducing radiation exposure in the electrophysiology laboratory: it is more than just fluoroscopy times! Pacing Clin Electrophysiol 2015;38(1):136–45.

40. Doshi SK, Negus IS, Oduko JM. Fetal radiation dose from CT pulmonary angiography in late pregnancy: a phantom study. Br J Radiol 2008;81(968):653–8.

41. Moore W, Bonvento MJ, Lee D, et al. Reduction of fetal dose in computed tomography using anterior shields. J Comput Assist Tomogr 2015;39(2):298–300.

42. Tuzcu V, Kilinc OU. Implantable cardioverter defibrillator implantation without using fluoroscopy in a pregnant patient. Pacing Clin Electrophysiol 2012;35(9): e265–6.

43. Gudal M, Kervancioglu C, Oral D, et al. Permanent pacemaker implantation in a pregnant woman with the guidance of ECG and two-dimensional echocardiography. Pacing Clin Electrophysiol 1987;10(3 Pt 1):543–5.

44. Smith G, Clark JM. Elimination of fluoroscopy use in a pediatric electrophysiology laboratory utilizing three-dimensional mapping. Pacing Clin Electrophysiol 2007; 30(4):510–8.

45. Abello M, Peinado R, Merino JL, et al. Cardioverter defibrillator implantation in a pregnant woman guided with transesophageal echocardiography. Pacing Clin Electrophysiol 2003;26(9):1913–4.
46. Brent RL. Protection of the gametes embryo/fetus from prenatal radiation exposure. Health Phys 2015;108(2):242–74.
47. Saez TM, Aronne MP, Caltana L, et al. Prenatal exposure to the CB1 and CB2 cannabinoid receptor agonist WIN 55,212-2 alters migration of early-born glutamatergic neurons and GABAergic interneurons in the rat cerebral cortex. J Neurochem 2014;129(4):637–48.
48. ACOG Committee on Obstetric Practice. ACOG committee opinion. Number 299, September 2004 (replaces No. 158, September 1995). Guidelines for diagnostic imaging during pregnancy. Obstet Gynecol 2004;104(3):647–51.
49. Goland S, Elkayam U. Anticoagulation in pregnancy. Cardiol Clin 2012;30(3): 395–405.
50. Epstein AE, DiMarco JP, Ellenbogen KA, et al. 2012 ACCF/AHA/HRS focused update incorporated into the ACCF/AHA/HRS 2008 guidelines for device-based therapy of cardiac rhythm abnormalities: a report of the American College of Cardiology Foundation/American Heart Association Task Force on Practice Guidelines and the Heart Rhythm Society. J Am Coll Cardiol 2013;61(3):e6–75.
51. Epstein AE, DiMarco JP, Ellenbogen KA, et al. ACC/AHA/HRS 2008 guidelines for device-based therapy of cardiac rhythm abnormalities: a report of the American College of Cardiology/American Heart Association task force on practice guidelines (writing committee to revise the ACC/AHA/NASPE 2002 guideline update for implantation of cardiac pacemakers and antiarrhythmia devices) developed in collaboration with the American Association for Thoracic Surgery and Society of Thoracic Surgeons. J Am Coll Cardiol 2008;51(21):e1–62.
52. Russo AM, Chung MK. Is defibrillation testing necessary? Cardiol Clin 2014; 32(2):211–24.
53. Schipke JD, Heusch G, Fritzsche A, et al. Blood pressure and heart rate immediately after termination of short-term ventricular fibrillation. Resuscitation 2008; 79(3):404–9.

Management of Acute Kidney Injury in Pregnancy for the Obstetrician

Anjali Acharya, MBBS

KEYWORDS

- Acute kidney injury • Pregnancy-related acute kidney injury
- Atypical hemolytic uremic syndrome • Thrombotic microangiopathy • Preeclampsia
- Hypertensive disorders of pregnancy

KEY POINTS

- The physiologic changes in the kidney pose a challenge to the diagnosis of acute kidney injury in pregnancy.
- Assessment of baseline renal function and proteinuria early in prenatal care is essential for accurate diagnosis of pregnancy-related acute kidney injury.
- Identification of women at risk for acute kidney injury plays a crucial role in prompt diagnosis and prevention of acute kidney injury.
- Optimal management of women with pregnancy-related acute kidney injury requires a multidisciplinary team approach.
- It is prudent to limit renal biopsy to women with a suspicion of any condition that is severe enough to warrant urgent treatment or a change in management.
- The indications for starting renal replacement therapy in pregnancy-related acute kidney injury are the same as those in the nonpregnant population.

BACKGROUND

The incidence of pregnancy-related acute kidney injury (PR-AKI) varies widely across the world, with reported incidence of 1 in 20,000 pregnancies[1] to as much as 1 in 50 pregnancies.[2] Many factors contribute to this variation in incidence, such as lack of uniform defining criteria, physiologic changes in pregnancy that affect interpretation of laboratory tests, and regional differences in factors contributing to acute kidney injury (AKI). In addition, AKI (a term that has replaced acute renal failure) is often under-recognized until it is severe. Often there is a lack of information on baseline

The author has no financial conflict.
Jacobi Medical Center, Albert Einstein College of Medicine, 6E-23B, Building 1, Bronx, NY 10461, USA
E-mail address: Anjali.Acharya@NBHN.NET

prepregnancy serum creatinine (SCr) values in this population, which further poses a problem. The diagnostic accuracy of the currently accepted definition of AKI in the general population is not fully known in pregnancy and perhaps is inadequate.

Some nations report a bimodal distribution with an early peak of AKI as a consequence of septic abortions and a second peak later in pregnancy from hypertensive disorders of pregnancy, along with obstetric complications such as hemorrhage. Although the etiology of PR-AKI varies based on the country of origin, in most regions, including low-income countries, preeclampsia and eclampsia account for 5% to 20% of cases, with one study reporting 36% of PR-AKI to be from hypertensive disorders of pregnancy (**Box 1**).[2] The risk of PR-AKI is higher in the setting of early-onset (<32 weeks gestation) preeclampsia. Other major causes of PR-AKI in developing countries include sepsis and severe hemorrhage, whereas primary renal disease, thrombotic microangiopathy (TMA), and acute fatty liver of pregnancy (AFLP) are more common in the developed nations. Pregnancy may also unmask underlying primary renal disease or modify the course of preexisting renal disease.

Although overall a decrease in the incidence of PR- AKI has been reported, a substantial increase in AKI during pregnancy has been reported recently in the United States and Canada, with a higher increase reported in the United States. PR-AKI was also associated with a higher mortality rate, ranging from 17.4% of deaths during delivery hospitalization to 31.5% of deaths among postpartum hospitalizations in those with AKI.[3,4] This change could be attributed to several reasons such as, an increase in testing for the condition and lowering of the threshold for diagnosis, with the older literature relying a higher decline in glomerular filtration rate (GFR) to diagnose AKI.[5,6] A potential diagnostic ascertainment bias is further supported with an increased need for renal replacement therapy (RRT) seen among pregnant women with chronic kidney disease (CKD) and chronic hypertension who develop AKI.[4] Although risk factors such as diabetes, preeclampsia, and chronic hypertension predisposing women to PR-AKI have increased, the recent study by Mehrabadi[4] found that these factors contributed little to the increase in overall acute renal failure.

Although most women with AKI in pregnancy recover renal function, up to a third do not fully recover and can have serious long-term outcomes.[2,7,8] Some may require RRT, and, when this option is unavailable (as in many parts of the world), it may result in mortality. Maternal and fetal outcomes, thus, depend on optimal management of AKI.

Following a brief overview of physiology, this article provides an in-depth review of management of the spectrum of AKI occurring in pregnancy. Significant anatomic and physiologic changes occur in the kidneys during pregnancy and some of these changes begin soon after conception. Specific attention is given to current research and the newer therapeutic options.

Anatomic changes in pregnancy

The length of the kidney increases by 1 to 1.5 cm.

The volume of the kidney increases up to 30% because of changes in the vascular and interstitial spaces.

The urinary collecting system is dilated with hydronephrosis seen in up to 80% of pregnant women.

Hydronephrosis, although usually asymptomatic, predisposes women to serious ascending urinary tract infections. When severe, these infections may result in serious fetal complications and maternal complications such as septic shock and AKI.

Physiologic changes in the kidneys in pregnancy

Within weeks of conception, GFR increases by 40% to 60% and kidney blood flow by 80%.

These changes persist until the middle of the third trimester, whereas the creatinine production remains unchanged.

Total body water increases by 6 to 8 L, 4 to 6 L of which is extracellular and accounts for the edema of pregnancy.

This volume expansion depends on activation of the renin-aldosterone-angiotensin system.

There is cumulative sodium retention of up to 950 mmol on average.

Relaxin, a 6-kDa peptide produced by the corpus luteum, contributes to an increase in kidney blood flow, GFR, and solute clearance.

Effects of the gestational physiologic changes on laboratory parameters

An increase in clearance leads to a physiologic decrease in circulating creatinine, urea, and uric acid levels.

The average SCr level during pregnancy is 0.5 to 0.6 mg/dL and blood urea nitrogen level decreases to approximately 8 to 10 mg/dL.

Even a modest increase in SCr level to 1.0 mg/dL, although within the normal range, is reflective of kidney impairment.

An increase in protein excretion to 180 to 250 mg every 24 hours is seen in the third trimester because of an increase in filtered load combined with less efficient tubular reabsorption.[9,10]

Normal protein excretion in pregnancy is less than 260 mg every 24 hours, with 1 + protein on urine dipstick considered abnormal.[10]

Women with preexisting proteinuria may exhibit an exaggeration of protein excretion in the second and third trimesters.

Traditionally, elevated uric acid has been used as a marker in preeclampsia, but its predictive value for diagnosis and prognosis of this condition has been mixed.[11] However, a recent study looking at uric acid in patients with gestational hypertension found it to be an accurate predictor of presence and severity of preeclampsia.[12]

Definitions of pregnancy-related acute kidney injury

Definitions used in the literature vary from a mild increase in SCr level to the need for dialysis.

Consensus definitions have been put forth for the definition of AKI in the general population (http://kdigo.org/home/guidelines/).

Some investigators have used the Risk, Injury, Failure, Loss, and End stage (RIFLE) criteria focusing on the change in SCr or GFR levels and urine output.[13]

One prospective study reported a higher RIFLE stage in PR-AKI to be related to unfavorable renal outcomes.[14]

High RIFLE class has discriminative power in predicting risk of mortality from AKI in obstetric ICU patients.[15]

The Acute Kidney Injury Network criteria, which use urine output and a change in SCr value of 26.2 mmol/L or 0.3 mg/dL from baseline to define the presence of AKI, is being used more often in pregnancy.[16]

Physiologic changes in pregnancy limit the use of these criteria or consensus definitions in PR-AKI.

Use of serum cystatin C has not been well studied in PR-AKI and cannot be recommended.

There is a need for a definition with high diagnostic accuracy that will allow early detection of AKI.

In the author's opinion, because of an increased solute clearance and the plasma volume expansion seen during pregnancy, a significant decline in GFR or a greater increase in the absolute SCr value is required to satisfy the current Acute Kidney Injury Network criteria of a 0.3- mg/dL increase in SCr level. Therefore, the current SCr criteria used in the general population probably may underestimate the occurrence of PR-AKI.

In the general population with CKD, the Modification of Diet in Renal Disease formula is widely used and yields results that are corrected for body surface area. In pregnancy, because body surface area changes, the results may be inaccurate. In one study, the Modification of Diet in Renal Disease formula underestimated GFR by more than 40 mL/min. Other methods such as measurement of serum cystatin C–based formulas have not been proven useful in pregnancy. Creatinine clearance measured with 24-hour urine collection remains the best approximate of the gold standard of insulin clearance, and remains the most validated method for measuring renal function in pregnancy.

The following pregnancy-associated AKI causes (**Box 2**) are discussed in some detail below.

1. Preeclampsia
2. Hemolysis, elevated liver enzymes, and a low platelet count (HELLP) syndrome
3. AFLP
4. TMA
5. Acute cortical necrosis (ACN)
6. Glomerular Disease

Box 1
Etiology of PR-AKI by gestational age

As in the general population, the causes of AKI in pregnant women are divided into 3 groups: prerenal, intrarenal, and postrenal causes.

Prerenal AKI (functional AKI) or acute tubular necrosis in the context of hyperemesis gravidarum or septic abortion are common causes when AKI occurs in the earlier stage of pregnancy.

In the later stages of pregnancy, when AKI is more frequent, it is usually associated with preeclampsia and other hypertensive disorders of pregnancy, acute fatty liver of pregnancy, HUS, and sepsis.[17]

Box 2
Etiologies of PR-AKI

Prerenal Causes[a]

- Pregnancy-related conditions
  - Hyperemesis gravidarum
  - Vomiting caused by preeclampsia, HELLP, and AFLP
  - Hemorrhage
    - Missed abortion
    - Septic abortion
    - Placental abruption
    - Placental previa
    - Uterine atony
    - Bleeding during surgery
    - Uterine laceration
    - Uterine perforation

- Pregnancy-unrelated conditions
  - Vomiting caused by infections such as UTI or sepsis, gastroenteritis
  - Pyelonephritis
  - Diuretic use
  - Congestive heart failure

Renal causes

- Pregnancy-related conditions
  - ATN, ACN
    - Preeclampsia
    - HELLP
    - AFLP
    - Amniotic fluid embolism
    - Pulmonary embolism
  - TMA
    - HUS
    - Preeclampsia
    - HELLP
    - AFLP
    - DIC
    - Worsening of existing glomerular disease

- Pregnancy-unrelated conditions
  - ATN
  - De novo glomerular diseases
  - Acute interstitial nephritis

Postrenal causes

- Pregnancy-related conditions
  - Bilateral hydronephrosis in rare cases
  - Trauma to the ureters and bladder during cesarean section

- Pregnancy-unrelated conditions
  - Bilateral ureteral obstruction caused by stones or tumor
  - Tubular obstruction (calcium or uric acid crystal induced)
  - Obstruction at the bladder outlet

AKI in kidney allograft

- Acute rejection

- ATN

- Acute interstitial nephritis, calcineurin inhibitor toxicity, recurrent disease, infections such as cytomegalovirus or BK virus
- Postinfectious glomerulonephritis

[a] Can cause ATN and ACN.
From Acharya A, Santos J, Linde B, et al. Acute kidney injury in pregnancy—current status. Adv Chronic Kidney Dis 2013;20(3):217; with permission.

Preeclampsia is characterized by the new development of hypertension and either proteinuria or end-organ dysfunction after 20 weeks of gestation. Eclampsia, refers to the development of new-onset, generalized, tonic-clonic seizures or coma in a woman with preeclampsia. Both of these conditions are defined by the occurrence of fibrin and/or platelets thrombi in the microvasculature of organs, mainly the kidney and brain.

Hemolysis (with a microangiopathic anemia), elevated liver enzymes, and a low platelet count (HELLP) is considered by many, to be a severe form of preeclampsia, and may be seen in 10% to 20% of women with this condition. AKI caused by pre-eclampsia or eclampsia is rare in high-income countries, but can occur in 3% to 15% of cases of HELLP syndrome. It is a leading cause of PR-AKI, accounting for 40% to 60% of all cases.[18–20] PR-AKI in HELLP syndrome, even severe forms requiring dialysis, usually has a favorable renal outcome, with less than 10% of patients, progressing to CKD, except in those patients with preexisting hypertension or renal disease.[19,21,22]

Acute fatty liver of pregnancy is a rare condition, occurs in the third trimester of pregnancy, and is associated with preeclampsia in more than one-half of women, resulting in AKI in some. Differentiating it from HELLP may be difficult, but evidence of hepatic insufficiency, such as hypoglycemia or encephalopathy, and abnormalities in coagulation studies point toward AFLP. It may recur after pregnancies, especially if associated with long-chain 3-hydroxyacyl CoA dehydrogenase deficiency mutations.[23,24] Supportive care and delivery of the fetus are the only treatments available.

Although rare in developed countries, ACN is responsible for a significant number of cases of AKI in parts of the world in which deliveries are remote from large cities and proper obstetric care is unavailable. ACN is usually seen when there is a catastrophic obstetric emergency such as placental abruption with massive hemorrhage, amniotic fluid embolism, disseminated intravascular coagulation (DIC), or any condition leading to severe renal ischemia. Women usually present with oliguria or anuria after the inciting event. Renal imaging shows hypoechoic areas on ultrasound or hypodense areas on computed tomography scan.

Significant breakthroughs have occurred in our understanding of the pathogenesis of TMA syndromes (**Box 3**), which led to a reclassification of this disorder[25] mainly into complement dysregulation TMA, ADAMTS13 (a disintegrin and metalloprotease with thrombospondin type 1 motif 13 repeats)–deficient TMA, and TMA linked to other mechanisms (verotoxin and vascular endothelial growth factor deficiency), with a clear overlap between all these forms. This classification is more helpful for choosing the appropriate treatment than the older terms hemolytic uremic syndrome (HUS) and thrombotic thrombocytopenia purpura (TTP). These syndromes require urgent treatment based on the pathophysiology, with TMAs

> **Box 3**
> **Thrombotic microangiopathy syndromes**
>
> *The primary TMA syndromes*
>
> TTP; hereditary or acquired
>
> Shiga toxin-mediated HUS
>
> Drug-induced TMA syndromes
>
> Complement-mediated TMA (hereditary or acquired)
>
> Rare hereditary disorders of vitamin B12 metabolism or factors involved in hemostasis.
>
> *Secondary TMA—Caused by systemic disorders*
>
> Pregnancy-associated syndromes (eg, severe preeclampsia/HELLP syndrome)
>
> Severe hypertension
>
> Systemic infections and malignancies
>
> Autoimmune disorders such as systemic lupus erythematosus or antiphospholipid antibody syndrome
>
> Complications of hematopoietic stem cell or organ transplantation

associated with systemic disorders requiring therapy directed at the underlying disorder. TMA and other etiologies of AKI may occur in the transplanted kidney during pregnancy and require input and close monitoring from the transplant nephrologist (**Table 1**).

> *Pregnancy-related thrombotic microangiopathy*
>
> Etiology of pregnancy-related TMA (P-TMA) is similar to other types of TMA.
>
> P-TMA may be associated with ADAMTS13 deficiency, complement dysregulation, or other mechanisms.
>
> The timing of presentation seems to vary with the type of TMA.
>
> ADAMTS13 deficiency–related P-TMA occurs mainly during the second and third trimesters of pregnancy.[26]
>
> There is a progressive decrease in ADAMTS13 level and a parallel increase in von Willebrand factor antigen during normal pregnancy[27,28] with ADAMTS13 activity/von Willebrand factor antigen ratio reaching a nadir during the second and third trimesters.
>
> This potentiates the inhibitory effect of anti-ADAMTS13 autoantibodies, leading to TMA.
>
> P-TMA caused by complement pathway dysregulation occurs mainly (80% of cases) during the postpartum period.
>
> Infections and bleeding, which frequently complicate the postpartum period, may trigger complement activation leading to TMA.

Complement pathway dysregulation may be involved in the pathogenesis of pregnancy complications beyond atypical HUS (aHUS). It has been recently linked to autoimmune (lupus/antiphospholipid syndrome–associated preeclampsia) and the antiphospholipid syndrome–associated obstetric complications and nonimmune

Table 1
Differential diagnosis of acute kidney injury with Thrombotic microangiopathy during pregnancy

Disease Manifestations and Management	Severe Preeclampsia/ HELLP	AFLP	TTP/ HUS	SLE/ APLS	aHUS
Timing of onset					
2nd trimester	+	+	++	+	+
3rd trimester	++	++	+	+	+
Postpartum	+	-	+	+	++
Signs and symptoms					
Fever	-	-	+	+	+
HTN	+++	++	+	++	+
Neurologic symptoms	+	+	++	+	-
Purpura	-	-	++	+	++
Laboratory abnormalities					
AKI	+	++	+++	++	+++
Hemolytic anemia	++	+	+++	++	+++
Thrombocytopenia	++	+	+++	+	+++
Transaminitis	++	+++	+	-	+
DIC	+	++	-	+	-
Elevated PT	++	+++	-	-	-
Hypoglycemia	-	++	-	-	-
ADAMTS13 deficiency	+	-	++	-	+
Treatment					
Delivery/supportive	+++	+++	-	-	-
Plasmapheresis	-	-	+++	+	+++
Steroids	+a	+a	+/-	+++	-

+ indicates mild/occasionally; ++ indicates moderate/sometimes; +++ indicates severe/always; +/− indicates limited data.
Abbreviations: HTN, hypertension; PT, prothrombin time; SLE/APLS, systemic lupus erythematosus/antiphospholipid syndrome.
a Indicated for fetal lung maturation.
From Acharya A, Santos J, Linde B, et al. Acute kidney injury in pregnancy—current status. Adv Chronic Kidney Dis 2013;20(3):218; with permission.

preeclampsia.[29] Complement blockade is effective in ameliorating preeclampsia features in a murine model.[30–32] Complement gene mutations similar to those seen in aHUS have been identified in some forms of HELLP syndrome.[33]

Management of Pregnancy-related Acute Kidney Injury Requires a Multidisciplinary Approach

Although baseline assessment of renal function is not part of routine practice, having a baseline assessment of renal function is invaluable. This strategy aids in early identification of those at risk and helps make an accurate and timely diagnosis of PR-AKI (**Fig. 1**).

Diagnostic testing and treatment varies based on the suspected underlying diagnosis and the clinical scenario.

Breakthroughs in our understanding of the pathogenic mechanisms underlying many of the pregnancy-associated conditions, such as imbalance of angiogenic

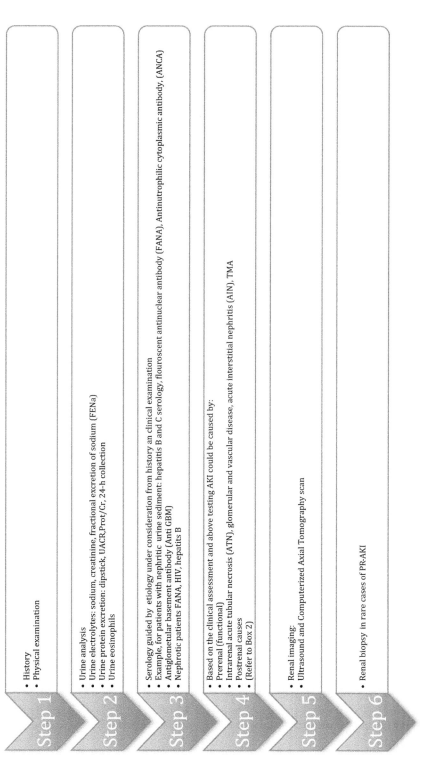

Step 1
- History
- Physical examination

Step 2
- Urine analysis
- Urine electrolytes: sodium, creatinine, fractional excretion of sodium (FENa)
- Urine protein excretion: dipstick, UACR,Prot/Cr, 24-h collection
- Urine eosinophils

Step 3
- Serology guided by etiology under consideration from history an clinical examination
- Example, for patients with nephritic urine sediment: hepatitis B and C serology, flouroscent antinuclear antibody (FANA), Antinutrophilic cytoplasmic antibody, (ANCA)
- Antiglomerular basement antibody (Anti GBM)
- Nephrotic patients FANA, HIV, hepatits B

Step 4
- Based on the clinical assessment and above testing AKI could be caused by:
- Prerenal (functional)
- Intrarenal acute tubular necrosis (ATN), glomerular and vascular disease, acute interstitial nephritis (AIN), TMA
- Postrenal causes
- (Refer to Box 2)

Step 5
- Renal imaging;
- Ultrasound and Computerized Axial Tomography scan

Step 6
- Renal biopsy in rare cases of PR-AKI

Fig. 1. Basic flow chart for PR-AKI workup.

factors in preeclampsia and pathogenetic mechanisms in thrombotic microangiopathies, hold promise and will undoubtedly enable strides in management of these conditions in the near future.

Tools for evaluation of a patient with pregnancy-related acute kidney injury

Evaluation of a pregnant patient with AKI is similar to that in the general population.

Prerenal, intrarenal, and postrenal causes of AKI are sought, based on history and physical examination.

Urinalysis and urine electrolytes are evaluated using the general principles of evaluating AKI.[13]

These parameters, particularly the use of urine electrolytes, need exploration in pregnancy because many physiologic mechanisms promote sodium reabsorption and natriuresis at different stages of pregnancy.

Although proteinuria is removed from the recent American Congress of Obstetricians and Gynecologists definition of preeclampsia, it plays an important role in the diagnosis of primary glomerular disease and in severe and superimposed preeclampsia.

The distinction between renal disease and preeclampsia is extremely important because it affects clinical management.

Proteinuria can be assessed by using the urinary dipstick method, 24-hour urine collection, and protein/creatinine ratio on a random sample.

Urine albumin/creatinine ratio (ACR) can be performed using an automated analyzer, allowing immediate point-of-care testing.

Ultrasound and Computerized Axial Tomography scan of the kidney as required.

Renal biopsy

Evaluation of proteinuria

Twenty-four–hour urine collection, although the most accurate for quantifying urinary protein, is cumbersome for the patient and has the possibility of incomplete collection.

Obstetric caregivers are using the protein/creatinine ratio more frequently.

Many studies have confirmed the reliability of spot protein/creatinine ratio in pregnancy and it has become accepted as the test of choice for quantifying proteinuria in pregnancy.[34–36]

ACR has the potential to supplant urinary dipstick as a rapid and accurate screening method for proteinuria in routine obstetric care.[37]

Although ACR and protein/creatinine ratio are well correlated we recommend that clinicians keep the cost in consideration and use the test with which they are familiar.[38]

Role of renal biopsy during pregnancy

There is reluctance to perform kidney biopsies in pregnancy because of the potential risk of complications such as major bleeding, severe obstetric complications, and early preterm deliveries.

The risk/benefit ratio varies according to gestational age.

Prior studies of renal biopsies in preeclampsia show that histologic changes do not reflect the severity of preeclampsia.

The risks and advantages of empirical therapeutic approaches versus kidney biopsy must be considered on a case-by-case basis.

It is prudent to limit the procedure to women with a suspicion of any condition that is associated with rapid worsening of renal function and is severe enough to warrant urgent treatment or a change in therapy.

In cases of TMA, kidney biopsy does not help identify the etiology of the TMA.[39]

The most common lesion in women with HELLP-associated AKI is glomerular endotheliosis, similar to the lesions in preeclampsia and not that of TMA.

Novel noninvasive diagnostic approaches

These tests may change the indications for kidney biopsy in pregnancy in the future.

The angiogenic factors such as soluble fms-like tyrosine kinase-1, placental growth factor, and soluble endoglin are used as diagnostic and predictive markers for preeclampsia[40,41]

Fms-like tyrosine kinase-1/placental growth factor ratio[28,42] is used to differentiate renal disease from preeclampsia.

Anti-PLA2R (M-type phospho-lipase A_2 receptor) for detection and monitoring disease activity in membranous nephropathy[43]

Soluble urokinase-type plasminogen activator receptor to diagnose focal segmental glomerulosclerosis

Analyzing the patterns of proteinuria and identifying discriminating proteins using proteomic techniques

Other novel serum or urine markers of glomerular diseases, preeclampsia, and acute kidney injury that were not available earlier[76–79]

Strategies for prevention of pregnancy-related acute kidney injury

Address predisposing factors such as hyperemesis gravidarum in a timely fashion to avoid functional renal injury.

It is important to minimize the use of nonsteroidal anti-inflammatory drugs especially in women at risk for AKI and to avoid them in those with established AKI.

Avoid unnecessary medications or withdraw medications that may be suspicious of causing acute interstitial nephritis. Proton pump inhibitors are associated with increased risk of AKI from acute interstitial nephritis, in the general population.

Ascending infections from urinary tract infection (UTIs) in pregnancy is not uncommon. Pregnant women may become quite ill and are at risk for both medical and obstetric complications from pyelonephritis.

Infectious Diseases Society of America recommends screening all pregnant women for asymptomatic bacteriuria at least once in early pregnancy, especially in women at high risk or those with known anatomic renal anomalies.

Treat UTI with appropriate antibiotics after obtaining urine culture. Progression to pyelonephritis not only has detrimental effects on the fetus but also increases risk of AKI in the mother.

Refer to US Food and Drug Administration (FDA) drug class before prescribing.

Treatment of Pregnancy-Related Acute Kidney Injury

Because of the heterogeneity of the etiology of PR-AKI, therapy must be tailored to the underlying condition. Strategies are presented as supportive care and targeted therapies.

Supportive care

Optimal fluid management and the selection of the specific type of fluid should be based on indications and keeping in mind contraindications and aiming to minimize toxicity.

Volume repletion with isotonic crystalloid solutions is indicated in women with blood loss.

The rate and type of fluids used for volume correction depends on the severity of volume depletion. Isotonic solutions are used for initial resuscitation when hypovolemia is present. Balanced or physiologic solutions are gaining favor based on recent studies in the general population, for maintenance.

Concurrent abnormalities in other electrolytes, such as serum sodium, and the presence of underlying kidney or cardiac disease also influence the choice and rate of fluid administration.

Close monitoring for signs and symptoms of electrolyte abnormalities is essential in those with PR-AKI.

Hypermagnesemia may develop in patients with preeclampsia and eclampsia who have AKI when magnesium sulfate is being administered. This is especially a concern in those with oliguria or anuria. Frequent assessment of serum magnesium level is recommended.

Use of Renal Replacement Therapy in Pregnancy-related Acute Kidney Injury

The reported use of RRT in PR-AKI ranges widely depending on the population reported.

One study from the developed world reported less than 1 in 10,000 to 15,000 pregnancies needing RRT; another from a developing nation found that up to 60% of their PR-AKI patients required RRT.[44,45]

Both intermittent hemodialysis and peritoneal dialysis have been used successfully.[46]

For critically ill and hemodynamically unstable women with PR-AKI, continuous RRT modalities should be considered. Continuous RRT has theoretic benefits of lower hemodynamic and volume shifts.

Data on timing of initiation (**Box 4**) are lacking, but a lower threshold for initiating RRT has been proposed in PR-AKI, similar to that in pregnant women with CKD. This is in order to decrease the unwanted effects of uremia on the fetus, such as polyhydramnios, developmental delay, and preterm birth.[13,47,48]

Box 4
Indications for starting renal replacement therapy in pregnancy-related acute kidney injury are similar to those in the nonpregnant population

Acidosis

Uremia

Electrolyte disturbance, such as hyperkalemia, hypermagnesemia and hypercalcemia that are refractory to medical management

Fluid overload

Intoxications

Targeted Therapy for Pregnancy-related Acute Kidney Injury

In cases of acute tubular necrosis (ATN), there is no specific therapy, and supportive care is practiced while the injury runs its course. Oliguria indicates more severe injury and requires diuretic use to increase urine output. This may delay the need for RRT but does not prevent ATN or shorten the duration of renal failure and is not recommended for this purpose (KIDIGO 2012). In patients with ATN, a positive fluid balance is an independent predictor of increased mortality in several prospective ICU studies.[49]

Acute interstitial nephritis, which is characterized by an inflammatory infiltrate in the kidney interstitium, is most commonly caused by drugs. Onset of AKI is temporally related to the initiation of a new drug. Withdrawal of the drug usually results in improvement of renal function in 5 to 7 days, but treatment with glucocorticoids is necessary in some. Other less frequent etiologies include infection, sarcoidosis, or uveitis syndrome and require appropriate workup.

There is no specific therapy for acute cortical necrosis. Supportive care is provided, and RRT is required in many cases. Partial or complete recovery may be seen in 20% to 40% of women.[50]

Glomerular disease may be preexisting or may develop de novo during pregnancy. Treatment is based on expert opinion, as little evidence-based data are available. Differentiating from preeclampsia is important, and many of these women subsequently have superimposed preeclampsia. In biopsy-proven glomerulonephritis, steroid and immunosuppressive therapy may be warranted. Use of immunosuppression in pregnancy is only indicated for life-threatening maternal illness and agents with the most desirable safety profile and FDS drug class are used.

The mainstay of treatment in pregnancies complicated by preeclampsia/eclampsia, HELLP syndrome, and AFLP is delivery of the fetus[51] guided by the gestational age, maternal and fetal condition, and the severity of preeclampsia. Corticosteroids should be considered if preterm delivery is likely. Control of blood pressure plays an important role to reduce maternal morbidity.

In the last decade, our management of hypertension in pregnancy has dramatically improved. Although there is ongoing debate on what level of hypertension to initiate therapy, treatment of severe hypertension with systolic blood pressure $\geq$160 mm Hg or diastolic blood pressure $\geq$110 mm Hg is always recommended to reduce the risk of maternal complications such as posterior reversible encephalopathy syndrome and stroke. Recent data suggest that treatment may be associated with maternal benefits without excess risk to the fetus.[52,53]

Although all antihypertensive drugs cross the placenta, there are many effective antihypertensive agents with an acceptable safety profile in pregnancy and during breast feeding. The choice of drug depends on the acuity and severity of hypertension and whether parenteral or oral therapy is used; angiotensin-converting enzyme inhibitors, angiotensin II receptor blockers, and direct renin inhibitors are contraindicated in pregnancy because of their effects on fetal development.

The other crucial therapy is the use of magnesium sulfate with an aim to prevent and treat seizures. The kidneys are the main route of excretion of magnesium, and dose adjustment is necessary when PR-AKI develops. In women with established PR-AKI, additional serum magnesium level monitoring every 6 hours is recommended to avoid neuromuscular and cardiovascular toxicity. Severe magnesium toxicity may require RRT.

Apart from delivery of the fetus, the use of steroids and plasma exchange for treatment of severe HELLP syndrome is controversial.[54,55] As the spectrum of pregnancy disorders linked to complement dysregulation/activation expands and the link confirmed, complement inhibition may represent a potential treatment for severe HELLP syndrome.

Pregnancy is a potent trigger for TMA in predisposed women and P-TMA is considered a secondary form of TMA that is associated with a high morbidity and mortality (up to 10%).[56] It accounts for 8% to 18% of all cases of TMA.[26,57–59] In the French aHUS registry, 1 of 5 women presented with aHUS at the time of pregnancy.[26]

Treatment of ADAMTS13 deficiency–related pregnancy-related thrombotic microangiopathy

Plasma therapy aims to restore a significant enzymatic activity (>10%) through: clearance of autoantibodies using plasma exchanges (PEX); restoration of ADAMTS 13 with fresh frozen plasma infusions in case of constitutional ADAMTS13 deficiency

PEX should be initiated as soon as possible.[60] both in established cases and when it is not possible to differentiate between preeclampsia, HELLP, and AFLP.

PEX is performed daily until a platelet count of greater than $150 \times 10^9/L$ is achieved for at least 3 days and until the serum lactate dehydrogenase level normalizes.

For TTP presenting in the first trimester, regular plasma exchange with close monitoring may allow for continuation of pregnancy.

Use of corticosteroids is not well supported.

Delivery is recommended in cases that do not respond to PEX.[61]

Concern for fetal toxicity and long-term effects on the neonates limits the use of rituximab, a B-cell–depleting antibody that is a second-line agent for TTP.[62,63]

The FDA has given rituximab a pregnancy label C.

Its use during pregnancy should be decided on a case-by-case basis depending on the potential benefits and risks of such treatment.

Treatment of complement dysregulation thrombotic microangiopathy

Aim to rapidly inhibit complement cascade activation using complement modulators.

Early use probably improves renal recovery.

Response to plasma therapy may not be optimal.

Eculizumab, a monoclonal humanized IgG that prevents the generation of C5a, and C5b, which initiates the formation of the membrane attack complex[64,65] and blocks the common terminal activation is currently the only available agent.

The standard eculizumab regimen includes 4 weekly 900-mg infusions followed by 1200-mg infusions every 2 weeks.

C5 inhibition can be easily monitored using total complement hemolytic assay with an aim of keeping it less than 20%.

Its prohibitive cost makes treatment impractical in many parts of the world.

Precautions before use of eculizumab

C5 inhibition increases the risk of infections with meningococcus.

Antimeningococcal vaccine should be administered before the start of eculizumab.

Additional oral antibiotic prophylaxis may be required during the period of eculizumab treatment and while waiting for the vaccine to take effect.

Pregnancy can increase the overall risk of TMA relapse, and a relapse rate of around 30% has been reported.[63,66]

The monitoring of ADAMTS13 levels during pregnancy may help identify patients at high risk of TMA relapse. Some investigators have even advocated the use, early in pregnancy, of PEX in pregnant women with known ADAMTS13 deficiency, to maintain an enzymatic activity greater than 10%.[67] However, there are no clear evidence-based guidelines for prophylactic treatment of ADAMTS13 deficiency TMA during pregnancy.

Complement dysregulation is not a contraindication for pregnancy, but genetic testing of patients to identify their potential risk of P-TMA is encouraged. Prepregnancy counseling of patients with complement gene abnormalities is crucial. The risk of recurrence varies based on the type of genetic mutation (eg, high in *CFH* and C3 mutations versus lower in CFI and membrane-cofactor protein).

A major limitation in improving outcome of AKI has been the lack of common standards for diagnosis and classification. The best way to improve outcomes of PR-AKI is prevention and early detection.

SUMMARY

In all, the incidence of P-AKI has probably decreased, but its fetal and maternal morbidity remain unacceptably high.

Pregnancy hypertensive complications, notably HELLP syndrome, are the leading cause of P-AKI.

P-TMA is a clinically challenging cause of P-AKI.

Several breakthroughs in our understanding of different mechanisms underlying P-TMA and preeclampsia have already led to a better treatment of these patients.

REFERENCES

1. Stratta P, Besso L, Canavese C, et al. Is pregnancy-related acute renal failure a disappearing clinical entity? Ren Fail 1996;18(4):575–84.
2. Prakash J, Niwas SS, Parekh A, et al. Acute kidney injury in late pregnancy in developing countries. Ren Fail 2010;32(3):309–13.
3. Mehrabadi A, Liu S, Bartholomew S, et al. Hypertensive disorders of pregnancy and the recent increase in obstetric acute renal failure in Canada: population based retrospective cohort study. BMJ 2014;349:g4731.
4. Mehrabadi A. Investigation of a rise in obstetric acute renal failure in the United States, 1999-2011. Obstet Gynecol 2016;127(5):899–906.
5. Mehta RL, Kellum JA, Shah SV, et al. Acute Kidney Injury Network: report of an initiative to improve outcomes in acute kidney injury. Crit Care 2007;11(2):R31.
6. Levey AS, Becker C, Inker LA. Glomerular filtration rate and albuminuria for detection and staging of acute and chronic kidney disease in adults: a systematic review. JAMA 2015;313(8):837–46.
7. Sibai BM, Villar MA, Mabie BC. Acute renal failure in hypertensive disorders of pregnancy. Pregnancy outcome and remote prognosis in thirty-one consecutive cases. Am J Obstet Gynecol 1990;162(3):777–83.
8. Vikse BE. Pre-eclampsia and the risk of kidney disease. Lancet 2013;382(9887): 104–6.
9. Higby K, Suiter CR, Phelps JY, et al. Normal values of urinary albumin and total protein excretion during pregnancy. Am J Obstet Gynecol 1994;171(4):984–9.
10. Airoldi J, Weinstein L. Clinical significance of proteinuria in pregnancy. Obstet Gynecol Surv 2007;62(2):117–24.

11. Johnson RJ, Kanbay M, Kang DH, et al. Uric acid: a clinically useful marker to distinguish preeclampsia from gestational hypertension. Hypertension 2011; 58(4):548–9.

12. Roberts JM, Bodnar LM, Lain KY, et al. Uric acid is as important as proteinuria in identifying fetal risk in women with gestational hypertension. Hypertension 2005; 46(6):1263–9.

13. Gammill HS, Jeyabalan A. Acute renal failure in pregnancy. Crit Care Med 2005; 33(Suppl 10):S372–84.

14. Arrayhani M, El Youbi R, Sqalli T. Pregnancy-related acute kidney injury: experience of the nephrology unit at the university hospital of fez, morocco. ISRN Nephrol 2013;2013:109034.

15. Kamal EM, Behery MM, Sayed GA, et al. RIFLE classification and mortality in obstetric patients admitted to the intensive care unit with acute kidney injury: a 3-year prospective study. Reprod Sci 2014;21(10):1281–7.

16. Gurrieri C, Garovic VD, Gullo A, et al. Kidney injury during pregnancy: associated comorbid conditions and outcomes. Arch Gynecol Obstet 2012;286(3):567–73.

17. Machado S, Figueiredo N, Borges A, et al. Acute kidney injury in pregnancy: a clinical challenge. J Nephrol 2012;25(1):19–30.

18. Drakeley AJ, Le Roux PA, Anthony J, et al. Acute renal failure complicating severe preeclampsia requiring admission to an obstetric intensive care unit. Am J Obstet Gynecol 2002;186(2):253–6.

19. Gul A, Aslan H, Cebeci A, et al. Maternal and fetal outcomes in HELLP syndrome complicated with acute renal failure. Ren Fail 2004;26(5):557–62.

20. Haddad B, Barton JR, Livingston JC, et al. HELLP (hemolysis, elevated liver enzymes, and low platelet count) syndrome versus severe preeclampsia: onset at < or =28.0 weeks' gestation. Am J Obstet Gynecol 2000;183(6):1475–9.

21. Sibai BM, Ramadan MK, Usta I, et al. Maternal morbidity and mortality in 442 pregnancies with hemolysis, elevated liver enzymes, and low platelets (HELLP syndrome). Am J Obstet Gynecol 1993;169(4):1000–6.

22. Selcuk NY, Odabas AR, Cetinkaya R, et al. Outcome of pregnancies with HELLP syndrome complicated by acute renal failure (1989-1999). Ren Fail 2000;22(3): 319–27.

23. Wilcken B, Leung KC, Hammond J, et al. Pregnancy and fetal long-chain 3-hydroxyacyl coenzyme A dehydrogenase deficiency. Lancet 1993;341(8842): 407–8.

24. Schoeman MN, Batey RG, Wilcken B. Recurrent acute fatty liver of pregnancy associated with a fatty-acid oxidation defect in the offspring. Gastroenterology 1991;100(2):544–8.

25. Fakhouri F, Fremeaux-Bacchi V. Does hemolytic uremic syndrome differ from thrombotic thrombocytopenic purpura? Nat Clin Pract Nephrol 2007;3(12): 679–87.

26. Fakhouri F, Roumenina L, Provot F, et al. Pregnancy-associated hemolytic uremic syndrome revisited in the era of complement gene mutations. J Am Soc Nephrol 2010;21(5):859–67.

27. Mannucci PM, Canciani MT, Forza I, et al. Changes in health and disease of the metalloprotease that cleaves von Willebrand factor. Blood 2001;98(9):2730–5.

28. Verlohren S, Galindo A, Schlembach D, et al. An automated method for the determination of the sFlt-1/PlGF ratio in the assessment of preeclampsia. Am J Obstet Gynecol 2010;202(2):161.e1-11.

29. Salmon JE, Heuser C, Triebwasser M, et al. Mutations in complement regulatory proteins predispose to preeclampsia: a genetic analysis of the PROMISSE cohort. PLoS Med 2011;8(3):e1001013.

30. Shamonki JM, Salmon JE, Hyjek E, et al. Excessive complement activation is associated with placental injury in patients with antiphospholipid antibodies. Am J Obstet Gynecol 2007;196(2):167.e1-5.

31. Redecha P, Tilley R, Tencati M, et al. Tissue factor: a link between C5a and neutrophil activation in antiphospholipid antibody induced fetal injury. Blood 2007;110(7):2423–31.

32. Qing X, Redecha PB, Burmeister MA, et al. Targeted inhibition of complement activation prevents features of preeclampsia in mice. Kidney Int 2011;79(3): 331–9.

33. Fakhouri F, Jablonski M, Lepercq J, et al. Factor H, membrane cofactor protein, and factor I mutations in patients with hemolysis, elevated liver enzymes, and low platelet count syndrome. Blood 2008;112(12):4542–5.

34. Cote AM, Brown MA, Lam E, et al. Diagnostic accuracy of urinary spot protein:-creatinine ratio for proteinuria in hypertensive pregnant women: systematic review. BMJ 2008;336(7651):1003–6.

35. Cheung HC, Leung KY, Choi CH. Diagnostic accuracy of spot urine protein-to-creatinine ratio for proteinuria and its association with adverse pregnancy outcomes in Chinese pregnant patients with pre-eclampsia. Hong Kong Med J 2016;22(3):249–55.

36. Nischintha S, Pallavee P, Ghose S. Correlation between 24-h urine protein, spot urine protein/creatinine ratio, and serum uric acid and their association with feto-maternal outcomes in preeclamptic women. J Nat Sci Biol Med 2014;5(2):255–60.

37. Wilkinson C, Lappin D, Vellinga A, et al. Spot urinary protein analysis for excluding significant proteinuria in pregnancy. J Obstet Gynaecol 2013;33(1): 24–7.

38. Cade TJ, de Crespigny PC, Nguyen T, et al. Should the spot albumin-to-creatinine ratio replace the spot protein-to-creatinine ratio as the primary screening tool for proteinuria in pregnancy? Pregnancy Hypertens 2015;5(4):298–302.

39. Abraham KA, Kennelly M, Dorman AM, et al. Pathogenesis of acute renal failure associated with the HELLP syndrome: a case report and review of the literature. Eur J Obstet Gynecol Reprod Biol 2003;108(1):99–102.

40. Sunderji S, Gaziano E, Wothe D, et al. Automated assays for sVEGF R1 and PlGF as an aid in the diagnosis of preterm preeclampsia: a prospective clinical study. Am J Obstet Gynecol 2010;202(1):40.e1-7.

41. Hadker N, Garg S, Costanzo C, et al. Financial impact of a novel pre-eclampsia diagnostic test versus standard practice: a decision-analytic modeling analysis from a UK healthcare payer perspective. J Med Econ 2010;13(4):728–37.

42. Rolfo A, Attini R, Nuzzo AM, et al. Chronic kidney disease may be differentially diagnosed from preeclampsia by serum biomarkers. Kidney Int 2013;83(1): 177–81.

43. Fresquet M, Jowitt TA, Gummadova J, et al. Identification of a major epitope recognized by PLA2R autoantibodies in primary membranous nephropathy. J Am Soc Nephrol 2015;26(2):302–13.

44. Najar MS, Shah AR, Wani IA, et al. Pregnancy related acute kidney injury: A single center experience from the Kashmir Valley. Indian J Nephrol 2008;18(4):159–61.

45. Clark SL. Handbook of critical care obstetrics. Boston: Blackwell Scientific Publications; 1994.

46. Chou CY, Ting IW, Lin TH, et al. Pregnancy in patients on chronic dialysis: a single center experience and combined analysis of reported results. Eur J Obstet Gynecol Reprod Biol 2008;136(2):165–70.

47. Holley JL, Reddy SS. Pregnancy in dialysis patients: a review of outcomes, complications, and management. Semin Dial 2003;16(5):384–8.

48. Dragun D. Acute kidney failure during pregnancy and postpartum. Management of acute kidney problems. Heidelberg (Germany): Springer-Verlag; 2010. p. 445–58.

49. Grams ME, Estrella MM, Coresh J, et al. Fluid balance, diuretic use, and mortality in acute kidney injury. Clin J Am Soc Nephrol 2011;6(5):966–73.

50. Matlin RA, Gary NE. Acute cortical necrosis. Case report and review of the literature. Am J Med 1974;56(1):110–8.

51. Lindheimer MD, Taler SJ, Cunningham FG. Hypertension in pregnancy. J Am Soc Hypertens 2010;4(2):68–78.

52. Abalos E, Duley L, Steyn DW. Antihypertensive drug therapy for mild to moderate hypertension during pregnancy. Cochrane Database Syst Rev 2014;(2):CD002252.

53. Magee LA, von Dadelszen P, Rey E, et al. Less-tight versus tight control of hypertension in pregnancy. N Engl J Med 2015;372(5):407–17.

54. Katz L, de Amorim MM, Figueiroa JN, et al. Postpartum dexamethasone for women with hemolysis, elevated liver enzymes, and low platelets (HELLP) syndrome: a double-blind, placebo-controlled, randomized clinical trial. Am J Obstet Gynecol 2008;198(3):283.e1-8.

55. Eckford SD, Macnab JL, Turner ML, et al. Plasmapheresis in the management of HELLP syndrome. J Obstet Gynaecol 1998;18(4):377–9.

56. Vesely SK, George JN, Lammle B, et al. ADAMTS13 activity in thrombotic thrombocytopenic purpura-hemolytic uremic syndrome: relation to presenting features and clinical outcomes in a prospective cohort of 142 patients. Blood 2003;102(1):60–8.

57. Veyradier A, Obert B, Houllier A, et al. Specific von Willebrand factor-cleaving protease in thrombotic microangiopathies: a study of 111 cases. Blood 2001;98(6):1765–72.

58. Morigi M, Galbusera M, Gastoldi S, et al. Alternative pathway activation of complement by Shiga toxin promotes exuberant C3a formation that triggers microvascular thrombosis. J Immunol 2011;187(1):172–80.

59. Noris M, Caprioli J, Bresin E, et al. Relative role of genetic complement abnormalities in sporadic and familial aHUS and their impact on clinical phenotype. Clin J Am Soc Nephrol 2010;5(10):1844–59.

60. George JN. How I treat patients with thrombotic thrombocytopenic purpura: 2010. Blood 2010;116(20):4060–9.

61. Scully M, Hunt BJ, Benjamin S, et al. Guidelines on the diagnosis and management of thrombotic thrombocytopenic purpura and other thrombotic microangiopathies. Br J Haematol 2012;158(3):323–35.

62. Fakhouri F, Vernant JP, Veyradier A, et al. Efficiency of curative and prophylactic treatment with rituximab in ADAMTS13-deficient thrombotic thrombocytopenic purpura: a study of 11 cases. Blood 2005;106(6):1932–7.

63. Scully M, McDonald V, Cavenagh J, et al. A phase 2 study of the safety and efficacy of rituximab with plasma exchange in acute acquired thrombotic thrombocytopenic purpura. Blood 2011;118(7):1746–53.

64. Kaplan M. Eculizumab (Alexion). Curr Opin Investig Drugs 2002;3(7):1017–23.

65. Woodruff TM, Nandakumar KS, Tedesco F. Inhibiting the C5-C5a receptor axis. Mol Immunol 2011;48(14):1631–42.
66. Kremer Hovinga JA, Vesely SK, Terrell DR, et al. Survival and relapse in patients with thrombotic thrombocytopenic purpura. Blood 2010;115(8):1500–11 [quiz: 1662].
67. Scully M, Starke R, Lee R, et al. Successful management of pregnancy in women with a history of thrombotic thrombocytopaenic purpura. Blood Coagul Fibrinolysis 2006;17(6):459–63.

Obesity and the Critical Care Pregnant Patient

Garrett K. Lam, MD, FACOG[a,b],*

KEYWORDS

- Obesity (morbid, super) • Maternal mortality • BMI
- National Health and Nutrition Examination Survey

KEY POINTS

- Obesity puts the gravid patient at risk for serious health problems such as diabetes in pregnancy, hypertensive diseases, and obstructive sleep apnea.
- The antepartum issues that are influenced by obesity all contribute to cardiovascular health problems, which are linked to a higher rate of maternal mortality.
- Obese gravidas, compared with normal-weight gravidas, experience an increased number of intrapartum difficulties, such as labor dystocia, and prolonged operative course.
- Obese gravidas also experience more complications in the immediate postnatal and puerperal recovery periods.
- Anesthetic management of the obese pregnant patient is made problematic by the physiologic changes in body habitus, some of which may require advanced critical care and support.

CASE PRESENTATION

A 27-year-old gravida 2 para 1001 presents at 38 0/7 weeks for repeat cesarean section. Her medical history is significant for superobesity. Her prepregnancy weight was 560 lbs (254 kg). She is 5′3″ tall (1.6 m), giving her a total body mass index (BMI) of 99.2 kg/m^2 at intake appointment.

This pregnancy has been complicated by gestational diabetes, for which she initially started metformin. However, for the last 3 weeks, she has been on subcutaneous insulin (currently 40 U of long-acting insulin and 20 U of immediate-acting insulin

Disclosure: Dr G.K. Lam has served, or is currently serving as a physician advisor and/or consultant for Sequenom, Clinical Innovations, Perkin Elmer Diagnostics, Qiagen, Sera Prognostics and Smart Human Dynamics. He does not have any stock or ownership in these companies, and has received honoraria for past service to some of these companies. He will not refer to any of the products produced by these companies in this publication.
[a] Department of Obstetrics and Gynecology, University of Tennessee College of Medicine Chattanooga, 979 East 3rd Street, Suite C-720, Chattanooga, TN 37403, USA; [b] Regional Obstetrical Consultants Chattanooga, TN, USA
* Department of Obstetrics and Gynecology, University of Tennessee College of Medicine Chattanooga, 979 East 3rd Street, Suite C-720, Chattanooga, TN 37403.
E-mail address: Garrett.Lam@erlanger.org

Obstet Gynecol Clin N Am 43 (2016) 767–778
http://dx.doi.org/10.1016/j.ogc.2016.07.012
0889-8545/16/© 2016 Elsevier Inc. All rights reserved.

with each meal). She has required steady dose increases to maintain euglycemia. She has experienced fluctuating bouts of hypoglycemia in between her predominant hyperglycemic episodes, which led to her current set insulin dosing at each meal.

Her past medical history is significant for a previous pulmonary embolism owing to a deep venous thrombosis, both of which occurred spontaneously, during the puerperal period of her last pregnancy. She was tested for thrombophilias, all of which were negative for significant findings. Her laboratory tests show a homozygous MTHFR defect without an elevated homocysteine level.

Her past obstetric history was significant for a previous cesarean section at 40 weeks gestation after prolonged labor (per the attending note: "failure to descend"). The infant weighed 7 lb 4 oz at 40 weeks. That pregnancy was otherwise uncomplicated.

On day of delivery, her admission physical now shows her weight to be 612 lbs (277.6 kg). The patient states she started feeling contractions last evening, which have progressed to the point where her contractions are now occurring every 8 to 10 minutes. Her blood glucose values before admission have fluctuated between 68 and 170 mg/dL.

Current medications include insulin, and enoxaparin, which was replaced by twice daily heparin injections starting 1 week ago.

The cesarean section is performed under combined spinal epidural anesthesia that results in the delivery of a 4785 g infant. The surgeons enter the peritoneal cavity through a vertical, supraumbilical incision, and the infant is extracted through a posterior, fundal classical uterine incision. The total operative time is longer than 2.5 hours.

Postnatally, the patient is restarted on heparin, but her dosing is changed by different providers, likely owing to her large volume of distribution. She is also started on warfarin (Coumadin) at the end of postoperative day 1.

On postoperative day 2, she notes a headache that runs from the top of her head to the back of her neck, which is temporarily alleviated with oral narcotics, promethazine (Phenergan) and caffeine. However, the headache persists. The anesthesia service consults, but declines blood patch placement owing to her anticoagulation. Of note, she continues on both warfarin and heparin throughout her postpartum course, which is extended as an inpatient owing to her symptoms and the fact that she cannot consistently reach her target international normalized ratio value.

On postoperative day 6, the patient exhibits mental status changes: somnolence, unintelligible mumblings, and falls to her knees once. No specific focal neurologic signs are discerned. Neurologic consultants order a computed tomography scan, but her size makes the imaging study impossible. A naloxone (Narcan) challenge is given without improvement. Unfortunately, patient mental status declines and she becomes obtunded.

The patient is transferred to the intensive care unit and intubation is required. Aggressive efforts to reverse anticoagulation are empirically started, but the patient shows papilledema, loss of corneal and doll's eye reflexes, and absent gag response. An electroencephalogram done after reversal of sedation shows absent cortical activity and an apnea test confirms no brain stem response. The decision is made to withdraw life support on postoperative day 8.

INTRODUCTION

Obesity has long been a subject of intermittent study. The medical literature characterizing the period prevalences of obesity in industrialized nations may be traced for more than 35 years,[1] showing a gradual increase of 8% within populations over that time. In more recent times, data collected from industrialized countries have shown that rates of obesity are rising dramatically, especially over the past 10 to 15 years.

Data collected by the Centers for Disease Control's Behavioral Risk Surveillance Study showed that from 1991 to 2002, the rates of obesity in various states jumped 10% to 12%. Although these data may be criticized because they were based on phone interviews of selected participants, to obtain their self-reported weights, this similar increase was observed in smaller scale studies of the US population.[2–4] The most recent data from the National Health and Nutrition Education Survey (from the Centers for Disease Control and Prevention) on obesity alarmingly showed that more than one-third of American adults (34.9%), and specifically 36.1% of women, were obese in 2011 to 2012.[5] Similarly, the combined proportion of overweight and obese patients in the Canadian population jumped from 40% in 1992% to 53% in 2004.[6] Sebire and associates[7] in 2001 performed a retrospective review of more than 287,000 gravidas in the UK, and calculated a population rate of 27.5% for women being overweight, and an 18.5% rate of obesity.

Further studies specific to the trends of obesity among the female population show race and socioeconomic status have substantial influence on disease prevalence. The US Department of Health and Human Services released their subanalysis of data from the National Health and Nutrition Education Survey from 2005 to 2008:

- Among women, the rate of obesity was inversely related to level of education and personal income.[8,9]
- Non-Hispanic black and Hispanic women had the highest rates of age-adjusted obesity (47.8% and 42.5% respectively), followed by non-Hispanic whites (32.6%) and then non-Hispanic Asians (10.8%).

Clearly, the increasing pace of prevalence and severity of obesity among the population signifies more than an epidemiologic problem; rather, obesity has become a health crisis.

DEFINITION

A definitive prevalence rate of obesity within a general population is unknown given that obesity is not clearly defined. Should the definition be made strictly against a weight threshold? Previous studies have set a weight limit of 90 kg in men and 80 kg in women—is that accurate? Would an analysis of body fat versus muscle mass be more relevant to assess health and physical fitness? Such questions characterize the ambiguity that obscure the ability to define an exact prevalence of obesity in pregnancy is even more difficult to define: Given that pregnancy is a physiologic state where steady weight gain of 10 to 18 kg is expected for a "normal weight" woman, is it reasonable and fair to set a weight threshold to define obesity in pregnancy?

Per the World Health Organization, BMI is the most clinically sound metric to define normal versus obese individuals. BMI is a calculation that is inherently understood and easily reproducible: BMI = weight (kilograms) divided by the patient's height (meters squared). The World Health Organization and Institute of Medicine have established of range of BMI values that not only characterize an individual's weight (normal vs overweight vs obese), but further subcategorizes obesity into grades (**Table 1**). Of note, recent surgical literature now lists new descriptors of grade III obesity: morbid obesity (BMI >40 kg/m^2), super obesity (BMI >50 kg/m^2), and even super-super obesity (BMI >60 kg/m^2).[8]

Table 1
The International classification of adult overweight and obesity according to BMI

Classification	BMI (kg/m^2) Principal Cutoff Points
Normal range	18.50–24.99
Overweight	≥25.00
Preobese	25.00–29.99
Obese	≥30.00
Obese class I	30.00–34.99
Obese class II	35.00–39.99
Obese class III	≥40.00

Of note, new terms introduced in the bariatric surgery literature equate "morbid obesity" to class III, "super obesity" to BMI greater than 50 kg/m^2, and "super-super obesity" to BMI greater than 60 kg/m^2.

Multiple studies on maternal obesity describe morbid effects on both fetus and mother. This review focuses specifically on the circumstances that would critically impinge on the maternal condition.

IMPACT ON ANTEPARTUM HEALTH
Diabetes

Many studies have confirmed higher rates of diabetes, whether gestational or preexisting, in obese gravidas compared with the general obstetric population. Indeed, Torloni and colleagues[10] in their literature review were able to identify a linear risk of a 1% increase in risk of diabetes for every increase of 1 kg/m^2 with a BMI of greater than 30. Glucose intolerance of any type has the potential to adversely impact maternal outcome, however, preexistent diabetic conditions seem to have more magnified effects on the mother. The pregnant diabetic population was surveyed in the UK in 2007. The study found that women with preexisting diabetic morbidity experienced increased risk for complications in pregnancy (combined effects of preterm delivery, cesarean section and hypoglycemic episodes (odds ratio, 2.6; 95% confidence interval, 1.3–4.9) compared with nondiabetics.[11]

The sequelae of diabetes in pregnancy may best be grouped around the categories of glycemic control (hyperglycemia vs hyperglycemia), diabetic ketoacidosis (DKA), gastroparesis, microvascular complications (ie, nephropathy), and macrovascular damage (ie, coronary artery disease). All of these issues will impact the health of the obese gravida.

Hypoglycemia (low blood sugars <68 mg/dL) versus severe hypoglycemia (any episode where low blood sugar requires external assistance, including diabetic coma) was studied in various countries. In the UK, the prevalence rate for recurrent hypoglycemic episodes in pregnancy was 61%, with severe hypoglycemia occurring in 25%.[11]

The prevalence of DKA in a diabetic pregnancy is low (1%–2%). DKA is thought to mainly occur in women with preexistent type 1 DM, particularly in the second and third trimesters; however, it may also occur in patients with late onset/type II diabetes and even in rare cases of gestational diabetes.[12] The maternal mortality rate in pregnancy is not known; however, the metabolic consequences to the mother are familiar, as manifested by nausea/emesis, hyperventilation, altered mental status, and dehydration with polyuria. Most telling is the deterioration of the fetus into metabolic acidosis that may result in stillbirth.

The cause of delayed gastric emptying of gastroparesis is likely multifactorial, of which autonomic dysfunction is only a contributing factor. The treatment of gastroparesis is therefore difficult. The resultant symptoms of nausea, bloating, and vomiting may result in malnutrition, poor blood glucose control, and multiple hospitalizations that may lead to depression.

Diabetic nephropathy equates to microvascular damage from diabetes that is defined by proteinuria (>300 mg/24 hours in the preconception period or the first half of pregnancy, or anytime protein excretion >3 g/24-hour period). It is thought to be present in approximately 5% of pregnancies, but the incidence varies depending on the patient's age and duration of diabetes. The pathogenesis is believed to be from initial glomerular hyperperfusion (from increased capillary pressure), which over time, causes deterioration of kidney function. In pregnancy, diabetic nephropathy has been associated with increased risk of preeclampsia, preterm delivery, and fetal growth issues.[13]

Interestingly, it would be sensible that more severe levels of obesity would proportionally worsen the severity of diabetes, thus increasing maternal morbidity. This assumption is not always borne out in the literature. Harper and colleagues[14] assessed the impact of obesity on the perinatal outcomes of diabetic women (gestational or type II) versus their euglycemic counterparts. They reviewed risks for outcomes such as severe preeclampsia, maternal birth trauma (third- and fourth-degree perineal lacerations), and length of antepartum and postpartum stays. There was no significant difference in any of those morbidities between the 2 groups.[14] Overall, the fact remains: diabetes in pregnancy is associated with obesity. No matter the severity of diabetes, the disease puts mothers at high risk for conditions that can make them critically ill. These patients require careful observation and considerable effort to monitor their health.

Hypertensive Diseases

BMI and maternal weight are both independent risk factors for hypertensive diseases in pregnancy such as preeclampsia. O'Brien and colleagues[15] conducted a metaanalysis of 13 studies, totaling more than 1.4 million pregnant women, and found that preeclampsia risk consistently doubled for every 5 to 7 kg/m^2 increase in BMI. Another epidemiologic study suggests that obesity is the leading attributable risk for preeclampsia in the United States (compared with diabetes, chronic hypertension, etc), resulting in about 30% of cases.[16] No evidence exists that obesity increases the severity of preeclampsia, but all forms of preeclampsia (early onset [<32 weeks], severe preeclampsia, HELLP [hemolysis, elevated liver enzymes, low platelets] syndrome, and onset near term) are manifested more often in obese women compared with their normal-weight counterparts.[17]

Given that not all obese women develop preeclampsia, it is implied that morbidity is not linked solely to weight, so how does obesity increase the risk for preeclampsia? Some postulate that the metabolic and physiologic changes associated with obesity are the true culprits. Insulin resistance predisposes toward increased adipose tissue deposition, which, in animal models, decreases vascular response to endothelium vasodilators.[18] Other studies have shown that insulin resistance and subsequent obesity reduces availability of nitric oxide to decrease sympathetic tone and oxidative stress in the vasculature, and that adipose tissue increases expression of angiotensinogen,[19] further worsening hypertension.

Adipose tissue also releases inflammatory factors that impact vascular reactivity by modulating endothelial function. C-reactive protein is released from adipose tissue, and the total levels of C-reactive protein are higher in obese subjects, many of who eventually develop preeclampsia.[20] Tumor necrosis factor alpha is also produced by adipocytes. It is also increased in preeclamptic patients and augments insulin resistance, thus synergistically acting with C-reactive protein to affect endothelial cell activity and increase oxidative stress.[21]

Knowledge of these biochemical and physiologic issues are important to the clinician's ability to care for the obese gravida, because it allows them to predict specific morbidities and make preparations to monitor the patient appropriately.

Obstructive Sleep Apnea

Additional to preeclampsia, obstructive sleep apnea (OSA) in pregnancy is increasingly recognized as a major effect of obesity that potentially adversely impacts a gravid woman's cardiovascular health. OSA is defined as the severe reduction or absence of airflow during sleep, despite respiratory effort. Patients become hypoxemic and stressed from the periods of reduced airflow, experience frequent awakening and repeated sympathetic stimulation, and develop hypertension. To date, no comprehensive prospective study has been done to clearly define the prevalence of OSA in pregnant women. Part of the problem is that no method of diagnosis has been accepted universally. Pien and associates[22] performed a small prospective cohort study on OSA. They estimated the prevalence of OSA within a study population that was equally divided across normal weight women, versus those who were overweight, class I obese and class II or greater obese in all 3 trimesters of pregnancy. Their data confirmed that OSA increased with BMI, with a corrected prevalence calculated at 8.4% in the first trimester and 19.7% in the third trimester.[22]

Patients with untreated OSA, in large part owing to their obesity, trend toward expression of adverse conditions such as increased insulin resistance, increased severity of systemic hypertension, coronary artery disease, mild pulmonary hypertension, cardiac arrhythmia, stroke (hemorrhagic and ischemic), and perioperative complications (difficulty with awakening from anesthesia or difficult intubation). These sequelae of OSA will certainly impact the clinical course of the obese gravida. Data based on discharge coding link OSA in pregnancy to obesity, and demonstrate increased expression of various cardiovascular morbidities such as eclampsia, cardiomyopathy, pulmonary embolism, and nosocomial mortality.[23]

The Collective Effect of Obesity and Comorbidities on Cardiovascular Health

Overall, the multitude of morbidities all dovetail into the central issue of impaired cardiovascular health. How that impairment affects the obese gravida is a question that was investigated by a team of researchers in California. The California Maternal Quality Care Commission conducted an in-depth review on the incidences and types of cardiovascular disease that contributed to the pregnancy-related mortality in California.

The California Pregnancy-Associated Mortality Review retrospectively examined a case series of cardiovascular-related deaths in pregnant women from 2002 through 2006, a period when the rate of maternal mortality increased markedly. There were 864 total deaths that occurred during pregnancy or within 1 year after birth; 257 deaths were deemed immediately related to conditions in the pregnancy, and 64 of these were owing to cardiovascular disease. Of the patients in this group, 37.5% were obese and 20.3% had a concomitant diagnosis of hypertension or preeclampsia during pregnancy. The incidence of cardiovascular pregnancy-related deaths in California was 2.35 deaths per 100,000 live births.[24]

Of interest in this study, 84% of women who died from cardiovascular disease presented with symptoms of decreased cardiopulmonary function during pregnancy or in the immediate postpartum period. The most frequent complaints included shortness of breath, palpitations, chest pain, wheezing, or fatigue. It was determined that many of these cases experienced a delay in diagnosis because neither the patient or the practitioner responded to the clinical warning signs found in the history and physical examination in a timely fashion (patient and health care provider factors contributed to 70.3% and 68.8% of cardiovascular disease). It is thought that those same symptoms are seen nonspecifically in normal pregnancy, and may have caused people to be less attuned to the underlying issues. In retrospect, the reviewers felt there was a "good to strong chance to alter the outcome" in 23.8% of the cardiovascular deaths that occurred.[24]

THE IMPACT OF OBESITY ON INTRAPARTUM MANAGEMENT
Impairment of Ultrasound Accuracy

The practitioner must be wary of the increased risks for macrosomia, prolonged labor, and possible shoulder dystocia in the obese patient, but how realistic are these risks? The literature contains studies which show that "maternal BMI obscures visualization of fetal anatomy by ultrasound, regardless of gestational age," and therefore "accurate prediction of birth weight is extremely difficult."[25] Meuller-Heubach[26] reported on pregnancy outcome after ultrasound diagnosis of fetal macrosomia. They studied 242 women with estimated fetal weights at least 4000 g or greater-than-90% for-gestational-age. Eighty-six were delivered within 3 days of ultrasound, with only 48% (41 women) having a birthweight that were within 500 g of the estimated fetal weight. Out of these 242 women, only 5 cases of shoulder dystocia were recorded, with no birth trauma.[26] Another retrospective study by Parry and coworkers[27] compared the cesarean delivery rate for neonates "falsely diagnosed with macrosomia," versus those who were "correctly diagnosed as *nonmacrosomic*." They found that the rate of cesarean delivery was significantly higher in the falsely diagnosed group (42.3%) versus those who were correctly diagnosed (24.3%), producing a relative risk of 1.74 (CI 1.09-2.78) for confidence interval.[27]

Changes in Labor and Increased Risk of Cesarean Section

Obese women are more likely to experience dysfunctional labor. Multiple studies have shown that the obese parturient experiences a slower progression in the first stage of labor. When labor curves are plotted for obese women (BMI $\geq$30) versus those with lesser BMIs, obese patients took a statistically significant longer amount of time to progress in the early part of labor, and had an overall longer duration in the first stage of labor.[28]

These factors, along with other known problems of intrapartum management (ie, difficulty of consistent external fetal monitoring and contraction monitoring) all contribute to an increased risk for cesarean section. Interestingly, obesity itself seems to be an independent risk factor for operative delivery, aside from these other contributing factors. The metaanalysis that Poobalan and associates[29] performed showed that cesarean section risk is increased by 50% in overweight women compared with those with normal BMI, and more than doubled in the obese population.

The greatest risk for critical care comes from the circumstances surrounding the operative delivery itself. The obese patient may experience critical delay in starting the procedure on time, which may lend to a more urgent procedure. Logistical issues such as bed transfer of the morbidly obese patient, having the requisite sized bed that is properly rated for the patient's weight in the operating room, proper sized equipment to perform the procedure, and the extra personnel needed to move the patient will all contribute to the delay. In this author's experience, the standard operating room table has the capacity to support 350 to 500 lbs. A special table for bariatric patients is wider and may support up to 1000 lbs (A. Royer, Director of Surgical Services, Chattanooga, TN, personal communication, 2016), but requires advanced notice to reserve its use.

The cesarean delivery itself may bring other issues that complicate the course of the obese patient. Experience and analysis have documented that obese patients experience longer duration of surgery, require operative techniques that could increase the risk for infection, necessitate consideration for alternative types of incision, and possess an inherent risk for venous thromboembolism (VTE). Professional opinion has noted that obese gravidas seem to experience more intraoperative blood loss (ie >1000 mL) than seen in normal weight patients. It is suggested that lapses in surgical technique or inability to achieve adequate hemostasis due to the need for deeper dissection through large layers of fatty tissue, the increased presence of perfusing vessels within the adipose tissue, and the poor visualization posed by large amounts of tissue.[30] Interestingly, there have not been studies that have definitively shown that utilization of transfusion from intraoperative blood loss has increased.

Concerns for Anesthesia

Administration of anesthesia to the obese patient necessitates extra consideration to avoid potentially critical complications. The successful administration of regional anesthesia depends on accurate epidural or subarachnoid placement of a catheter or needle. Unfortunately, the additional corporeal tissue makes identification of proper landmarks difficult, and the use of longer needles and catheters are a necessity. As a result, epidural failure rates are higher in obese women compared with normal weight counterparts (42% vs 6%).[31] Physiologically, the weight of the pannus compresses the vena cava, causing venous distension. This issue, combined with the larger amounts of epidural fat, will cause capillary and venous distension in the epidural space, spreading the local anesthetic cephalad. A greater-than-expected level of neurologic impairment puts the patient at risk for respiratory depression and hypotension. Overall, regional anesthesia carries substantial risk to the patient. In a review by Hawkins,[32] 25% of obstetric anesthesia–related deaths were associated with regional blockade, with 70% of these cases from epidural blocks and the remaining 30% from spinal anesthesia.

General anesthesia is also fraught with risk. The obese gravida carries a greater risk for aspiration given the presence of larger gastric volumes that are further augmented by the gastrointestinal slowing caused by progesterone. Respiratory difficulties may not only be caused by aspiration, but from the difficulty of intubation. Obese parturients, particularly the morbidly obese, will likely have poor Mallampati scores given the typical habitus of shorter necks and wider neck circumferences (predictive of difficult intubation). Vallejo's article[33] also notes that the typically enlarged breasts of obese patients, along with the increased adipose deposition in the upper airway, weigh down the chest and constrict the laryngeal diameter. Both of these issues make visualization for intubation difficult, and ventilation of the patient under anesthesia hard to handle. As a result, obese patients are at least 10 times more likely to fail endotracheal intubation than the general population (1 in 280–750 vs 1 in 2230).[33]

The gravid uterus is already known to upwardly displace the diaphragm, which decreases functional residual capacity in pregnant women. The increased weight of fatty tissue, along with the resultant larger muscle mass, increases the overall oxygenation and metabolic needs of the obese patient. These factors result in an increase in minute ventilation and oxygen demand, which can exceed the oxygenation during tidal breathing. Overall, the obese patient is more prone to rapid oxygen desaturation and resultant hypoxemia (**Fig. 1**).

Overall, providing the obese patient with safe and effective anesthesia can be daunting. The best practice is to notify the consulting anesthesiologist early. This author recommends outpatient consultation before admission to labor and delivery if possible, or early notification of the anesthesiologist upon arrival of the patient to the floor. Early placement of an intravenous line and the epidural catheter, before active labor, should be entertained.

THE IMPACT OF OBESITY ON POSTPARTUM COMPLICATIONS

Among the most concerning issues experienced by obese parturients are venous thromboembolism (VTE), postpartum wound infection, and possibly postpartum hemorrhage (PPH). Many of these patients face prolonged recovery in bed owing to difficulty with rising out of bed and ambulation. They may also have received vertical skin incisions, which are much more painful and at greater risk for seroma formation or opening.

Pregnancy alone significantly increases VTE risk given the hormonally induced procoagulative state, increased venous capacitance, and the increased production of factors VII, VIII, and X, as well as von Willebrand factor. Obesity further magnifies this risk: Edwards and colleagues[34] retrospectively reviewed the cases of 683 obese women, who were matched to 660 women with a BMI of less than 26. The incidence of VTE was 2.5% in the obese group compared with 0.6% in the control group. Currently, the Royal College of Obstetricians and Gynecologists in the UK recommends thromboprophylaxis with low molecular weight heparin for 3 to 5 days after delivery (vaginal included) for women greater than 35 years of age with a prepregnancy BMI of greater than 30 and/or current weight of greater than 90 kg. They further recommend thromboprophylaxis before surgery and for 3 to 5 days after cesarean section for those with a prepregnancy BMI of greater than 30 or weight of greater than 80 kg.[35] The American College of Obstetricians and Gynecologists currently recommends mechanical and

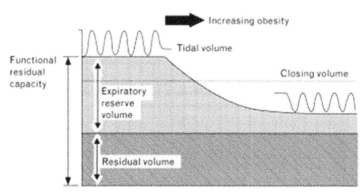

Fig. 1. Diagram of respiratory function in pregnant women in relation to increasing obesity. (*Adapted from* Vallejo MC. Anesthetic management of the morbidly obese parturient. Curr Opin Anaesthesiol 2007;20(3):178; with permission.)

pharmacologic thromboprophylaxis, using either unfractionated or low-molecular-weight heparin, in women at "high risk for VTE" after cesarean delivery only. This includes those with a BMI of greater than 50 kg/m^2.[36]

The obese patient also has a higher risk for wound infection, regardless of the type of delivery, cesarean incision, perineal/episiotomy repair, or endometritis. As mentioned, the greater amounts of adipose tissue are supported by an arcade of capillary vessels, thus predisposing to hematomas and seromas. Fastidious use of aseptic practices, minimizing operative times, and consistent use of sufficient antibiotics will help to reduce these risks. Although general agreement exists that obese individuals likely need greater doses of antibiotics (given larger volumes of distribution), standardized dosing is lacking. Bratzler and colleagues[37] submitted recommendations on behalf of the Surgical Infection Prevention Guideline Writers Workgroup. They advocated using 2 g of cefazolin for women with a BMI of less than 120 kg/m^2 and 3 g IV for those with a BMI of greater than 120 kg/m^2. If the surgery is longer than 2 hours, redosing is appropriate. Those who are penicillin allergic should receive a combination of clindamycin 900 mg with gentamicin 5/mg/kg of actual body weight.[37]

The evidence supporting increased risk for PPH in obese patients is mixed. Theoretically, the previous data presented for the longer labors experienced by obese patients, the potential for increased use of oxytocin, and the greater likelihood for macrosomia should all contribute to a greater risk for PPH. Indeed, Sebire and colleagues'[7] general population review of obese patients in the UK described a 44% increased risk for PPH. However, subsequent studies have not distinctively ascertained that this risk exists, perhaps owing in part to the greater usefulness of surgical delivery in our modern society, which abrogates the issue of prolonged labor. At this time, recommendations are that the practitioner should be aware of progress in labor and be prepared to take action in the event of PPH. No other specific recommendations have been established at this time.

SUMMARY

Clearly, the obese gravida has many potential points of care from which she may devolve into a critical situation. Preexistent conditions such as diabetes and hypertensive diseases (such as preeclampsia) might detrimentally impact cardiovascular health, which has been shown to result in increased maternal mortality. Both diabetes and OSA are associated with hypertension, and factors that could lead to acidosis (metabolic causes from DKA, respiratory from hypercapnea and hypoxia in OSA).

The physical composition of the obese gravida creates points of obstruction in care. Ultrasound imaging is compromised, anesthetic administration is problematic, and the physical increase in weight make for longer operative times, adjustments in technique, and suboptimal management during the procedure. All of these factors potentially increase the risk for morbidity from routine procedures such as vaginal and cesarean deliveries. These morbidities, among them anesthesia complications, wound infection and opening, and VTE, are sequelae that may lead to deterioration of health such that care in the critical care unit may be advisable. The keys to maximizing the outcome for an obese patient are foreknowledge of potential conditions, organization of the proper resources, and assurance that both patient and practitioner have access to the requisite level of care. The thoughtful arrangement of the care team, complete with the requisite tools, will reduce the chance the obese patient ends up for a prolonged stay in the critical care unit.

REFERENCES

1. Torrance GM, Hooper MD, Reeder BA. Trends in overweight and obesity among adults in Canada (1970-1992): evidence from national surveys using measured height and weight. Int J Obes Relat Metab Disord 2002;26:797–804.
2. Remington PL, Brownson R. Fifty Years of progress in chronic disease epidemiology and control. Centers for Disease Control. Behavioral risk factor surveillance system. Available at: http://www.cdc.gov/brfss. Accessed February, 2016.
3. Ehrenberg HM, Dierker L, Milluzzi C, et al. Prevalence of maternal obesity in an urban center. Am J Obstet Gynecol 2002;187(5):1189–93.
4. LaCoursiere DY, Bloebaum L, Duncan JD, et al. Population-based trends and correlates of maternal overweight and obesity, Utah 1991-2001. Am J Obstet Gynecol 2005;192(3):832–9.
5. Centers for Disease Control. National Health and Nutrition Survey on obesity 2011-2012. Available at: http://www.cdc.gov.nchs/nhanes.html. Accessed January 30, 2016.
6. Statistics Canada. Adult obesity in Canada measured height and weight 2005. Available at: http//:www.statcan.gc.ca/pub/82-620-m/2005001/article/adults-adults/8060. Accessed February, 2015.
7. Sebire NJ, Jolly M, Harris JP, et al. Maternal obesity and pregnancy outcome: a study of 287,213 pregnancies in London. Int J Obes Relat Metab Disord 2001; 25(8):1175–82.
8. Ogden C, Lamb M, Carroll M, et al. Obesity and socioeconomic status in adults: United States, 2005-2008. NCHS Data Brief no. 50. Hyattsville (MD): National Center for Health Statistics; 2010.
9. Sturm R. Increases in morbid obesity in the USA: 2000-2005. Public Health 2007; 121(7):492–6.
10. Torloni MR, Betrán AP, Horta BL, et al. Prepregnancy BMI and the risk of gestational diabetes: a systematic review of the literature with meta-analysis. Obes Rev 2009;10(2):194–203.
11. Confidential Enquiry into Maternal and Child Health. Diabetes in pregnancy: are we providing the best care? Findings of a national enquiry: England, Wales and Northern Ireland. London: CEMACH; 2007.
12. Parker JA, Conway DL. Diabetic ketoacidosis in pregnancy. Obstet Gynecol Clin North Am 2007;34:533–43.
13. Singh R. Pregnancy in women with diabetic nephropathy. Clinical Queries: Nephrology 2012;1(2):168–71.
14. Harper LM, Renth A, Cade WT, et al. Impact of obesity on maternal and neonatal outcomes in insulin-resistant pregnancy. Am J Perinatol 2014;31(5):383–8.
15. O'Brien TE, Ray JG, Chan WS. Maternal body mass index and the risk of pre-eclampsia: a systematic overview. Epidemiology 2003;14:368–72.
16. Bodnar LM, Ness RB, Markovic N, et al. The risk of preeclampsia rises with increasing prepregnancy body mass index. Ann Epidemiol 2005;15(7):475–82.
17. Catov JM, Ness RB, Kip KE, et al. Risk of early or severe pre-eclampsia related to pre-existing conditions. Int J Epidemiol 2007;36(2):412–9.
18. Galili O, Versari D, Sattler KJ, et al. Early experimental obesity is associated with coronary endothelial dysfunction and oxidative stress. Am J Physiol Heart Circ Physiol 2007;292(2):H904–11.
19. Dandona P, Aljada A, Chaudhuri A, et al. Metabolic syndrome: a comprehensive perspective based on interactions between obesity, diabetes, and inflammation. Circulation 2005;111(11):1448–54.

20. Wolf M, Kettyle E, Sandler L, et al. Obesity and preeclampsia: the potential role of inflammation. Obstet Gynecol 2001;98(5 Pt 1):757–62.
21. Conrad KP, Benyo DF. Placental cytokines and the pathogenesis of preeclampsia. Am J Reprod Immunol 1997;37(3):240–9.
22. Pien GW, Pack AI, Jackson N. Risk factors for sleep-disordered breathing in pregnancy. Thorax 2014;69:371–6.
23. Louis JM, Mogos MF, Salemi JL. Obstructive sleep apnea and severe maternal-infant morbidity/mortality in the United States, 1998-2009. Sleep 2014;37:843–8.
24. Hameed AB, Lawton ES, McCain CL, et al. Pregnancy-related cardiovascular deaths in California: beyond peripartum cardiomyopathy. Am J Obstet Gynecol 2015;213(3):379.e1-10.
25. Thornburg LL, Barnes C, Glantz JC, et al. Sonographic birth-weight prediction in obese patients using the gestation-adjusted prediction method. Ultrasound Obstet Gynecol 2008;32(1):66–70.
26. Delpapa EH, Mueller-Heubach E. Pregnancy outcome following ultrasound diagnosis of macrosomia. Obstet Gynecol 1991;78(3 Pt 1):340–3.
27. Parry S, Severs CP, Sehdev HM, et al. Ultrasonographic prediction of fetal macrosomia. Association with cesarean delivery. J Reprod Med 2000;45(1):17–22.
28. Norman SM, Tuuli MG, Odibo AO, et al. The effects of obesity on the first stage of labor. Obstet Gynecol 2012;120(1):130–5.
29. Poobalan AS, Aucott LS, Furung T, et al. Obesity as an independent risk factor for elective and emergency caeserean delivery in nulliparous women-systematic review and meta-analysis of cohort studies. Obes Rev 2009;10:28–35.
30. Porreco R. Cesarean delivery of the obese woman. Uptodate. Available at: http://www.uptodate.com/contents/cesarean-delivery-of-the-obese-woman. Accessed April 4, 2016.
31. Schneider MC. Anaesthetic management of high-risk obstetric patients. Acta Anaesthesiol Scand Supp 1997;111:163–5.
32. Hawkins JL. Maternal mortality: anesthetic implications. Int Anesthesiol Clin 2002;40:1–11.
33. Vallejo MC. Anesthetic management of the morbidly obese parturient. Curr Opin Anaesthesiol 2007;20(3):175–80.
34. Edwards LE, Hellerstedt WL, Alton IR, et al. Pregnancy complications and birth outcomes in obese and normal-weight women: effects of gestational weight change. Obstet Gynecol 1996;87(3):389–94.
35. Nelson-Piercy C. Thromboprophylaxis during pregnancy, labour and after vaginal delivery. RCOG Guideline No. 37, 2004.
36. James A, Committee on Practice Bulletins-Obstetrics. ACOG Practice bulletin no. 123: thromboembolism in pregnancy. Obstet Gynecol 2011;118(3):718–22.
37. Bratzler DW, Houck PM, Surgical Infection Prevention Guidelines Writers Workgroup, et al. Antimicrobial prophylaxis for surgery: an advisory statement from the National Surgical Infection Prevention Project. Clin Infect Dis 2004;38(12):1706–15.

Amniotic Fluid Embolism

Amir A. Shamshirsaz, MD, Steven L. Clark, MD*

KEYWORDS

- Amniotic fluid embolism • Cardiorespiratory arrest • Pregnancy
- Disseminated intravascular coagulopathy • Maternal death

KEY POINTS

- Amniotic fluid embolism remains one of the most devastating conditions in obstetrics practice with reported mortality of 20% to 60%.
- The pathophysiology seems to involve an abnormal maternal response to fetal tissue exposure associated with breaches of the maternal–fetal physiologic barrier during parturition.
- This response seems to involve activation of proinflammatory mediator similar to systemic inflammatory response syndrome.
- Treatment is mainly supportive and involves the delivery of the fetus when indicated, respiratory support (usually in the form of endotracheal intubation and mechanical ventilation), and hemodynamic support with the judicious use of fluids, vasopressors, inotropes, and, in some cases, pulmonary vasodilators. Rapid initiation of treatment, aided by a high index of clinical suspicion, is essential.

INTRODUCTION

Amniotic fluid embolism (AFE) is a catastrophic syndrome typically occurring during labor and delivery or immediately postpartum. Despite its recognition as a distinct entity for almost 100 years, the syndrome remains one of the most enigmatic and devastating conditions in obstetrics practice. Although rare, AFE has a high case fatality rate and remains a leading cause of maternal mortality in industrialized countries.[1–5] AFE is classically characterized by hypoxia, hypotension or hemodynamic collapse, and coagulopathy. Despite numerous attempts to develop animal models, AFE remains incompletely understood. Over the last 2 decades, more rigorous research efforts have greatly improved our understanding of this condition.

HISTORIC CONSIDERATIONS

The first case report of AFE was published in a 1926 Brazilian medical journal.[6] The condition was not widely recognized until 1941 when Steiner and Lushbaugh[7] described

Department of Obstetrics and Gynecology, Texas Children's Hospital, Baylor College of Medicine, 6651 Main Street, 10th Floor, Houston, TX 77030, USA
* Corresponding author.
E-mail address: Steven.Clark@bcm.edu

Obstet Gynecol Clin N Am 43 (2016) 779–790
http://dx.doi.org/10.1016/j.ogc.2016.07.001
0889-8545/16/© 2016 Elsevier Inc. All rights reserved.

obgyn.theclinics.com

fetal mucin and squamous cells during postmortem examination of the pulmonary vasculature in women who had unexplained obstetric death. Despite widely disparate clinical presentation, these authors viewed all patients with such findings as having died of a unique clinical syndrome, regardless of clinical presentation. These authors concluded that the patients had died as a result of "pulmonary embolism by amniotic fluid," giving rise to the term *amniotic fluid embolism*.[7] In a follow-up report by Liban and Raz in 1961,[8] cellular debris was also observed in the kidney, liver, spleen, pancreas, and brain of several such patients, although the exact route of squamous cells from the venous to the arterial circulation was not discussed.

The pathognomonic nature of the pulmonary findings described by Steiner and Lushbaugh[7] went largely unchallenged for several decades. As a result, numerous case reports appeared in the medical literature describing an incredible variety of presumed clinical presentations of "amniotic fluid embolism" based solely on the finding of fetal cells or other debris in the pulmonary arteries at autopsy.[9,10] However, a critical review of the clinical details provided in the original description found that 7 of the 8 index patients seem to have died of conditions such as sepsis or hemorrhage from undiagnosed uterine rupture, and the cause was labeled as "amniotic fluid embolism" based solely on pulmonary histologic findings.[7,9,10]

In the 1980s, the pulmonary artery catheter was introduced into critical care obstetrics. As a result, more frequent examination of pulmonary artery histologic specimens during life became possible. Several reports in the 1980s documented identical pulmonary pathologic findings in pregnant women with a variety of conditions unrelated to AFE.[9–11] These findings cast doubt on the validity of cases reported between 1941 and 1985 in which the diagnosis of AFE was based on pathologic findings alone.

Several experimental animal models yielded conflicting results regarding the pathologic potential of intravascular amniotic fluid and the pathophysiologic underpinnings of AFE (**Table 1**).[9,10,12–14] These studies generally involved a description of pathophysiologic changes resulting from the injection of whole or filtered human amniotic fluid or meconium into the central circulation of various animal species.[12–14] Most studies assumed a simple, mechanical mechanism of injury that can be summarized as follows: amniotic fluid is somehow forced into the maternal circulation, which results in obstruction of pulmonary arterial blood flow as amniotic fluid cellular debris is filtered by the pulmonary capillaries. Such obstruction leads to hypoxia, right ventricular heart failure, and death. However, the only 2 such studies carried out in primates using autologous or homologous amniotic fluid showed no adverse physiologic effects at all despite the infusion in one series of a volume of amniotic fluid that would represent 80% of the entire uterine volume.[12,13] Perhaps the fairest evaluation of these studies would be to conclude that the injection of large amounts of amniotic fluid or fetal fecal material from one species into the central circulation of small mammals of a different species sometimes causes adverse physiologic effects; the relevance of this observation to the human syndrome of AFE is dubious at best. An objective evaluation of this body of evidence finds quite clearly that the entrance of homologous amniotic fluid into the central circulation of primates and humans is generally innocuous, even in large volumes.[12–14]

The modern era of AFE investigation was heralded in the 1980s with the publication of several studies made possible by the development of clinical techniques for pulmonary artery catheterization of critically ill women, basic science investigations of maternal–fetal physiology, and the establishment of the first systematic case registry of AFE.[2,11,14,15] These studies found several surprising results that led to reevaluation and rejection of earlier theories of pathogenesis.

Table 1
Animal models of amniotic fluid embolism

Study Author, Year	Animal	Anesthetized	Pregnant	Filtered AF	Whole AF	AF Species	Hemodynamic Changes	Coagulopathy[a]
Steiner & Lushbaugh,[7] 1941	Rabbit or dog	No	No	No	Yes	Human	Not examined (death)	No
Cron, 1952	Rabbit	No	No	Not examined	Yes	Human	Not examined (death)	No
Schneider, 1953	Dog	No	No	Not examined	Yes	Human	Not examined (death)	Yes
Jacques, 1960	Dog	Yes	No	Not examined	Yes	Human or dog	Yes	Yes
Halmagyi, 1962	Sheep	Yes	No	No	Yes	Human	Yes	No
Attwood, 1965	Dog	Yes	No	Yes	Yes	Human	Yes	Yes
Stolte et al,[13] 1967	Monkey	Yes	Yes	No	No	Human or Monkey	No	No
Macmillan, 1968	Rabbit	No	No	No	Yes	Human	Not examined (death)	No
Reis, 1969	Sheep	Yes	Yes	Yes	Yes	Sheep	Yes	No
Dutta, 1970	Rabbit	Yes	No	Not examined	Yes	Human	Not examined (death)	No
Adamsons et al,[12] 1971	Monkey	Yes	Yes	Not examined	No	Monkey	No	No
Kitzmiller, 1972	Cat	Yes	No	No	Yes	Human	Yes	No
Spence, 1974	Rabbit	No	Yes	No	No	Rabbit	No	No
Reeves, 1974	Calf	No	No	Not examined	Yes	Calf	Yes	Not examined
Azegami et al,[25] 1986	Rabbit	No	No	No	Yes	Human	Not examined (death)	No
Richard, 1988	Rat[b]	Yes	No	Yes	No	Human	Coronary flow	Not examined
Hankins et al,[20] 1993	Goat	Yes	Yes	Yes	Yes	Goat	Yes	No
Petroianu, 1999	Minipig	Yes	Yes	Yes	Yes	Minipig	Not examined	Yes
Rannou, 2011	Rabbit	Yes	Yes	Yes	No	Rabbit	No	Yes

Abbreviation: AF, amniotic fluid.
[a] In most patients.
[b] Isolated heart preparation.
From Clark SL. Amniotic fluid embolism. Obstet Gynecol 2014;123:337–48; with permission.

INCIDENCE

Although uncommon in the general population, in the population of women who have died during pregnancy, AFE is common, and in the population of women who die after unexpected cardiovascular collapse during labor, AFE is statistically the most likely diagnosis.[2,5,9,16] The incidence of AFE, including both fatal and nonfatal cases, ranges between 1 in 12,953 deliveries in the United States[17] to 1 in 50,000 deliveries in the United Kingdom.[18] The true incidence and mortality rates of AFE are confounded by several factors:

1. The clinical definition of AFE varies across reports.
2. The signs and symptoms of AFE overlap with other more common obstetric complications such as hemorrhagic shock caused by postpartum hemorrhage.
3. Many of the population-based studies relying on hospital discharge diagnostic codes do not ascertain the clinical diagnosis of AFE from the medical record.
4. There is not a gold standard test for the diagnosis of AFE.
5. The diagnosis of AFE is often a diagnosis of exclusion.

PATHOPHYSIOLOGY

The hemodynamic alterations occurring with classic AFE are incompletely understood but seem to involve a complex sequence of pathophysiologic reactions resulting from abnormal activation of proinflammatory mediators similar to the systemic inflammatory response syndrome (SIRS).[9,10,14] Romero and colleagues[19] hypothesized infection/sepsis as an etiology of AFE based on 2 cases of proposed AFE in which elevated maternal plasma tumor necrosis factor–α levels were present before the clinical AFE event (**Fig. 1**). Cases in which transesophageal echocardiography was rapidly available and some carefully constructed animal models suggest the presence of an initial, transient period of pulmonary and systemic hypertension as a consequence of such inflammatory mediator activation.[20,21] In human subjects, who survive long enough after AFE event for evaluation of myocardial performance, depression of left ventricular function with normal pulmonary arterial pressures are the dominant longer-term hemodynamic alterations.[15,16,22]

Pulmonary manifestations of hypoxia seem to result from an initial period of profound shunting often followed (in survivors) by lung injury patterns consistent with acute respiratory distress syndrome (ARDS).

Coagulopathy is the third leg of the classic triad of signs and symptoms comprising the AFE syndrome.[10,14] Patients whose initial manifestations do not include fatal cardiac arrest often subsequently have coagulopathy. A few patients were reported who had acute, severe disseminated intravascular coagulation without any clinical evidence of primary cardiopulmonary dysfunction or antecedent hemorrhage.[10,14,23] The nature of disseminated intravascular coagulation in AFE is not completely understood. Amniotic fluid has been found to induce both platelet aggregation and the release of platelet factor III as well as activate factor X and the complement factors in vitro.[10,14] Amniotic fluid is also the source of tissue factor, which initiates the coagulation cascade.[23] However, investigators found high levels of tissue factor pathway inhibitor during late pregnancy, which would inhibit the procoagulant activation and may actually contribute to the rarity of this condition.[24] We suspect that the coagulopathy of AFE and that seen with massive placenta abruption share a similar pathophysiologic mechanism.[24] Both conditions presumably release thromboplastic material of fetal/placental origin into the maternal circulation. However, this connection remains unproven.

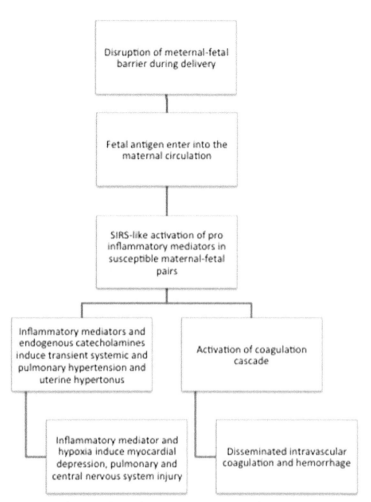

Fig. 1. Proposed mechanism of AFE. (*From* Clark SL Amniotic Fluid Embolism. Obstet Gynecol 2014; 337–48; with permission.)

When one considers the spectrum of clinical and laboratory manifestations of classic AFE syndrome, the similarities of AFE and conditions such as anaphylactic shock or endotoxin-mediated septic shock are striking.[10,14,19]

In these and similar conditions, various foreign antigens trigger an abnormal maternal host response with the subsequent release of endogenous mediators, which initiate the pathophysiology of each specific clinical syndrome. In an animal model of AFE, death was prevented by pretreatment of the animals with a leukotriene inhibitor.[25] Thus, it seems that AFE is, from a pathophysiologic standpoint, similar to the SIRS or septic shock, in which abnormal host response rather than the intrinsic nature of the inciting antigen is primarily responsible for clinical manifestations.[26]

Because the pathophysiology of this syndrome is not embolic in nature and seems to be unrelated to normal amniotic fluid, and given the apparent relationship of this condition to SIRS and other endogenous mediator release, the term *amniotic fluid embolism* is likely a misnomer.[14,23] In 1995, a new term was proposed emphasizing the anaphylacticlike clinical manifestations of the syndrome, *anaphylactoid syndrome of pregnancy*.[14] Although this term makes sense from a clinical and physiologic standpoint, it has not been widely adopted. Accordingly, the original term, *amniotic fluid embolism* (AFE), is used throughout this article.

RISK FACTORS

A review of multiple registry series found a wide range of conflicting conclusions regarding the presence of identifiable risk factors for AFE.[14,18,23] In general, reported risk factors for AFE include situations in which the exchange of fluids between the maternal and fetal compartments is more likely, such as cesarean delivery, instrumental delivery, cervical trauma, placenta previa, and abruption.[14,18,23] Association of induction of labor and AFE is inconsistently reported.[14,23] Abnormalities of uterine tone are described commonly in cases of AFE. However, based on investigations of maternal–fetal exchange, the frequency of oxytocin or other uterine simulants use, and the rarity of AFE, most investigators struggle to find a causative link between induction medications and AFE.[9,10,14] As early as 1976, investigations into maternal–fetal oxygen transport during uterine contractions found a complete cessation of uteroplacental exchange as intrauterine pressures exceed 40 mm Hg.[27] Thus, a contraction, especially a hypertonic contraction, is least likely event during all of labor or induce entrance of amniotic fluid and fetal tissue into the maternal circulation.[14] Other reported risk factors include advanced maternal age and parity, male fetus, eclampsia, polyhydramnios, and multiple gestations.[23,28]

CLINICAL MANIFESTATION

As with any condition resulting from a complex interaction between foreign antigens and a host of potential endogenous inflammatory mediators, the clinical manifestations of AFE are not uniform, and variation exists within the general triad of hypotension, hypoxia, and coagulopathy.[23] The analysis of the national registry found that 70% of cases of AFE occur during labor, 11% after a vaginal delivery, and 19% during a cesarean delivery.[14] Although AFE typically occurs during labor and delivery or immediately postpartum, rare cases of AFE have been reported after early pregnancy termination, transabdominal amniocentesis, trauma, and saline amnioinfusion.[29,30] **Table 2** shows the signs and symptoms with AFE. In its classic form, a woman in labor or shortly after vaginal or cesarean delivery sustains acute dyspnea, desaturation, or dyspnea followed by sudden cardiovascular collapse or arrest. These symptoms are commonly followed by the development of coagulopathy (83% of patients).[14] Coagulopathy may be the cause of death despite successful resuscitation of cardiopulmonary collapse and expert management of bleeding and component replacement.[23] In the US national registry, 75% of patients who presented with hemorrhage and isolated coagulopathy died despite appropriate resuscitative efforts.[14] In women sustaining cardiac arrest, any of the 3 classic lethal patterns of dysrhythmia, including ventricular fibrillation, asystole, and pulseless electrical activity, have been described, probably reflecting different mechanisms of arrest, including hypoxia, direct myocardial depression, and exsanguination from severe coagulopathy.[14] In women who survive the initial hemodynamic collapse and coagulopathy, lung injury and ARDS are often seen. In women whose initial course involves cardiac arrest, hypoxic brain injury is common and not uncommonly occurs out of proportion to the duration of the arrest.[23]

In cases occurring before delivery, electronic fetal monitoring shows decelerations, loss of variability, or terminal bradycardia as oxygenated blood is shunted away from

Table 2 Signs and symptoms noted in patients with amniotic fluid embolism		
Sign or Symptom	**Number**	**%**
Hypotension	43	100
Fetal distress	30	100
Pulmonary edema or ARDS	28	93
Cardiopulmonary arrest	40	87
Cyanosis	38	83
Coagulopathy	38	83
Dyspnea	22	49
Seizure	22	48
Atony	11	23
Bronchospasm	7	15
Transient hypertension	5	11
Cough	3	7
Headache	3	7
Chest pain	1	2

From Clark SL, Hankings GD, Dudley DA, et al. Amniotic fluid embolism: analysis of a national registry. Am J Obstet Gynecol 1995;172:1158–69; with permission.

the uterus, and catecholamine-induced uterine hypertonus causes a further decline in uterine perfusion (**Fig. 2**).[14,23]

Because of the vast overlap of AFE symptoms with other disease, consideration of differential diagnosis of AFE is warranted. **Box 1** shows a differential diagnosis for possible AFE.

DIAGNOSIS

The diagnosis of AFE is primarily based on the clinical observations. The classic triad of sudden onset of hypoxia, hypotension, and coagulopathy with on onset during labor

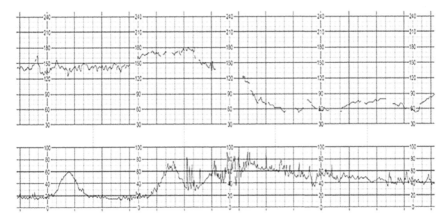

Fig. 2. Fetal heart rate tracing in a woman with AFE. Note spontaneous uterine tachysystole in conjunction with fetal heart rate deceleration several minutes before maternal cardiovascular collapse. (*From* Clark SL, Hankins DV, Dudley DA, et al. Amniotic fluid embolism: analysis of the national registry. Am J Obstet Gynecol 1995;172:1158–69; with permission.)

Box 1
Differential diagnosis for women presenting with possible amniotic fluid embolism

Pulmonary thromboembolism

Transfusion reaction

Hemorrhage

Anaphylaxis

High spinal anesthesia

Placenta abruption

Air embolism

Peripartum cardiomyopathy

Myocardial infarction

Eclampsia

Septic shock

Uterine rupture

---

and delivery within 30 minutes postpartum forms the hallmark of AFE diagnosis.[14,23] However, in some cases of AFE, one or more components of this triad may be minimal or absent.[31,32] In such cases, the diagnosis is more difficult, and one should consider other possible differential diagnoses as mentioned in **Box 1**.

Although the detection of fetal squamous cells in the maternal pulmonary circulation was considered diagnostic of AFE, more recent studies showed the same findings in various critical illness including complicated preeclampsia, cardiac disease, and septic shock using pulmonary artery catheterization.[9,11,14] Although available data do suggest a fetal origin for some of these squamous cells, identification of indistinguishable adult squamous cells in similar samples drawn from critically ill adult men suggests a component of desquamation from vascular access lines and ports as well.[11] Based on these studies, detection of squamous cells in the pulmonary artery bed in pregnant patients is not helpful for diagnosis of AFE. Such studies are not generally useful in either the diagnosis or exclusion of this condition.[9–11]

Several investigators have proposed more specific laboratory findings to confirm the diagnosis of AFE. The proposed laboratory investigations include tryptase, urinary histamine, insulinlike growth factor–binding protein–1, various markers of complement activation and postmortem immunohistologic staining for Sialyl Tn antigen, zinc coproporphyrin, or other evidence of pulmonary mast cell degranulation.[9,10,23,33,34] Data collection from patients whose diagnosis is not based on strict, objective, predetermined clinical criteria must be viewed with skepticism, particularly when the 'control' group consists of normal pregnant women rather than critically ill women in whom acute-phase reactant levels would be expected to increase, regardless of the diagnosis. Although the search for specific histologic or laboratory markers of AFE continues, this condition remains primarily a clinical diagnosis.

MANAGEMENT

Management of AFE is directed at the support of acute multisystem dysfunction. Initial diagnostic testing to consider in a patient whose differential diagnosis includes AFE is summarized in **Box 2**. The primary management goal includes rapid maternal

---

Box 2
Initial diagnostic testing suggested for a woman presenting with signs and symptoms of AFE

Complete blood count with platelets

Blood type and antibody screening

Serum electrolytes

Arterial blood gas

Cardiac enzymes

Coagulation profile (prothrombin time, partial thromboplastin time, international normalized ratio, and fibrinogen)

12-lead electrocardiogram

Echocardiogram

Chest radiograph

---

cardiopulmonary stabilization with treatment of hypoxia and maintenance of vascular perfusion. This management may require endotracheal intubation to maintain adequate oxygen saturation.

After cardiac arrest, initial resuscitation does not require a specific diagnosis of AFE.[23] Standard Basic Life Support and Advanced Cardiac Life Support algorithms should be applied. The involvement of a multidisciplinary team including anesthesia, respiratory therapy, maternal fetal medicine, and critical care departments should be considered. The management of cardiac arrest is beyond the scope of this article and has been discussed in another article (See Bennett and colleagues' article, "Cardiac Arrest and Resuscitation Unique to Pregnancy," in this issue).

Coagulopathy and ensuing hemorrhage are managed by aggressive blood and component replacement; widely available massive transfusion protocols are often helpful.[35]

The initial phase of AFE consists mainly of right ventricular failure. This failure can be verified using transthoracic or transesophageal echocardiography, if available.[17] Immediately after presentation, echocardiography may show a severely dilated and hypokinetic right ventricle (acute cor pulmonale) with deviation of the interventricular septum into the left ventricle.[17,28] Focus should be on avoiding hypoxia, hypercapnia, and acidosis, as these conditions increase pulmonary vascular resistance and lead to deterioration of the right ventricle failure.[17,36] Initial intervention may include agents such as dobutamine and milrinone, which may improve right ventricular output, and drugs aimed at decreasing pulmonary vascular resistance such as sildenafil, inhaled or intravenous prostacyclin, and inhaled nitric oxide.[36] Although the use of these agents makes sense given our current understanding of pathophysiology, no evidence exists of actual outcome improvement, and these drugs may not be readily available during the acute phase of the disease. Hypotension in this phase should be treated with preload optimization and vasopressors such as norepinephrine or vasopressin.[36] After an initial phase of right ventricular failure, left ventricular failure ensues and predominates. Excess fluid administration should be avoided in the setting of a massively dilated right ventricle, because it will increase the overdistension of the right ventricle and may increase the risk of right myocardial infarction and later pulmonary edema.[36] Increased distention of the right ventricle will also displace the interventricular septum to the left, which further compromises the cardiac output because of left ventricular obliteration.[36] Left-sided heart failure should be treated by optimizing cardiac preload and the use of vasopressors in cases of refractory hypotension to maintain coronary perfusion pressure. Also, by adding inotropes (dobutamine or milrinone), left ventricular contractility will improve. Severe pulmonary congestion not responsive to diuretic therapy may require fluid removal through dialysis.

If the fetus is undelivered and at a viable gestational age ($\geq$23 weeks), prompt delivery is generally indicated. Although scattered, anecdotal case reports exist in which delivery seems to have improved the maternal condition, and although such an effect is physiologically plausible as a result of the release of venocaval obstruction by the gravid uterus, a conclusion that in any individual case delivery would have altered the maternal outcome would be unjustified. Given the dismal maternal prognosis associated with AFE and cardiac arrest even after prompt delivery, and an ascertainment bias that favors case reports of apparent miraculous, but vanishingly rare maternal recovery after delivery with AFE, an objective, evidence-based assessment of this issue must conclude that delivery confers no maternal benefit.[14,23]

OUTCOME

Estimates of maternal mortality vary greatly and seem to largely depend on criteria required for the inclusion of cases as true AFE.[10,14,31,34] Series restricted to patients in whom all classic signs and symptoms of AFE are present suggest mortality rates exceeding 60%.[14] In cases complicated by cardiac arrest, the survival rate is even worse, with most series reporting that fewer than 25% of adults sustaining in-hospital cardiac arrest of any origin are discharged alive.[37] On the other hand, when less sick patients are included, particularly in population-based, death certificate, or discharge code–dependent series in which many patients do not actually have AFE, reported mortality rates are much lower, in some cases less than 20%.[10,31,32] Although it is clear that expert critical care management will improve the likelihood of survival in some women, prognosis ultimately seems to be more closely linked to disease severity and the occurrence of concomitant cardiac arrest than to any specific treatment modality.

RECURRENCE RISK

The recurrence rate of AFE is difficult to define because of the rarity of the condition and high mortality rate. Multiple cases of eventful subsequent pregnancies and no cases of recurrence have been reported.[28] Patients should be cautioned, however, that the available sample size precludes definitive conclusion regarding recurrence risk.

SUMMARY

Despite many new research developments in this field, the precise etiology and pathogenesis of AFE remain unclear. There is currently no gold standard diagnostic test or specific therapy for AFE. AFE remains a diagnosis of exclusion, dependent on bedside evaluation and judgment. Treatment is mainly supportive and involves the delivery of the fetus when indicated, respiratory support (usually in the form of endotracheal intubation and mechanical ventilation), and hemodynamic support with the judicious use of fluids, vasopressors, inotropes, and, in some cases, pulmonary vasodilators. Rapid initiation of treatment, aided by a high index of clinical suspicion, is essential. AFE is an unpredictable and rare event, and its study at any single obstetrics institution is impractical. Future research efforts will be depend on collaborative efforts by national and international programs.

REFERENCES

1. Chang J, Elam-Evans LD, Berg CJ, et al. Pregnancy-related mortality surveil-lance–United States, 1991–1999. MMWR Surveill Summ 2003;52(2):1–8.
2. Clark SL, Belfort MA, Dildy GA, et al. Maternal death in the 21st century: causes, prevention, and relationship to cesarean delivery. Am J Obstet Gynecol 2008; 199(1):36.e1-5 [discussion: 91–2.e7–11].
3. Roberts CL, Algert CS, Knight M, et al. Amniotic fluid embolism in an Australian population-based cohort. BJOG An Int J Obstet Gynaecol 2010;117(11): 1417–21.
4. Hogberg U, Joelsson I. Amniotic fluid embolism in Sweden. Gynecol Obstet Invest 1985;20:130–7.
5. Stolk KH, Zwart JJ, Schutte J, et al. Severe maternal morbidity and mortality from amniotic fluid embolism in the Netherlands. Acta Obstet Gynecol Scand 2012; 91(8):991–5.
6. Meyer J. Embolia pulmonary amniocaseosa. Bras Med 1926;2:301–3.
7. Steiner PE, Lushbaugh CC. Landmark article, Oct. 1941: Maternal pulmonary embolism by amniotic fluid as a cause of obstetric shock and unexpected deaths in obstetrics. By Paul E. Steiner and C. C. Lushbaugh. JAMA 1986;255(16): 2187–203.
8. Liban E, Raz S. A clinicopathologic study of fourteen cases of amniotic fluid em-bolism. Am J Clin Pathol 1969;51(4):477–86.
9. Clark SL. New concepts of amniotic fluid embolism: a review. Obstet Gynecol Surv 1990;45(6):360–8.
10. Dildy GA, Belfort MA, Clark SL. Anaphylactoid syndrome of pregnancy (amniotic fluid embolism). In: Belfort M, Saade G, Foley M, et al, editors. Critical Care Ob-stetrics. 5th edition. Oxford (UK): Whiley-Blackwell; 2010. p. 466–74.
11. Clark SL, Pavlova Z, Greenspoon J, et al. Squamous cells in the maternal pulmo-nary circulation. Am J Obstet Gynecol 1986;154(1):104–6.
12. Adamsons K, Mueller-Heubach E, Myers RE. The innocuousness of amniotic fluid infusion in the pregnant rhesus monkey. Am J Obstet Gynecol 1971;109(7): 977–84.
13. Stolte L, van Kessel H, Seelen J, et al. Failure to produce the syndrome of amni-otic fluid embolism by infusion of amniotic fluid and meconium into monkeys. Am J Obstet Gynecol 1967;98(5):694–7.
14. Clark SL, Hankins GD, Dudley DA, et al. Amniotic fluid embolism: analysis of the national registry. Am J Obstet Gynecol 1995;172(4 Pt 1):1158–67 [discussion: 1167–69].
15. Clark SL, Montz FJ, Phelan JP. Hemodynamic alterations associated with amnio-tic fluid embolism: a reappraisal. Am J Obstet Gynecol 1985;151(5):617–21.
16. Clark SL, Cotton DB, Gonik B, et al. Central hemodynamic alterations in amniotic fluid embolism. Am J Obstet Gynecol 1988;158(5):1124–6.
17. Abenhaim HA, Azoulay L, Kramer MS, et al. Incidence and risk factors of amniotic fluid embolisms: a population-based study on 3 million births in the United States. Am J Obstet Gynecol 2008;199(1):1–8.
18. Knight M, Tuffnell D, Brocklehurst P, et al. Incidence and risk factors for amniotic-fluid embolism. Obstet Gynecol 2010;115(5):910–7.
19. Romero R, Kadar N, Vaisbuch E, et al. Maternal death following cardiopulmonary collapse after delivery: Amniotic fluid embolism or septic shock due to intrauter-ine infection? Am J Reprod Immunol 2010;64(2):113–25.

20. Hankins GDV, Snyder RR, Clark SL, et al. Acute hemodynamic and respiratory effects of amniotic fluid embolism in the pregnant goat model. Am J Obstet Gynecol 1993;168(4):1113–30.

21. Shechtman M, Ziser A, Markovits R, et al. Amniotic fluid embolism: early findings of transesophageal echocardiography. Anesth Analg 1999;89(6):1456–8.

22. Girard P, Mal H, Laine JF, et al. Left heart failure in amniotic fluid embolism. Anesthesiology 1986;64(2):262–5.

23. Clark SL. Amniotic fluid embolism. Obstet Gynecol 2014;123(2 Pt 1):337–48.

24. Sarig G, Klil-Drori AJ, Chap-Marshak D, et al. Activation of coagulation in amniotic fluid during normal human pregnancy. Thromb Res 2011;128(5):490–5.

25. Azegami M, Mori N. Amniotic fluid embolism and leukotrienes. Am J Obstet Gynecol 1986;155(5):1119–24.

26. Rangel-Frausto MS, Pittet D, Costigan M, et al. The natural history of the systemic inflammatory response syndrome (SIRS). A prospective study. JAMA 1995; 273(2):117–23.

27. Towell ME. Fetal acid-base physiology and intrauterine asphyxia. In: Goodwin JW, Godden JO, Chance GW, editors. Perinatal medicine. Balrimore (MD): Williams & Wilkins; 1976. p. 200.

28. Pacheco LD, Saade G, Hankins GD, et al. SMFM clinical guidelines No. 9: amniotic fluid embolism: diagnosis and management. Am J Obstet Gynecol 2016. http://dx.doi.org/10.1016/j.ajog.2016.03.012.

29. Hasaart TH, Essed GG. Amniotic fluid embolism after transabdominal amniocentesis. Eur J Obstet Gynecol Reprod Biol 1983;16(1):25–30.

30. Ray BK, Vallejo MC, Creinin MD, et al. Amniotic fluid embolism with second trimester pregnancy termination: a case report. Can J Anaesth 2004;51(2): 139–44.

31. Knight M, Berg C, Brocklehurst P, et al. Amniotic fluid embolism incidence, risk factors and outcomes: a review and recommendations. BMC Pregnancy Childbirth 2012;12:7.

32. Gilbert WM, Danielsen B. Amniotic fluid embolism: decreased mortality in a population-based study. Obstet Gynecol 1999;93(6):973–7.

33. Benson MD. Current concepts of immunology and diagnosis in amniotic fluid embolism. Clin Dev Immunol 2012;2012:946576.

34. Conde-Agudelo A, Romero R. Amniotic fluid embolism: an evidence-based review. Am J Obstet Gynecol 2009;201(5):445.e1-13.

35. Pacheco LD, Saade GR, Costantine MM, et al. An update on the use of massive transfusion protocols in obstetrics. Am J Obstet Gynecol 2016;214(3):340–4.

36. Duarte AG, Thomas S, Safdar Z, et al. Management of pulmonary arterial hypertension during pregnancy: a retrospective, multicenter experience. Chest 2013; 143(5):1330–6.

37. Clark SL. Successful pregnancy outcomes after amniotic fluid embolism. Am J Obstet Gynecol 1992;167(2):511–2.

Trauma and Considerations Unique to Pregnancy

Christy Pearce, MD, MS[a,b,*], Stephanie R. Martin, DO[a,c]

KEYWORDS

- Trauma • Pregnancy • Protocol • Physiology

KEY POINTS

- Fifty percent of fetal losses occur after "minor trauma."
- Proper seat belt use in pregnancy reduces adverse fetal outcomes in motor vehicle crashes.
- Clinical signs of hemorrhage and shock are delayed in pregnant women.
- Prioritize maternal stability before fetal assessment.
- Displace the gravid uterus to prevent aortocaval compression.

INTRODUCTION

Trauma complicates 6% to 7% of all pregnancies and requires multidisciplinary education and training for both trauma and obstetric (OB) teams to achieve the best outcome. The importance of this is emphasized by the statistics, which show trauma to be the leading cause of non-OB maternal death that also results in an annual loss of 4000 fetuses.[1,2] Although the great majority of OB trauma is considered minor, this statement can be misleading, because 50% of fetal losses occur in what is often considered to be minor trauma. Only 4 per 1000 OB trauma cases lead to inpatient admission; however, the delivery rate after admission is 24% to 38%.[2–6]

Systems such as the Injury Severity Score and Revised Trauma Score exist in the trauma arena to categorize patients and attempt to quantify risk of adverse outcome. Higher scores reflect greater injury. However, these systems have not been found to be applicable to outcomes in OB cases. A population-based study of 10,000 pregnant women examined outcomes in relation to Injury Severity Score. Women were categorized by those who required delivery at the time of their trauma admission and those who were delivered at a later time. An Injury Severity Score of greater than 10 was

[a] Southern Colorado Maternal Fetal Medicine, Colorado Springs, CO, USA; [b] Outreach Services, Centura South State, Colorado Springs, CO, USA; [c] Maternal Fetal Medicine Services, Centura South State, Colorado Springs, CO, USA
* Corresponding author. Outreach Services, Centura Southstate, Southern Colorado Maternal Fetal Medicine, 6071 East Woodmen Road, Suite 440, Colorado Springs, CO 80923.
E-mail address: cpearce@southerncoloradomfm.com

Obstet Gynecol Clin N Am 43 (2016) 791–808
http://dx.doi.org/10.1016/j.ogc.2016.07.008
0889-8545/16/© 2016 Elsevier Inc. All rights reserved.

obgyn.theclinics.com

associated with the highest risk of adverse outcome; however, those dyads with a score of less than 10 remained at increased risk of abruption, uterine rupture, and maternal and fetal death.[3] Owing to the limitations of these scoring systems and trauma providers' lack of consistent OB experience, it is important to understand mechanisms for certain adverse maternal and fetal/neonatal outcomes incurred as a result of trauma, as well as caveats to pregnancy physiology that make some injuries more likely and detection of maternal compromise more difficult.

MATERNAL AND FETAL RISK

Common pregnancy-associated risks in trauma include preterm contractions, preterm labor, preterm delivery, abruption, fetal and neonatal death, and uterine rupture. Motor vehicle crashes (MVCs) are the most common source of OB trauma (two-thirds of all cases), followed by falls, intimate partner violence (IPV), assault, and suicide.[1,7–10]

Although the severity of the MVC is associated most strongly with adverse outcomes, even minor collisions can result in fetal demise.[10,11] Correct seat belt use and air bag deployment decrease the risk of maternal injury and fetal loss.[12–15] However, even with this, at a speed of 20 mph, the risk of adverse fetal event is still as high as 12%.[11] IPV often escalates during pregnancy and is thought to exist in 20% of pregnancies. IPV can take many forms (falls, MVCs, gunshot wound, stabbing, strangulation, blunt trauma) and should be screened for in all trauma patients.[16,17]

Blunt trauma can occur as a result of falls, MVC, or assault. Upper abdominal injuries include risks to the spleen and liver.[18,19] The bowel is less often injured as a result of blunt trauma because it is shielded by the gravid uterus. Although rare, uterine rupture can occur (most often posterior and fundal) with a fetal mortality rate approaching 100%. Fetal injury can also occur and may not be perceptible until after delivery. Fetal–maternal hemorrhage occurs in up to 10% of blunt trauma cases.[1,6,9,18,20]

Penetrating abdominal trauma most often occurs as a result of gunshot, stabbing, assault, or attempted suicide. A larger uterus, owing to late gestational age or multiple gestation, is more likely to sustain injury. Bowel injury is somewhat prevented by the gravid uterus, but should be more strongly suspected in upper abdominal stab wounds.[21] Gunshot wound injuries are variable and determined by distance from the gun, entry point, unseen visceral path, and exit point.

Pelvic fracture is most often seen as a result of MVC or serious fall. Open pelvic fracture is associated with increased risk for bowel injury, other maternal structural injury, and maternal and fetal death.[22] Fetal head injuries can occur as a result of pelvic fracture when the fetus is vertex. If a fracture is deemed stable and the pelvic inlet and outlet are not compromised, vaginal delivery can still be attempted.

Abruption occurs in 7% of trauma cases, most of which are considered "minor."[1,9,23–25] When the uterus decelerates owing to a sudden stop, the continued inertia of the amniotic fluid can create negative pressure on the uteroplacental interface. This inertia, along with shearing force and stretching at the uteroplacental interface, can create separation and resultant retroplacental bleeding. Abruption most often occurs as the result of an MVC, but can occur in any setting with the right combination of intrauterine inertia and shearing force. It may not be apparent clinically until more than 24 hours after trauma.[23,26] Abruption is associated with worse neonatal outcomes than gestational age–matched controls, including death, cerebral palsy, intraventricular hemorrhage, asphyxia, and periventricular leukomalacia.[27] Classically, an abruption presents as vaginal bleeding with abdominal or back pain, although 10% may be concealed (no vaginal bleeding). The amount of vaginal bleeding is not necessarily predictive of the size of the abruption. Coagulopathy can develop in 10% of abruptions, with other bleeding from trauma further increasing that risk.[28] Abruptions may be challenging to detect. The absence of pain or bleeding does not exclude abruption. Ultrasound imaging will detect a relatively small portion of abruptions. This is addressed later in the article.

Preterm labor is also commonly associated with trauma. Multiple etiologies include direct uterine injury, maternal hypoxia, or bleeding, which stimulate contractions. Morbidity and mortality from preterm delivery increases as gestational age decreases. Stillbirth risk is increased in trauma and may be a result of undetected or delayed abruption, fetal distress, or fetal–maternal hemorrhage. Some fetuses may be at higher risk of this, including those with preexisting uteroplacental insufficiency. If a stillbirth is encountered at initial evaluation, there is typically no urgency for delivery, and maternal stabilization should occur first.

PHYSIOLOGY CAVEATS

The physiologic adaptations to pregnancy are important to understand when evaluating and treating pregnant trauma patient (**Table 1**). Many of these adaptions are detectable as early as the first trimester. It is the obstetrician's role to relay this information to the trauma team both in education, simulation, and in actual trauma scenarios.

Cardiovascular adaptations are summarized in **Fig. 1**. These include a 20% to 50% increase in blood volume with resultant increase in stroke volume and cardiac output and decrease in systemic vascular resistance.[32] Clinical signs of hemorrhage and shock can be delayed in pregnant women owing to these cardiovascular adaptations. Once a pregnant patient develops tachycardia and hypotension in response to hemorrhage, at least 20% of her blood volume has been lost. Mortality is increased in pregnant women with blood loss so great as to cause tachycardia and hypotension.[25] Postpartum trauma patients are at increased risk for pulmonary edema owing to the immediate increase in cardiac output (80%) with autotransfusion of uterine/placental blood flow and mobilization of extravascular fluid compounded with any injuries sustained as a part of their trauma.[33]

Plasma volume increases to a greater proportion than red blood cell mass, resulting in a dilutional anemia in 20% to 60% of pregnant women.[34–36] This dilutional anemia leads to a decreased in hemoglobin relative to the nonpregnant states. However, it does not generally result in a true anemia. Anemia in pregnancy is defined by the

Table 1		
Laboratory changes in pregnancy		
Parameter	**Pregnant**	**Nonpregnant**
Fibrinogen (mg/mL)	400–650	150–400
Hemoglobin (g/dL)	>11	14 ± 2
AST (U/L)	10–30	7–40
ALT (U/L)	6–32	0–40
pH	7.4–7.46	7.38–7.42
P_{CO_2} (mm Hg)	26–32	38–45
P_{O_2} (mm Hg)	75–106	70–100
HCO_3 (mmol/L)	18–21	24–31
O_2 saturation (%)	95–100	95–100

Data from Refs.[28–31]

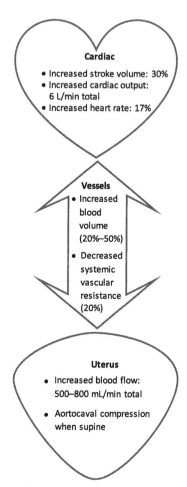

Cardiac
- Increased stroke volume: 30%
- Increased cardiac output: 6 L/min total
- Increased heart rate: 17%

Vessels
- Increased blood volume (20%–50%)
- Decreased systemic vascular resistance (20%)

Uterus
- Increased blood flow: 500–800 mL/min total
- Aortocaval compression when supine

Fig. 1. Cardiovascular changes in pregnancy.

Centers for Disease Control and Prevention as a hemoglobin of less than 11 g/dL in the first and third trimesters, and less than 10.5 g/dL in the second trimester.[29] Anemia results in a lower arterial O_2 content; however, O_2 delivery is maintained owing to increased cardiac output. Pregnant women, therefore, depend on cardiac output for O_2 delivery more so than nonpregnant women.[37] If there is compromise of O_2 delivery (decreased gas exchange, respiratory illness, blood loss) then a pregnant woman can become compromised quickly, particularly surrounding the time of labor and delivery. O_2 delivery must be optimized before proceeding with delivery in a compromised patient.

Most (95%) pregnant women will demonstrate a systolic flow murmur of aortic or pulmonic origin. Any murmur greater than 2/4 or any diastolic murmur is abnormal.[38] owing to the superior, latera, and anterior displacement of the heart in the thorax, pregnant women can falsely seem to have cardiomegaly on chest radiography.[39]

Uterine blood flow represents a large portion of maternal cardiac output. Trauma teams need to be aware of the potential for massive blood loss via the uterus, placenta, and engorged uterine and ovarian veins.[40] The gravid uterus can rest on the great vessels as they return to the heart, creating aortocaval compression in the supine position as early at 20 weeks' gestation (sooner in multiple gestations). This can reduce cardiac output by 25% to 30%, leading 8% of pregnant women to develop hypotension, bradycardia, and syncope/presyncope.[40,41]

Respiratory changes are summarized in **Fig. 2**. These include an increased O_2 consumption of 20% to 30%, increased tidal volume, decreased functional residual capacity, and decreased CO_2 levels. As gestation advances, there is continued upward displacement of the diaphragm (up to 4 cm) decreasing the functional residual capacity (air left in the lungs after exhalation).[42] The decreased functional residual capacity allows for more alveolar collapse and decreased gas exchange. The chest diameter increases by 2 cm.[42] Pregnant women are at increased risk for pulmonary edema owing to increases in plasma volume and cardiac output in the setting of decreased oncotic pressure. Owing to compensated respiratory alkalosis, a high normal or slightly elevated carbon dioxide level is a much more concerning finding in a pregnant woman.

The liver has not been shown to be enlarged as a result of pregnancy, and therefore hepatomegaly in a pregnant trauma patient should be considered abnormal and undergo evaluation. Estrogen and pregnancy increase fibrinogen and coagulation factor synthesis in the liver. Fibrinogen levels double in pregnancy.[43] There is a 20% to 100% increase in factors VII, VIII, IX, and X, and von Willebrand factor.[43] Factor XI decreases slightly, and the free protein S levels show a 60% to 70% decrease.[44] Low or low normal fibrinogen typically signals consumptive coagulopathy and must be addressed rapidly.

Alkaline phosphatase levels are highly elevated in pregnancy owing to placental production and reach 2 to 3 times baseline by the third trimester.[30] Glomerular filtration rate is increased by 50% after conception, whereas blood urea nitrogen and serum creatinine decrease as a result. Owing to pregnancy physiology, accurate calculation of the glomerular filtration rate via the Cockcroft-Gault and Modification of Diet in Renal Disease formulas is limited.[45] Values of 0.9 mg/dL for creatinine and

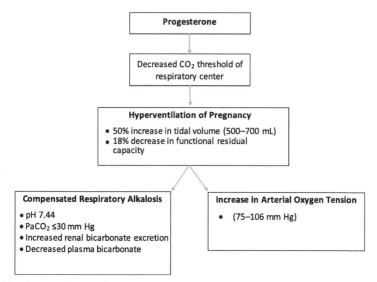

Fig. 2. Respiratory changes in pregnancy.

14 for blood urea nitrogen are suspect for underlying pathology in pregnant women, although they may not be outside the normal laboratory reference ranges.

MANAGEMENT OF TRAUMA

Core Advance Trauma Life Support protocols should be followed in the evaluation of a pregnant trauma patient, because these steps are proven to improve outcomes. Better maternal outcomes increase the chance of fetal survival and well-being. However, there are several modifications and additions to these protocols to allow for the simultaneous care of 2 patients (a mother and a fetus). See **Fig. 3** for a summary. If there is advance warning of an OB trauma arrival, a member of the OB team can save valuable time for the patient and fetus by obtaining as much information as possible before their arrival. Quick access to accurate records to determine gestational age, amount of prenatal care, fetal number, and other comorbidities is invaluable. Activation of an OB trauma alert also gives the team time to ready the OB ultrasound equipment, a precipitous delivery pack, a cesarean delivery (CD) pack,

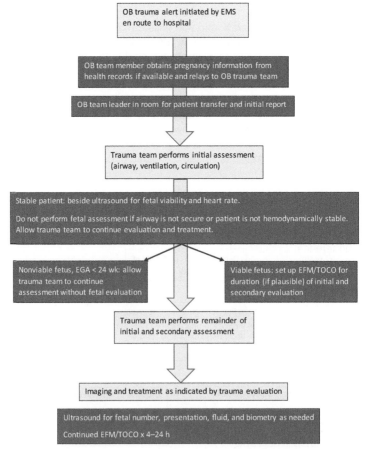

Fig. 3. Obstetric (OB) modifications to trauma protocol (*dark blue*). EFM, external fetal monitoring; EGA, estimated gestational age; EMS, emergency medical services; TOCO, tocodynamometer.

and mobilize the neonatal intensive care unit (NICU) team. If indicated, the trauma team can place an operating room (OR) on hold for any anticipated maternal injuries. En route, the emergency medical services (EMS) transport team can update everyone involved with maternal vital signs, airway status, Glasgow coma score, and other measures as available.

Initial Evaluation

If the patient is brought to a trauma bay in the emergency department for major trauma evaluation, the trauma team should be allowed to perform the initial assessment and determination of stability. This typically includes the ABCDEs (airway and c-spine protection, breathing and ventilation, circulation and hemorrhage control, disability, and exposure). Do not perform a fetal assessment if the maternal airway is not secure or the patient is not hemodynamically stable. A low threshold for early intubation should be considered given the fetal dependence on maternal oxygenation. If not ventilated, supplemental O_2 should be provided. If maternal spinal injury is not a concern, place the back board on a slight leftward tilt (15°) or place wedge under the right hip. Initial efforts of the OB team should focus on displacing the uterus and obtaining gestational age information while maternal stability is assessed.

Once initial stability is ensured by assessment of the airway, ventilation, and circulation, the obstetrician can quickly assess the fetus with beside ultrasound imaging. Meanwhile, the trauma team can continue to assess the patient and secure intravenous lines. If respiratory and hemodynamic stability cannot be confirmed before the Focused Assessment with Sonography in Trauma scan or chest/pelvis radiographs, these should be performed before OB ultrasound. Although the viability and well-being of the fetus is important to determine, the team cannot act on any information gained by ultrasound examination if the mother is not fit for intervention such as emergent CD. Communication between the trauma team leader and the OB team leader will be key in determining this timing. If the estimated gestational age is known and viability is assumed, then an initial quick determination of viability and heart rate via ultrasound is sufficient.

Monotonous

If the estimated gestational age is not known, then a quick assessment with biometry (head circumference, biparietal diameter, abdominal circumference, and or femur length; **Figs. 4–7**)[46] or cerebellar measurement can assist in making this determination. After this, if the maternal clinical scenario permits, further assessment of fetal number, presentation, placentation, and amniotic fluid is indicated.

If the fetus is nonviable (owing to stillbirth or by early estimated gestational age), allow the trauma team to complete maternal stabilization and resuscitative efforts. It is important to recognize that, if the fetus is demised, the precipitating factor may be owing to concealed intrauterine or retroperitoneal hemorrhage. If the fetus is viable and the clinical scenario is appropriate, work with trauma team to set up external fetal monitoring (EFM) and tocodynamometer (TOCO) monitoring while they continue their evaluation. EFM can also act as a supplemental maternal vital sign during the secondary evaluation. Adequate uterine perfusion is required to provide fetal oxygenation and a gestational age–appropriate EFM tracing. A decrease in uterine perfusion owing to maternal hypotension, hemorrhage, and so on could be signaled by an increase in uterine contractions or fetal heart rate decelerations. A member of the OB team should be with the patient while on EFM/TOCO at all times.

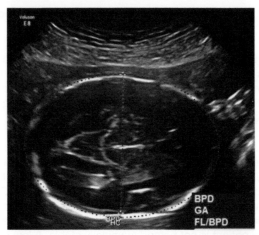

Fig. 4. Correct determination of fetal head measurements to estimate gestational age. Bi-parietal diameter (BPD): Section through the fetal head containing the thalamus and third ventricle. Calvarium must be smooth and symmetric. Place calipers from outside to inside of calvarium. Head circumference (HC): BPD requirements in a plane that contains the cavum septum pellucidi and the tentorial hiatus. Place ellipse to calvarial edges, not skin edges.

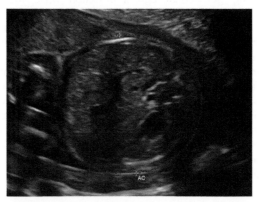

Fig. 5. Correct determination of fetal abdominal circumference (AC) to estimate gestational age. Section where the right and left portal veins are continuous with one another. Lower ribs are symmetric. Ellipse measures skin edge. Avoid significant transducer pressure to keep AC round. Stomach is almost always seen.

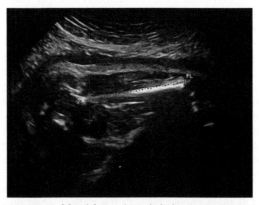

Fig. 6. Correct determination of fetal femur length (FL) to estimate gestational age. Obtain long axis view of the femur by viewing the cartilaginous femoral head, greater trochanter, and lateral condyle. Place calipers at junction of cartilage and ossified bone.

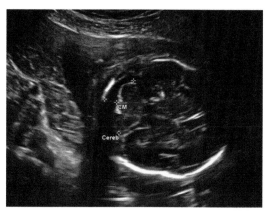

Fig. 7. Correct determination of fetal transverse cerebellar diameter to estimate gestational age. Measure widest section of "dumbbell" in the posterior fossa. Cereb, cerebellum; CM, cisterna magna.

Operating Room Monitoring

Often trauma patients will require continued evaluation and emergent treatment in the OR. If the fetus is known to be viable or OB assessment has not occurred, the obstetrician should accompany the team to the OR to perform fetal assessment there when feasible. This information will be valuable to the trauma and anesthesia teams. Intermittent fetal heart rate and viability monitoring can be performed (pending patient positioning) in the OR with sterile ultrasound probe cover. Again, monitoring should only occur if there is a safe opportunity for fetal intervention. Surgical intervention including exploratory laparotomy should not be avoided or delayed if indicated. The patient should be positioned to allow for uterine displacement.

Maternal Code

Typically, in a maternal code situation, the OB provider can delegate responsibility of running the maternal code to the trauma team. However, the obstetrician and their understanding of pregnancy physiology plays a very significant role. The obstetrician supports the resuscitative team in not deviating from appropriate advanced cardiac life support algorithms simply because the patient is pregnant. Even cardioversion indications are the same for pregnant and nonpregnant patients; therefore, pregnancy should not alter this or any portion of the advanced cardiac life support algorithm. Cardiopulmonary resuscitation can only provide 30% of cardiac output with a patient in the supine position. However, aortocaval compression from the gravid uterus (>20-week size) limits effective circulation. Unfortunately, placing the patient in tilt to relieve this compression makes chest compressions even more ineffective. Providing manual displacement of the uterus should be considered.

In the setting of a viable fetus or multiple gestations with suspected deleterious aortocaval compression, once a code is called, CD (perimortem CD) should be initiated if possible within 4 minutes. This timing balances opportunity to revive the mother without delivery, increase neonatal survival, and improve likelihood of effective perfusion with cardiopulmonary resuscitation.[47] A sterile field and OR are not required, and attempts to obtain these will only delay delivery. A resuscitation team for the neonate should be notified of impending delivery at the time of code. Clear, efficient communication among the multidisciplinary team involved in the code is key before proceeding with perimortem CD. Complete discussion of this topic occurs elsewhere (See Bennett T, Katz VL, Zelop CM: Cardiac Arrest and Resuscitation Unique to Pregnancy, in this issue).

Indications for delivery based on maternal respiratory compromise are not as clear cut. Most of what we know comes from ventilated patients critically ill with pneumonia. Delivery has been shown to decrease Fio_2 requirement, but not necessarily improve maternal outcomes.[48] However, maternal mortality may be increased by CD.[49–51] Therefore, if there is concern that CD would increase immediate mortality, then consideration should be given to no fetal monitoring until this risk is improved.

Secondary Evaluation

The secondary evaluation can typically continue in a simultaneous maternal and fetal fashion, with EFM of the fetus while the maternal evaluation continues. Secondary evaluation continues to assess for maternal and fetal injury as well as abruption, preterm labor, and fetal–maternal hemorrhage.

Radiologic diagnostic testing will almost always be indicated after significant trauma. Abdominal evaluation can initially be assessed via Focused Assessment with Sonography in Trauma scan or diagnostic peritoneal lavage. These do not rule out retroperitoneal, diaphragmatic, or solid organ injury that may be detected on computed tomography (CT) scanning. Radiographs may also be indicated to fully assess maternal injury. Diagnostic testing, including ionizing radiation, should proceed as indicated despite pregnancy. Attempts can be made to limit exposure, such as avoiding a pelvic plain radiograph if there is no tenderness or hip girdle instability or if a CT scan of the pelvis is already planned.

Theoretic fetal risks associated with ionizing radiation include cell death, teratogenesis, carcinogenesis, and induced genetic changes in germ cells lines. Cell death is thought to be an "all or none phenomenon" that occurs in early embryonic development.[52] Microcephaly and mental retardation risks increase after exposures of 10 to 20 rad.[53] Adverse pregnancy outcomes (anomalies, growth restriction, pregnancy loss) have not been seen with exposure of less than 5 rad. This is far below the exposure of an abdominal or chest CT (**Table 2**).[52] Radiographs carry a far lower radiation dose than CT. Carcinogenic risk to the fetus is difficult to

Table 2 Estimated fetal radiation exposure	
Radiology Exam	**Estimated Fetal Radiation Exposure (rad)**
Thoracic spine radiograph	<0.001
Chest (posteroanterior/lateral)	0.001
CT head	<0.01
Hip radiograph	0.13
Pelvis radiograph	0.17
Abdominal radiograph	0.24
Lumbar spine radiograph	0.34
CT abdomen/pelvis	1–2

Adapted from Cohn DC, Ramaswamy B, Blum K. Malignancy and pregnancy. In: Greene MF, Creasy RK, Resnik R, et al, editors. Creasy and Resnik's maternal-fetal medicine principles and practice. 6th edition. Philadelphia: Saunders Elsevier; 2009. p. 889.

estimate, but is thought to increase from a baseline childhood leukemia risk of 1 in 3000 children to 1 in 2000.[52]

MRI does not carry the risk of radiation exposure. Studies have shown no detrimental effects to pregnancy at 1.5 T or lower magnetic field. Unfortunately, there are no data for 2.5 T or higher fields.[54] Gadolinium-containing contrast is typically avoided unless necessary for an accurate diagnosis. Gadolinium crosses the placenta and remains in the amniotic fluid; however, no studies have shown adverse fetal or neonatal effects.[53]

Once the mother is stabilized, or perhaps even released from the emergency department or trauma care, continued OB evaluation will likely be indicated. Patients with minor trauma often undergo initial evaluation in OB triage and do not require assessment in the emergency department or activation of a trauma response team. For these patients and for those that have been released from the emergency department, this evaluation includes monitoring for abruption, preterm labor, and fetal distress. Abruption is not predicted by the severity of maternal injury and is difficult to detect in the absence of vaginal bleeding.[1,9,23–25] Abruption in the setting of MVC may not be clinically apparent until more than 24 hours after the event.[23,26] Ultrasound imaging, while often performed after trauma to rule out abruption, actually has a very low sensitivity (25%–50%) to detect abruption. If seen, a retroplacental bleed may seem to "jiggle" when the transducer moves it, a "Jello sign."[28] A normal ultrasound examination cannot rule out an abruption.[55–57] Detection must rely on clinical suspicion and examination. Contractions as a result of abruption, particularly in the setting of trauma, may not be noted on clinical examination, highlighting again the need for TOCO monitoring.[58]

EFM and TOCO have been studied extensively in their usefulness for detecting adverse outcomes in a trauma setting and, based on this analysis, the common 4-hour window of monitoring was established. In multiple studies, all adverse pregnancy outcomes were detected in those women with clinical evidence of abruption in the initial 4 hours of monitoring.[6,18,23,59] Stated differently, in 1 study, no adverse outcomes were seen in those patients without clinical evidence of abruption, or contractions less than every 15 minutes, during the 4-hour monitoring window.[9] The literature is less clear on the next step if there are contractions or other concerning findings in the initial four-hour window, but a 24-hour period of monitoring is generally accepted. During this time, betamethasone administration can also be initiated. Given the risk of preterm delivery and adverse outcomes in even cases of minor trauma, betamethasone administration should be considered in all patients admitted with trauma between 24 and 36 6/7 weeks.

If the patient is Rh negative, rho (D) immune globulin should be provided to the patient, even the setting of a negative Kleihauer-Betke test (KB). KB may be required to help calculate rho (D) immune globulin dose in those women with significant fetal–maternal hemorrhage. Outside of rho (D) immune globulin dose calculation, KB has not been shown to alter management because it has been found positive in the absence of abruption and negative in proven abruption.[23,26,60] Fetal anemia related to fetal–maternal hemorrhage can manifest as fetal tachycardia, fetal heart rate decelerations, or sinusoidal tracing on EFM. Therefore, EFM is much more likely to allow for appropriate fetal intervention over that of a KB.

Tetanus injection is safe in pregnancy and should be administered after the same indications as those for nonpregnant trauma patients. Pregnant women are at increased risk for venous thromboembolism, and if immobilized as a result of injuries sustained in trauma, prophylaxis with heparin or low-molecular-weight heparin should be considered.

Prevention

Certainly, the best treatment of trauma in pregnancy is primary prevention. Two of the largest contributors to trauma cases are MVC and IPV. As OB providers, we can initiate screening, education, and intervention toward prevention. One-third of women often stop wearing a seatbelt or wearing 1 correctly in pregnancy owing to discomfort, inconvenience, or fears of harming the pregnancy.[2] Study of seatbelt use in pregnancy has shown an 84% reduction in adverse fetal outcomes in those dyads protected by proper seat belt restraint.[11] All adult passengers, pregnant or not, are best protected by a 3-point restraint applied with shoulder belt across the shoulder and chest with lap belt low across the hip girdle and thighs (**Fig. 8**). Air bags are safe to use for pregnant women.[12–15]

OB provider visits may be the only opportunity a victim isolated by IPV has to reach out for or receive help. Often the perpetrator is with the victim in the examination room; therefore, attempts should be made to speak with a patient alone when screening for IPV. However, confrontation of a perpetrator can cause escalation of violence or retribution toward the victim. Therefore, other intervention options can be made available such as palm or shoe cards from the National Domestic Violence Hotline in the women's restroom (**Fig. 9**). Women can obtain these when providing routine prenatal urine sample. All OB patients should be screened for IPV or other abuse at prenatal care visits as well as trauma evaluations.

Preparation

Prevention is not always possible; therefore, preparation is tantamount to success in caring for pregnant trauma patients. All trauma centers with OB services should consider establishing an OB trauma protocol that involves team members from EMS, trauma, the emergency department, OB, NICU, and the OR (**Fig. 10**). Protocol

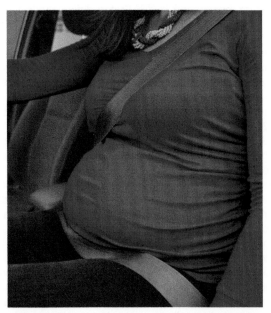

Fig. 8. Proper seat belt placement in pregnancy. Strap should lay across shoulder, between breasts, along the side of abdomen. Lap belt should be low across upper thighs and hip bones.

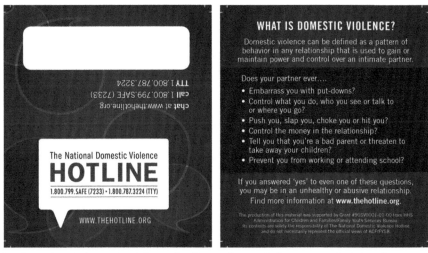

Fig. 9. National domestic violence hotline palm card. (*Courtesy of* National Domestic Violence Hotline, Austin, Texas. Available at: www.thehotline.org; with permission.)

should be developed as a collaborative effort among those on the team and regular cross-specialty education and multidisciplinary simulation instituted. Simulation helps to trouble shoot logistical problems with the protocol and an institution's handling of OB trauma in a no risk scenario. It also improves communication across and within specialties on the team and increases comfort level when in a real trauma scenario.[61]

Suggested Roles for Each Team

- EMS
  - Mechanism to activate OB trauma alert ahead of arrival.
  - Continued notification of all team members of estimated time of arrival, patient hemodynamic and respiratory status, pregnancy information including due date if known, fetal number, and pertinent patient history.
- Emergency department
  - Staging area large enough to accommodate EMS; trauma, OB, and NICU teams; portable ultrasound equipment, precipitous delivery and CD packs, and NICU warmer and supplies.
  - Team and capacity for handling nonpregnant trauma victims.
  - Access to blood bank and massive transfusion protocols.
- Trauma team
  - Advance Trauma Life Support trained with expertise in assessing and treating trauma victims.
- OB
  - Team of obstetrician, labor and delivery nurse(s), and an OB scrub technician.
  - Obstetrician capable of limited ultrasound assessment including fetal heart rate, fetal presentation, and limited biometry.
  - Ability to place and interpret EFM and TOCO, nurse staffing capable of one-on-one care while patient is not on the labor floor.
  - Ability to perform emergent CD.

- NICU team
  - ○ Neonatal intensivists and/or neonatal nurse practitioners capable of immediate neonatal resuscitation/stabilization including intubation.
  - ○ Expertise in assessment of gestational age if not known before delivery.
- OR with team and space large enough to accommodate:
  - ○ Polytrauma patient,
  - ○ Trauma team,
  - ○ Diagnostic imaging equipment,
  - ○ OB team (physician, nurse, scrub technician, portable ultrasound and/or fetal monitor), and
  - ○ NICU team (neonatal intensivists, nurse, respiratory therapist, NICU warmer, isolette for neonatal transport).

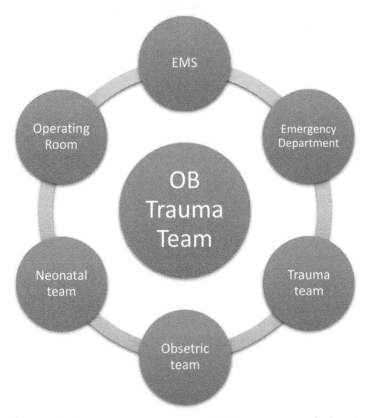

Fig. 10. Obstetrics (OB) trauma team components. EMS, emergency medical services.

SUMMARY

Trauma complicating pregnancy requires a multidisciplinary approach to provide the highest quality trauma care to 2 patients simultaneously. Care must incorporate knowledge of physiologic changes of pregnancy as well as risks unique to pregnancy.

Summary points
- Fifty percent of fetal losses occur in what if often considered to be minor trauma.
- Proper seat belt use in pregnancy reduces adverse fetal outcomes by 84% in MVC.

- Clinical signs of hemorrhage and shock are delayed in pregnant women, and mortality is increased when blood loss is sufficient to result in tachycardia and hypotension.
- Only perform fetal assessment if the mother has a secure airway and is hemodynamically stable.
- Have a low threshold for early intubation or supplemental oxygen.
- Displace the gravid uterus to prevent aortocaval compression.
- Diagnostic testing, including ionizing radiation, should proceed as indicated despite pregnancy.
- EFM/TOCO monitoring is indicated in most cases, when the fetus is viable, for 4 to 24 hours.
- Screen all trauma and pregnant patients for IPV.

REFERENCES

1. Connolly AM, Katz VL, Bash KL, et al. Trauma and pregnancy. Am J Perinatol 1997;14:331–6.
2. Pearlman MD, Phillips ME. Safety belt use during pregnancy. Obstet Gynecol 1996;88:1026–9.
3. El-Kady D, Gilbert WM, Anderson J, et al. Trauma during pregnancy: an analysis of maternal and fetal outcomes in a large population. Am J Obstet Gynecol 2004; 190:1661–8.
4. Williams JK, McClain L, Rosemurgy AS, et al. Evaluation of blunt abdominal trauma in the third trimester of pregnancy: maternal and fetal considerations. Obstet Gynecol 1990;75:33–7.
5. Kuo C, Jamieson DJ, McPheeters ML, et al. Injury hospitalizations of pregnant women in the United States, 2002. Am J Obstet Gynecol 2007;196:161.e1-e6.
6. Cahill AG, Bastek JA, Stamilio DM, et al. Minor trauma in pregnancy—is the evaluation unwarranted? Am J Obstet Gynecol 2008;198(2):208.e1-e5.
7. Weiss HB, Songer TJ, Fabio A. Fetal deaths related to maternal injury. JAMA 2001;286:1863–8.
8. Crosby WM. Traumatic injuries during pregnancy. Clin Obstet Gynecol 1983;26: 902–12.
9. Pearlman MD, Tintinalli JE, Lorenz RP. A prospective controlled study of outcome after trauma during pregnancy. Am J Obstet Gynecol 1990;162:1502–7.
10. Fischer PE, Zarzaur BL, Fabian TC, et al. Minor trauma is an unrecognized contributor to poor fetal outcomes: a population-based study of 78,552 pregnancies. J Trauma 2011;71:90–3.
11. Klinich KD, Flannagan CAC, Rupp JD, et al. Fetal outcome in motor-vehicle crashes: effects of crash characteristics and maternal restraint. Am J Obstet Gynecol 2008;198:450.e1-e9.
12. Automobile passenger restraints for children and pregnant women. ACOG technical bulletin number 151—January 1991 (replaces no. 74, December 1983). Int J Gynaecol Obstet 1992;37:305–8.
13. Pearlman MD, Viano D. Automobile crash simulation with the first pregnant crash test dummy. Am J Obstet Gynecol 1996;175(Pt 1):977–81.
14. Moorcroft DM, Stitzel JD, Duma GG, et al. Computational model of the pregnant occupant: predicting the risk of injury in automobile crashes. Am J Obstet Gynecol 2003;189:540–4.
15. Hyde LK, Cook LJ, Olson LM, et al. Effect of motor vehicle crashes on adverse fetal outcomes. Obstet Gynecol 2003;102:279–86.

16. Gazmararian JA, Lazorick S, Spitz AM, et al. Prevalence of violence against pregnant women. JAMA 1996;275:1915–20.

17. Chang J, Berg CJ, Saltzman LE, et al. Homicide: a leading cause of injury deaths among pregnant and postpartum women in the United States, 1991-1999. Am J Public Health 2001;95:471–7.

18. Goodwin TM, Breen MT. Pregnancy outcome and fetomaternal hemorrhage after noncatastrophic trauma. Am J Obstet Gynecol 1990;162:665–71.

19. Kuhlmann RS, Cruikshank DP. Maternal trauma during pregnancy. Clin Obstet Gynecol 1994;37:274–93.

20. Dhanraj D, Lambers D. The incidences of positive Kleihauer-Betke test in low-risk pregnancies and maternal trauma patients. Am J Obstet Gynecol 2004;190:1461–3.

21. Lavery JP, Staten-McCormick M. Management of moderate to severe trauma in pregnancy. Obstet Gynecol Clin North Am 1995;22:69–90.

22. Palmer JD, Sparrow OC. Extradural haematoma following intrauterine trauma. Injury 1994;25:671–3.

23. Dahmus MA, Sibai BM. Blunt abdominal trauma: are there any predictive factors for abruptio placentae or maternal-fetal distress? Am J Obstet Gynecol 1993;169:1054–9.

24. Schiff MA, Holt VL. The Injury Severity Score in pregnant trauma patients: predicting placental abruption and fetal death. J Trauma 2002;53:946–9.

25. Baerga-Varela Y, Zietlow SP, Bannon MP, et al. Trauma in pregnancy. Mayo Clin Proc 2000;75:1243–8.

26. Towery R, English TP, Wisner D. Evaluation of pregnant women after blunt injury. J Trauma 1993;35:731–5 [discussion: 735–6].

27. Givvs JM, Weindling AM. Neonatal intracranial lesions following placental abruption. Eur J Pediatr 1994;153:195–7.

28. Hull AD, Resnik R. Placenta previa, placenta accreta, abruptio placentae, and vasa previa. In: Greene MF, Creasy RK, Resnik R, et al, editors. Creasy and Resnik's maternal-fetal medicine principles and practice. 6th edition. Philadelphia: Saunders Elsevier; 2009. p. 725–37.

29. Centers for Disease Control and Prevention. Current trends: CDC criteria for anemia in children and childbearing-aged women. MMWR Morb Mortal Wkly Rep 1989;38:400–4.

30. Girling JC, Dow E, Smith JH. Liver function tests in preeclampsia: Importance of comparison with a reference range derived for normal pregnancy. BJOG 1997;104:246–50.

31. Dildy G, Clark SL, Phelan JP, et al. Maternal-fetal blood gas physiology. In: Dildy GA III, Belfort MA, Saade GR, et al, editors. Critical care obstetrics. 4th edition. New York: Blackwell; 2004.

32. Clark SL, Cotton DB, Lee W, et al. Central hemodynamic assessment of normal term pregnancy. Am J Obstet Gynecol 1989;161:1439.

33. Robson SC, Hunter S, Moore M, et al. Haemodynamic changes during the puerperium: a Doppler and M-mode echocardiographic study. BJOG 1987;94:1028.

34. Pritchard JA. Changes in the blood volume during pregnancy and delivery. Anesthesiology 1965;26:393.

35. Laros RK Jr, editor. Blood disorders in pregnancy. Philadelphia: Lea & Febiger; 1986.

36. Wiebe ER, Trouton KJ, Eftekhar A. Anemia in early pregnancy among Canadian women presenting for abortion. Int J Gynaecol Obstet 2006;94:60–1.

37. Barron W, Lindheeimer M. Medical disorders during pregnancy. St Louis (MO): CV Mosby; 1991. p. 234.
38. Limacher MC, Ware JA, O'Meara MED, et al. Tricuspid regurgitation during pregnancy: two-dimensional and pulse Doppler echocardiographic observations. Am J Cardiol 1985;55:1059.
39. Turner AF. The chest radiograph during pregnancy. Clin Obstet Gynecol 1975;18:65.
40. Homes F. Incidence of the supine hypotensive syndrome in late pregnancy. J Obstet Gynaecol Br Emp 1960;67:254.
41. Ueland K, Novy M, Peterson E, et al. Maternal cardiovascular dynamics: IV. The influence of gestational age on the maternal cardiovascular response to posture and exercise. Am J Obstet Gynecol 1969;104:856.
42. Whitty JE, Dombrowski MP. Respiratory changes in pregnancy. In: Greene MF, Creasy RK, Resnik R, et al, editors. Creasy and Resnik's maternal-fetal medicine principles and practice. 6th edition. Philadelphia: Saunders Elsevier; 2009. p. 927–48.
43. Brenme KA. Haemostatic changes in pregnancy. Best Pract Res Clin Haemotol 2003;15:153–68.
44. Paidas MJ, Kim DH, Lee MJ, et al. Protein Z, protein S levels are lower in in patients with thrombophilia and subsequent pregnancy complications. J Thromb Haemost 2005;3:497–501.
45. Smith MC, Moran P, Ward MK, et al. Assessment of glomerular filtration rate during pregnancy using the MDRD formula. BJOG 2008;115:109–12.
46. Galan HL, Pandipati S, Filly RA. Ultrasound evaluation of fetal biometry and normal and abnormal growth. In: Callen PW, editor. Ultrasonography in Obstetrics and Gynecology. 5th edition. Philadelphia: Saunders; 2007. p. 225–65.
47. Katz VL, Dotters DJ, Droegemueller W. Perimortem cesarean delivery. Obstet Gynecol 1986;68(4):571–6.
48. Tomlinson MW, Caruthers TJ, Whitty JE, et al. Does delivery improve maternal condition in the respiratory-compromised gravida? Obstet Gynecol 1998;91:108–11.
49. Jenkins TM, Troiano NH, Graves CR, et al. Mechanical ventilation in an obstetric population: characteristics and delivery rates. Am J Obstet Gynecol 2003;188: 549–52.
50. Mabie WC, Barton JR, Sibai BM. Adult respiratory distress syndrome in pregnancy. Am J Obstet Gynecol 1992;167:950–7.
51. Collop NA, Sahn SA. Critical illness in pregnancy. An analysis of 20 patients admitted to a medical intensive care unit. Chest 1993;103:1548–52.
52. ACOG Committee on Obstetric Practice. ACOG Committee Opinion. Number 299, September 2004 (replaces No. 158, September 1995). Guidelines for diagnostic imaging during pregnancy. Obstet Gynecol 2004;104(3):647–51.
53. Contag SA, Mertz HL, Bushnell CD. Migraine during pregnancy: is it more than a headache? Nat Rev Neurol 2009;5(8):449–56.
54. Sundgren PC, Leander P. Is administration of gadolinium-based contrast media to pregnant women and small children justified? J Magn Reson Imaging 2011; 34(4):750–7.
55. Glantz C, Purnell L. Clinical utility of sonography in the diagnosis and treatment of placental abruption. J Ultrasound Med 2002;21:837–40.
56. Sholl JS. Abruptio placentae: clinical utility of sonography in the diagnosis and treatment of placental abruption. Am J Obstet Gynecol 1987;156:40–51.
57. Jaffe MH, Schoen WC, Silver TM, et al. Sonography of abruptio placentae. Am J Roentgenol 1981;137:1049–54.

58. Warner MW, Salfinger SG, Rao S, et al. Management of trauma during pregnancy. Aust NZ J Surg 2004;74:125–8.

59. Rothenberger D, Quattlebaum FW, Perry JF, et al. Blunt maternal trauma: a review of 103 cases. J Trauma 1978;18:173–9.

60. Emery CL, Morway LF, Chung-Park M, et al. The Kleihauer-Betke test: clinical utility, indication, and correlation in patients with placental abruption and cocaine use. Arch Pathol Lab Med 1995;119:1032–7.

61. Gaba DM. The future vision of simulation in healthcare. Qual Saf Health Care 2004;13:i2–10.

Cardiac Arrest and Resuscitation Unique to Pregnancy

Terri-Ann Bennett, MD[a], Vern L. Katz, MD[b,c],
Carolyn M. Zelop, MD[d,e],*

KEYWORDS

- Maternal cardiac arrest • Maternal cardiopulmonary arrest • Maternal code
- Maternal resuscitation

KEY POINTS

- Physiologic changes in pregnancy require special consideration during resuscitative efforts.
- Cardiopulmonary resuscitation (CPR) should be performed with the mother in the supine position accompanied by manual left lateral uterine displacement.
- If cardiac arrest persists, delivery should be initiated at 4 minutes.
- Multidisciplinary teamwork is key to successful resuscitation.

Maternal cardiopulmonary arrest (MCPA) is a catastrophic event that can cause significant morbidity and mortality. Although maternal mortality is usually considered a developing world problem, it is important to note that the maternal mortality ratio (MMR) for the United States had doubled from 12 to 28 maternal deaths per 100,000 live births from 1990 to 2013, and US MMR in 2015 was 14. Meanwhile, the MMR of the developing world has had a 44% decrease.[1,2]

There are multiple reasons to explain this trend, including better ascertainment of cases and an increase in comorbidities of the pregnant population, particularly cardiovascular conditions, which rank number 1 among the etiologies.[3,4] However, it would be remiss not to thoroughly consider and evaluate how practices can be improved to save mothers' lives.

Conflicts of Interest: C.M. Zelop reports that she is a consultant for UpTodate on the same topic.
[a] Division of Maternal-Fetal Medicine, Department of Obstetrics and Gynecology, New York University Langone Medical Center, 560 1st Avenue, New York, NY 10016, USA; [b] Department of Obstetrics and Gynecology, Oregon Health and Science University, Portland, OR, USA; [c] Department of Human Physiology, University of Oregon, Eugene, OR, USA; [d] Division of Maternal-Fetal Medicine, Department of Obstetrics and Gynecology, The Valley Hospital, Ridgewood, NJ, USA; [e] Department of Obstetrics and Gynecology, New York University School of Medicine, New York, NY, USA
* Corresponding author. 12 Thistle Hollow, Avon, CT 06001.
E-mail address: cmzelop@comcast.net

Obstet Gynecol Clin N Am 43 (2016) 809–819
http://dx.doi.org/10.1016/j.ogc.2016.07.011
obgyn.theclinics.com

MCPA is an especially challenging clinical scenario for any provider, as it is an overall rare occurrence and involves 2 patients—mother and baby. A prepared, multidisciplinary team is necessary to perform basic and advanced cardiac life support specific to the anatomic and physiologic changes of pregnancy. These procedures should be initiated immediately and maneuvers performed simultaneously rather than sequentially.

PREVALENCE

According to the National Inpatient Sample of 1998 to 2011, approximately 1 in 12,000 (or 8.5 per 100,000) hospitalizations for delivery were complicated by maternal cardiac arrest.[5] Only 59% of women survived.[5]

ETIOLOGY

The cause of MCPA includes pregnancy-related and nonpregnancy-related etiologies. In the National Inpatient Sample, antepartum and postpartum hemorrhage accounted for the largest percentage of MCPA cases.[5] Other etiologies were heart failure, amniotic fluid embolism, sepsis, anesthesia complications, aspiration pneumonitis, venous thromboembolism, and eclampsia.[5] Other common etiologies include out-of-hospital trauma and domestic abuse.

The American Heart Association (AHA) has devised mnemonics to recognize etiologies of MCPA (**Box 1** and **Table 1**).[6,7]

MANAGEMENT

Imagine there is a 34-year-old African-American Gravida 1 Para 0 (G1P0) at 36 weeks with class B diabetes on insulin who is diagnosed with preeclampsia with severe features. She requires intravenous administration of antihypertensive agents given severe range of blood pressures. She is started on magnesium for maternal seizure prophylaxis, and an induction of labor is initiated with an insulin drip. Cytotec is used for cervical ripening followed by Pitocin for contraction augmentation. Artificial rupture of membranes is performed. She receives an epidural for pain management. The patient suddenly becomes bradycardic, then unresponsive, and asystole is detected. What is the next best step?

Box 1
Reversible causes of cardiac arrest

H
  Hypoxia
  Hypovolemia
  Hydrogen ion (acidosis)
  Hypo-/hyperkalemia
  Hypothermia

T
  Toxins
  Tamponade, cardiac
  Tension pneumothorax
  Thrombosis, pulmonary
  Thrombosis, coronary

From Neumar RW, Otto CW, Link MS, et al. Part 8: adult advanced cardiovascular life support: 2010 American Heart Association guidelines for cardiopulmonary resuscitation and emergency cardiovascular care. Circulation 2010;122(18 Suppl 3):S737; with permission.

Table 1	
Etiology of maternal cardiac arrest	
A	Anesthesia/accidents (trauma)
B	Bleeding
C	Cardiovascular
D	Drugs
E	Embolic
F	Fever
G	General nonobstetric causes (H/Ts)
H	Hypertension

Adapted from Jeejeebhoy FM, Zelop CM, Lipman S, et al. Cardiac arrest in pregnancy: a scientific statement from the American Heart Association. Circulation 2015;132(18):1763; with permission.

The recommendations for management of MCPA are based upon expert opinion, case reports, and extrapolated data from nonpregnant cardiac arrest patients. However, for successful resuscitative efforts, it is imperative to understand the anatomic and physiologic changes of pregnancy that must be accommodated when executing basic life support (BLS) and advanced cardiac life support (ACLS) (**Table 2**).

Principles of Maternal Resuscitation During a Cardiac Arrest

Although the components are listed sequentially, simultaneous execution is required for successful resuscitation.

Table 2	
Physiologic changes of pregnancy	
Cardiovascular	↑ Stroke volume ↑ Cardiac output ↑ Heart rate
Circulatory	↓ Systemic vascular resistance ↓ Mean arterial pressure ↓ Venous return ↑ Blood volume ↑ Red cell mass ↑ Procoagulants
Respiratory	*Elevation in diaphragm position* ↓ Expiratory reserve volume ↓ Residual volume ↓ Functional residual capacity ↑ Inspiratory capacity ↑ Tidal volume ↑ Minute Ventilation ↓ Total pulmonary resistance
Gastrointestinal	↓ Gastrointestinal tract motility ↓ Competence of lower esophageal sphincter
Renal	↑ Glomerular filtration rate
Metabolic	↑ Basal metabolic rate ↓ CO_2 ↓ HCO_3

First, call a maternal code blue

This multidisciplinary team should include obstetricians, anesthesiologists, neonatologists, nurses, the code team, and cart. The maternal code team should be knowledgeable about the alterations required for resuscitation of a pregnant woman and be well prepared for this challenging clinical scenario. This can be achieved through reliance upon clinical experiences, didactics, and simulation. Each member of the team should have an assigned role, such as a designated leader, rotating parties to perform cardiopulmonary resuscitation (CPR), and a recorder for documentation.

If the uterus is at the umbilicus, perform a left lateral displacement

In pregnancy, cardiac output increases up to 50%, and systemic vascular resistance decreases, leading to a decreased mean arterial pressure.[8–10] As the uterus enlarges, there is an increase in compression of the vessels in the pelvis and abdomen. The vena cava is obstructed at the level of the fundus, as early as 12 to 14 weeks, and is particularly profound when the parturient is in the supine position.[11,12] Aortocaval compression is substantial when the gravid uterus reaches the umbilicus, and can significantly affect cardiac output by decreasing venous return and increasing cardiac afterload. Postural changes can also cause profound hemodynamic changes. When a parturient is supine, there is a decrease in cardiac output and a postural hypotension, which can lead to fetal hypoxia.[12,13]

The efficiency of resuscitative vectors can be affected by the angle of inclination. The resuscitative force is almost halved from the supine (0-degree) to the tilted 90-degree angle.[14] The efficacy of chest compressions was assessed with a calibrated force transducer and concluded that 27-degrees was the optimal angle for lateral displacement.[14] Thus, in order to accomplish adequate venous return and effective resuscitation, for both mother and baby, uterine displacement of approximately 30-degrees is necessary.

Left uterine displacement (LUD) can be accomplished by several measures: tilting the bed, placing a wedge, or manually via the 1- or 2-hand technique (**Figs. 1–3**).[15]

In a systematic review, it was suggested that in order to accomplish high-quality chest compressions, it is best to maintain a supine position while achieving aortocaval decompression with a supine manual leftward uterine displacement.[6] In addition to possibly more efficient compressions, manual left uterine displacement may also allow for easier access to airway management and defibrillation.[6]

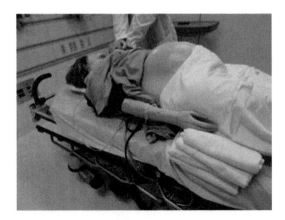

Fig. 1. 30° tilt.

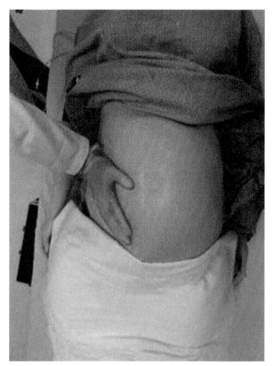

Fig. 2. 1-hand LUD.

Once aortocaval decompression is established, one can proceed to the C-A-C (compression-airway-circulation) protocol of CPR.

Initiate chest compressions

CPR should be performed in the same manner for pregnant and nonpregnant patients. The patient should be placed on a hard surface, and high-quality, uninterrupted, chest compressions should be initiated immediately after the diagnosis of cardiac arrest. Chest compressions should be performed at a rate of at least 100 per minute at a depth of at least 2 inches while allowing chest recoil between compressions.[6]

It was previously recommended that the hand placement for chest compressions in pregnant woman be more cephaled (2–3 cm higher on the sternum) to adjust for the suspected superior displacement of the heart secondary to elevated diaphragm from the gravid uterus. However, a recent MRI study revealed that there is no significant vertical displacement of the heart in the third trimester of pregnancy.[16] Due to the absence of data supporting a different approach in pregnancy, the AHA guidelines on cardiac arrest in pregnancy recommend the same hand position for the performance of chest compressions in pregnant women and nonpregnant adults.[6]

Defibrillation pads should be placed on the arrested parturient as soon as possible to determine if the rhythm is amenable to defibrillation. The newer biphasic models require lower voltage and are considered safe in all stages of pregnancy.[15] The energy required for defibrillation in the pregnant patient is the same as in the nonpregnant patient.[15,17] Automatic external defibrillators (AEDs) may be more practical and readily available in obstetric settings, because there is less familiarity with rhythm analysis. Fetal heart rate monitors should be removed early in the resuscitation process.

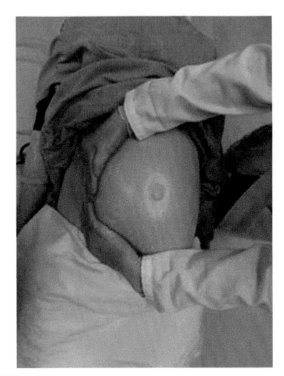

Fig. 3. 2-hand LUD.

Although there is only a theoretic risk of electrocution, it is the maternal status and not the fetal status that dictates clinical management.

Secure an airway

The anatomic and physiologic changes of pregnancy render the parturient a difficult airway, with a higher oxygen requirement and risk for hypoxemia. The elevation in estrogen levels promotes vascularity and increased interstitial fluid deposition in the larynx and pharynx. Thus, landmarks become distorted, leading to a greater risk of failed intubation.[18]

As the gravid uterus displaces the diaphragm more cephalad, there is a decrease in the functional residual capacity, increasing the tendency to desaturate more quickly during oxygen deprivation. Additionally, higher circulating levels of progesterone promote decreased gastrointestinal motility, and the gastric sphincter response is reduced, resulting in a greater likelihood of aspiration.[19] Thus, securing an airway during a maternal cardiopulmonary arrest is paramount.

When available, one should perform bag–mask ventilation of 100% oxygen by giving two breaths every 30 compressions.[6] This should be done by using the 2-hand technique to create a mask seal and providing a sufficient tidal volume to produce visible chest rise.[6] Ideally, intubation provides the best ventilation technique, but this should be performed with minimal interruption of CPR and by an experienced operator.

According to the American Society of Anesthesiologists (ASA), a portable storage unit that contains specialized equipment for difficult airway management should be readily available.[19,20] The content of this storage unit should include: rigid laryngoscope blades of alternate design and size, video laryngoscopic devices, endotracheal tubes of assorted size, endotracheal tube guides, supraglottic airways, flexible fiberoptic intubation equipment, equipment for a nonsurgical and surgical airway, and an exhaled carbon dioxide detector.[20,21] Only a small endotracheal tube measuring 6–7 mm is appropriate for intubation of the parturient.[6]

Obtain intravenous access

The demands of the growing fetus and metabolic processes of the gestating mother produce an increase in oxygen consumption. As the growing uterus leads to peripheral pooling of blood, there is a decrease in circulatory reserve in the parturient.[13] Additionally, the hemodynamic changes of pregnancy lead to a paradoxical increase in total blood volume and a dilutional anemia. This means that a substantial amount of hemorrhage can occur before this is reflected in the patient's vital signs or hemodynamic status.

The gravid uterus also leads to compression of the pelvic veins and can cause an increase in venous pressure below the uterus.[22] Given this increased pressure and poor venous return to the heart, intravenous lines in the lower extremities should be avoided.[23] Thus, 2 large bore intravenous lines should be placed immediately above the diaphragm. Intraosseous infusion in the humeri can provide alternative access.

Administer medications

The medications used for cardiac arrest in the nonpregnant patient are the same for the pregnant patient, and at the same doses. The vasopressor of choice is epinephrine, and 1 mg intravenously or intraosseous should be given early in the arrest period; this can be repeated every 3 to 5 minutes.[4–7] Toxicity and dosages to allow for the increase in glomerular fibrillation rate (GFR) of pregnancy are not considered during the resuscitative process. Vasopressin has become less important in the algorithm and may compromise uterine blood flow; it does not offer any benefits over epinephrine.[24]

If magnesium toxicity is suspected, one should discontinue magnesium infusion and administer calcium gluconate (10–30 mL of 10% solution) immediately, either intravenously or IO.

If acidosis or toxicity such as hyperkalemia is the etiology of the cardiac arrest, then sodium bicarbonate should be given. Otherwise, sodium bicarbonate is not routinely used, as it may lead to fetal carbon dioxide accumulation, resulting in fetal acidosis. In the setting of severe, systemic drug toxicity or poisoning, the poison control center and toxicologist should be contacted. If local anesthetic toxicity is suspected, then lipid rescue employing 20% lipid emulsion can be administered in addition to other ACLS interventions.[22,25,26]

Consideration of perimortem delivery

If cardiac arrest persists at 4 minutes, perform perimortem delivery, usually perimortem cesarean delivery (PMCD), also known as resuscitative delivery or hysterotomy.[27]

The concept of PMCD emerged in 1986 with recommendation to perform emergency cesarean delivery if resuscitative efforts were not successful after 5 minutes.[27] More recently, the AHA recommends initiating PMCD at the 4-minute mark, with fetal delivery within 5 minutes.[6] This has become known as the "5-minute rule".

In nonpregnant individuals, irreversible brain damage can occur in 4 to 6 minutes. In the pregnant state, the functional residual capacity is decreased, leading to an increase risk of hypoxia and eventual anoxia in the setting of maternal cardiopulmonary collapse. Given this decrease reserve, the pregnant woman is at a higher risk of anoxic brain injury.

Cardiac arrest leads to cessation of optimal blood flow throughout the body, with divergence to vital organs such as the heart and brain and away from nonvital organs such as the uterus.[22] And even during optimal CPR, cardiac output is only 30%.[22] Thus, maternal cardiac arrest not only affects blood flow to maternal vital organs, but can quickly lead to uteroplacental compromise and eventual fetal death.

A resuscitative delivery (hysterotomy) is performed to allow more effective maternal resuscitation and optimize maternal and fetal survival.[28] The medical literature of published cases of PMCD from 1985 to 2004 produced 38 cases of varying etiologies, gestational age, and timing of delivery.[29] This retrospective analysis provided support of delivery within 5 minutes by demonstrating that cesarean delivery did not cause deterioration in the maternal condition, and infants had a greater likelihood of intact survival.[29]

The 5-minute rule was reassessed in a retrospective literature review of maternal cardiac arrest cases between 1980 and 2010.[30] Eighty relevant papers generated 94 cases; only 75% of the cases documented time from arrest to delivery, and only 4 cases met the advocated 5-minute rule.[30] They found that neonatal survival was strongly associated with in-hospital maternal arrest and that maternal survival was improved if PMCD was performed with 10 minutes of maternal arrest.[30] This review concluded that PMCD provided maternal benefit in about one-third of cases and was without detriment in any case.[30]

The PMCD should be performed at the location of the arrest. Simulation studies have shown a decrease in the quality of CPR during transport to the operating room,[31] which is already compromised due to unrelieved aortocaval compression. Time should not be wasted with fetal monitoring, awaiting equipment, or abdominal preparation.

In order to decrease time to delivery, antiseptic (ie, betadine) should be poured over the abdomen, and the only essential instrument is a scalpel. Conventionally, it has been taught that a vertical skin incision is the fastest route; it also provides the advantages of exposure and access, especially when additional maneuvers and surgical techniques may be necessary. However, whichever incision with which the surgeon is most comfortable is likely to lead to the fastest incision to delivery time.

Alternative interventions

In the setting of ST elevation myocardial infarction, percutaneous coronary intervention is the preferred intervention, as fibrinolysis is relatively contraindicated in pregnancy.[19]

If return of spontaneous circulation (ROSC) is not accomplished after perimortem delivery, additional interventions may be considered. Direct cardiac massage performed after thoracotomy may provide enhanced organ perfusion.[27] Open cardiac massage may also be accomplished through the vertical abdominal incision. A simulation electrical model was used to characterize circulation during open- versus closed-chest CPR and demonstrated that direct cardiac compression was superior, generating greater perfusion throughout the CPR cycle.[32]

A transthoracic (TTE) or transesophageal (TEE) echocardiogram is an important tool to help elucidate potential cardiac causes of maternal cardiac arrest and assess potential benefit of cardiopulmonary bypass. Specifically, TTE is important for the cannulation process of extracorporeal membranous oxygenation (ECMO) and placement of intra-aortic balloon counterpulsation. The use of ECMO during or after CPR has been described in case reports and series, and its use in pregnancy is uncommon. Most publications on ECMO in pregnancy are in the setting of acute respiratory distress syndrome (ARDS) caused by H1N1.

A systematic review of the literature yielded 31 reports with 67 patients who had extracorporeal life support (ECLS) or ECMO during pregnancy or postpartum.[33] Overall, maternal survival was 80%, and fetal survival was 70%.[33] A subsequent systematic review of the literature produced 26 publications with 45 patients in whom ECLS/ECMO was used during pregnancy.[34] The survival rate was 77.8% for mothers and 65.1% for fetuses. These reviews concluded that ECLS was effective and relatively safe in pregnancy.[33,34] Only 1 of these patients had an indication of cardiac arrest.[35]

Delivery
A maternal cardiac arrest is not only a challenging academic and clinical scenario; there are also emotional implications for every participant involved in these cases. Thus, it is important to debrief with the entire team as soon as possible. Debriefing not only provides an extraordinary learning environment and a chance to review the case, but can also serve as an opportunity for the code team to open up about how their participation made (and continues to make) them feel. An MCPA is a relatively rare occurrence, but for those who have participated in a maternal code, the memory and lessons learned are palpable.

Now recall the patient presented at the beginning of this article. A maternal code was called; BLS and ACLS were immediately initiated. Resuscitative maneuvers and work-up of the maternal cardiac arrest were performed simultaneously. Manual left uterine displacement was established in the maternal supine position, and cardiac compressions were started while the patient was intubated. A defibrillator was applied and revealed no shockable rhythm. The laboratory findings were significant for a Cr of 4.5 mg/dL and a magnesium level of 18 mEq/L. The lead diagnosis was hypermagnesemia, and the patient was treated with calcium gluconate 1 g intravenously. She regained a pulse and survived this maternal cardiac arrest. A resuscitative delivery was not necessary, but a cesarean section was later performed for delivery of a live neonate.

SUMMARY

Maternal cardiac arrest is a rare but catastrophic event. Key interventions, performed simultaneously, may save the life of mother and baby:

- Call a maternal code
- Perform maternal left lateral uterine displacement
- Initiate chest compressions fast and hard (100/min)
- Open the airway and give 2 breaths per 30 compressions
- Obtain 2 large bore intravenous lines above the diaphragm
- Defibrillate if indicated
- If MCA persists, extract the fetus at 4 minutes to allow a resuscitative delivery by 5 minutes.

REFERENCES

1. Trends in maternal mortality: 1990 to 2013. Estimates by WHO, UNICEF, UNFPA, the World Bank and the United Nations Population Division. Geneva (Switzerland): World Health Organization; 2014.

2. Trends in maternal mortality: 1990 to 2015. Estimates by WHO, UNICEF, UNFPA, the World Bank and the United Nations Population Division. Geneva (Switzerland): World Health Organization; 2014.

3. Main EK, Menard MK. Maternal mortality: time for national action. Obstet Gynecol 2013;122(4):735–6.

4. Creanga AA, Berg CJ, Syverson C, et al. Pregnany-related mortality in the United States, 2006-2010. Obstet Gynecol 2015;125:5–12.

5. Mhyre JM, Tsen LC, Einav S, et al. Cardiac arrest during hospitalization for delivery in the United States, 1998-2011. Anesthesiology 2014;120:810.

6. Jeejeebhoy FM, Zelop CM, Lipman S, et al. Cardiac arrest in pregnancy: a scientific statement from the America Heart Association. Circulation 2015;132:1747.

7. Neumar RW, Otto CW, Link MS, et al. Part 8: adult advanced cardiovascular life support: 2010 American Heart Association guidelines for cardiopulmonary resuscitation and emergency cardiovascular care. Circulation 2010;122(Suppl 3): S729–67.

8. Tan EK, Tan EL. Alterations in physiology and anatomy during pregnancy. Best Pract Res Clin Obstet Gynaecol 2013;27:791–802.

9. San-Frutos L, Engels V, Zapardiel I, et al. Hemodynamic changes during pregnancy and postpartum: a prospective study using thoracic electrical bioimpedance. J Matern Fetal Neonatal Med 2011;24:1333–40.

10. Carbillon L, Uzan M, Uzan S. Pregnancy, vascular tone, and maternal hemodynamics: a crucial adaptation. Obstet Gynecol Surv 2000;55:574–81.

11. McLennan C, Minn M. Antecubital and femoral venous pressure in normal and toxemic pregnancy. Am J Obstet Gynecol 1943;45:568–91.

12. Kerr MG. The mechanical effects of the gravid uterus in late pregnancy. J Obstet Gynaecol Br Commonw 1965;72:513–29.

13. Ueland K, Novy MJ, Peterson EN, et al. Maternal cardiovascular dynamics. IV. The influence of gestational age on the maternal cardiovascular response to posture and exercise. Am J Obstet Gynecol 1969;104:856.

14. Rees GA, Willis BA. Resuscitation in late pregnancy. Anaesthesia 1988;43:347–9.

15. Vanden Hoek TL, Morrison LJ, Shuster M, et al. Part 12: cardiac arrest in special situations: 2010 American Heart Association guidelines for cardiopulmonary resuscitation and emergency cardiovascular care. Circulation 2010;122(Suppl 3): S829–61.

16. Holmes S, Kirkpatrick IDC, Zelop CM, et al. MRI evaluation of maternal cardiac displacement in pregnancy: implications for cardiopulmonary resuscitation. Am J Obstet Gynecol 2015;213:401.e1-5.

17. Nanson J, Elcock D, Williams M, et al. Do physiological changes in pregnancy change defibrillation energy requirements? Br J Anaesth 2001;87:237–9.

18. McDonnell NJ, Peach MJ, Clavisi OM, et al. Difficult and failed intubation in obstetric anaethesia: an observational study of airway management and complications associated with general anesthesia for cesarean section. Int J Obstet Anesth 2008;17:292.

19. American Heart Association. Cardiac arrest associated with pregnancy. Circulation 2005;112:150–3.

20. American Society of Anesthesiologists Task Force on Management of the Difficult Airway. Practice guidelines for management of the difficult airway: an updated report by the American Society of Anesthesiologists Task Force on Management of the Difficult Airway. Anesthesiology 2003;98:1269–77.

21. Practice guidelines for obstetric anesthesia: an updated report by the American society of anesthesiologists task force on obstetric anesthesia and the Society for Obstetric Anesthesia and Perinatology. Anesthesiology 2007; 124:27–300.

22. Suresh MS, Mason CT, Munnur U. Cardiopulmonary resuscitation and the parturient. Best Pract Res Clin Obstet Gynaecol 2010;24(3):383–400.

23. Crochetiere C. Obstetric emergencies. Anesthesiol Clin North America 2003; 21(1):111–25.
24. Bossmar T, Akerlund M, Fantoni G, et al. Receptors for and myometrial responses to oxytocin and vasopressin in preterm and term human pregnancy: effects of the oxytocin antagonist atosiban. Am J Obstet Gynecol 1994;171:1634–42.
25. Bern S, Weinberg G. Local anesthetic toxicity and lipid resuscitation in pregnancy. Curr Opin Anaesthesiol 2011;24:262–7.
26. Weinberg GJ. Treatment of local anesthetic systemic toxicity (LAST). Reg Anesth Pain Med 2010;35:188–93.
27. Lee RV, Rodgers BD, White LM, et al. Cardiopulmonary resuscitation of pregnant women. Am J Med 1986;81:311–8.
28. Rose CH, Faksh A, Traynor KD, et al. Challenging the 4 to 5 minute rule: from perimortem cesarean to resuscitative hysterotomy. Am J Obstet Gynecol 2015;213:653.
29. Katz V, Balderston K, DeFreest M. Perimortem cesarean delivery: were our assumptions correct? Am J Obstet Gynecol 2005;192:1916–21.
30. Einav S, Kaufman N, Sela HY. Maternal cardiac arrest and perimortem caesarean delivery: evidence or expert-based? Resuscitation 2012;83:1191–200.
31. Lipman SS, Wong JY, Arafeh J, et al. Transport decreases the quality of cardiopulmonary resuscitation during simulated maternal cardiac arrest. Anesth Analg 2013;116:162–7.
32. Babbs C. Hemodynamix mechanisms in CPR: a theoretical rationale for resuscitative thoracotomy in non-traumatic cardiac arrest. Resuscitation 1987;15:37–50.
33. Sharma NS, Wille KM, Bellot SC, et al. Modern use of extracorporeal life support in pregnancy and postpartum. ASAIO J 2015;61:110–4.
34. Moore SA, Dietl CA, Coleman DM. Extracorporeal life support during pregnancy. J Thorac Cardiovasc Surg 2016;151:1154–60.
35. Grimme I, Winter R, Kluge S, et al. Hypoxic cardiac arrest in pregnancy due to pulmonary haemorrhage. BMJ Case Rep 2012;2012:1–4.

Obstetric Transport

Julie Scott, MD*

KEYWORDS

- Obstetric transport • Perinatal regionalization of care • SBAR communication
- EMTALA

KEY POINTS

- Obstetric transport is a specialized medical transport that can occur for maternal, fetal, and even neonatal concerns.
- Perinatal regionalization of care provides a broader geographic availability of obstetric services with defined levels of maternal and neonatal care so that women can be transported to centers with increased resources and capabilities to reduce morbidity and mortality.
- The Emergency Medical Treatment and Active Labor Act provides regulatory guidance for care of laboring women who require transfer to a higher level of care.
- The Situation, Background, Assessment, and Recommendation communication is a tool that can quickly identify key pieces of medical information with recommendations given for mutual expectations of next steps.

INTRODUCTION AND HISTORICAL BACKGROUND

The concept of medical transport to provide life-and-limb-saving services has made dramatic changes throughout history. Before the modern era, health care providers typically attended the ill and infirm at the site of injury or place of rest in their homes. On the battlefield, medical care and services had to be immediately available before exsanguination occurred from injuries sustained during military action. Beasts of burden provided the necessary horsepower with cots and carriages to transport the medically needy.

The first motorized ambulance was electric and began service in 1899. It was a gift from 5 prominent businessmen to the Michael Reese Hospital in Chicago as published in the *New York Herald*. It traveled at the maximum speed of 16 miles per hour. A speaking tube extended from the driver to the doctor for direct communication.[1]

Modern medical transportation with its rules and regulations for emergency medical services (EMS) and patient stabilization was a rather late addition to medical care not occurring until the 1960s. Advances in the medical sciences were presidential

Division of Maternal Fetal Medicine, Obstetrics & Gynecology, University of Colorado, Aurora, CO, USA
* MSB B198-5, 12631 East 17th Avenue, Room 4001, Aurora, CO 80045
E-mail address: Julie.scott@ucdenver.edu

Obstet Gynecol Clin N Am 43 (2016) 821–840
http://dx.doi.org/10.1016/j.ogc.2016.07.013
0889-8545/16/© 2016 Elsevier Inc. All rights reserved.

obgyn.theclinics.com

endeavors with the government supporting the development of regional medical programs (RMPs), which included the development of specialized units of care, such as coronary care units, neonatal intensive care units, burn units, and cancer centers. Funding for RMPs expanded EMS services, and patients with specific needs (ie, burn patients) were routed to the facilities that could provide those services (ie, burn units). Thus, getting from point A to point B became easier as there were designated sites of specialty care. However, the ability to provide care en route was still marginal as personnel lacked the appropriate medical training or even the ability to provide advanced first aid.[2]

Trauma related to motor vehicle accidents during the 1960s was also considered a major public health crises leading President Johnson to create the President's Commission on Highway Safety. Concurrently, the National Academy of Sciences, National Research Council published a report entitled "Accidental Death and Disability: The Neglected Disease of Modern Society," which was critical of the quality of emergency medical care in the United States. Specifics of the report highlighted a lack of protocols for treatment, poorly trained medical personnel, lack of transportation services, lack of adequate communications support, abdication of responsibilities of political authorities, and lack of research in prehospital care as major areas of concern. Recommendations were made and incorporated in to the Highway Safety Act of 1966.[2]

EMS services continued to lag behind as medical services were advancing despite federal support. Medical pioneers were advancing care in the cardiac sciences with intravenous (IV) medications, defibrillation, and cardiopulmonary resuscitation and knew that rapid implementation of care would decrease morbidities and mortality. Key political leaders also saw the importance of prehospital EMS services and reintroduced legislation leading to the EMS Services Development Act of 1973. This act designated the Department of Health, Education, and Welfare as the lead EMS agency within the federal government authorizing for the development of a comprehensive EMS system nationally with a data collection component to evaluate programs implemented.[2]

Transport of OB patients is not specifically discussed or addressed in these early legislative actions. OB patients were often managed in their local care setting unless there was a serious illness or medical comorbidity. With the development of neonatal intensive care units (NICUs) that could provide a higher level of care to babies born prematurely, at lower birth weights, and potentially with correctable structural abnormalities, the consideration of maternal transport for fetal indications became more important and continues to be a leading reason for transport. Maternal transport for purely maternal indications is also evolving as a common reason to provide OB transport so that OB patients receive care and consultation, which cannot be provided or unavailable at the referring hospital (**Box 1**).

LEVELS OF MATERNAL AND NEONATAL CARE

The landmark publication "Toward Improving the Outcome of Pregnancy: Recommendations for the Regional Development of Maternal and Perinatal Health Services" released by a committee on perinatal health consisting of the March of Dimes, American Congress of Obstetricians and Gynecologists, American Academy of Family Physicians, American Academy of Pediatrics, and the American Medical Association defined levels of specialty care in perinatal medicine in the United States.[3] Its framework categorized care based on local resources and hospital capabilities allowing for collaborative efforts of hospital systems to provide risk-appropriate care at different levels with the ideal being that a woman and her child would receive care at the

Box 1
Maternal and neonatal indications for transport

Maternal

OB
- Eclampsia with subsequent neurologic sequelae-bleeding, deficit
- Hypertensive emergency without capabilities of IV antihypertensives and cardiac monitoring
- Acute fatty liver of pregnancy
- Massive hemorrhage without appropriate blood bank capabilities
- Puerperal sepsis

Cardiac
- Congenital anomalies-corrected and uncorrected
- Valvular heart disease with need for anticoagulation in labor
- Hypertensive emergencies
- Ischemia/Infarct
- Congestive heart failure with need for LVAD device, transplant
- Peripartum cardiomyopathy

Pulmonary
- Respiratory Insufficiency with potential need for intubation of OB patients
- Pulmonary embolism
- Severe asthma with need for subspecialty care
- Pulmonary hemorrhage
- Pulmonary hypertension
- OB patients with cystic fibrosis

Neurologic
- Stroke-ischemic and hemorrhagic
- Brain mass/cancer
- Aneurysm
- Subarachnoid hemorrhage

GI
- GI bleed
- Need for subspecialty diagnostics, including endoscopy, MRCP
- Cancer
- Acute hepatitis with or without fulminant liver failure
- Pancreatitis

Endocrine
- Diabetes including transport for IV insulin therapy for labor management and ketoacidosis
- Pheochromocytoma
- Thyroid storm
- Adrenal insufficiency/failure

Hematologic
- Aplastic crisis
- Severe thrombocytopenia with or without bleeding
- Coagulopathy
- New diagnosis of leukemia, lymphoma during pregnancy
- Venothromboembolism, including deep venous thrombosis and pulmonary embolism

Renal
- Renal failure with need for subspecialty care, diagnosis, and management
- Dialysis
- Hemolytic uremic syndrome

Autoimmune
- Systemic lupus erythematosus flare, multi-organ system failure
- Catastrophic antiphospholipid antibody syndrome with multi-organ involvement
- Severe Crohn disease or ulcerative colitis flare requiring multidisciplinary care

Infectious diseases
- Sepsis

Intensive care
- Cardiac support including pressor agents, assist devices
- Ventilatory support
- Multidisciplinary medical or surgical intensive care

Surgical
- Need for operation while pregnant, including cholecystectomy, appendectomy, trauma, mass/cancer, acute abdomen
- Care for necrotizing infection with subspecialty surgical care

Other
- Trauma
- Overdose/toxicology evaluation, ICU care
- Psychiatric emergencies
- Transplant services: acute fatty liver, fulminant hepatitis

Maternal-fetal

- Preeclampsia, severe preeclampsia, HELLP syndrome, and eclampsia

- Preterm labor

- Fetal growth restriction

- Preterm premature rupture of the membranes

- Multiple gestational

- OB bleeding, including antepartum bleeding and postpartum bleeding necessitating a higher level of care

- Infection/sepsis, including pyelonephritis, appendicitis, pancreatitis, cholecystitis, pneumonia, soft tissue/skin structures, osteomyelitis

Fetal/neonatal

- Prematurity

- Fetal growth restriction

- Fetal anomalies

- In utero therapies, including laser, transfusion, and surgical repair

- Known metabolic abnormalities requiring immediate therapy after birth

- Known genetic abnormalities requiring a higher level of NICU care

Other

- Capacity management/hospital divert

- Natural disaster

- Man-made disaster: shooting victims, bombings

Abbreviations: GI, gastrointestinal; HELLP, hemolysis, elevated liver enzymes, low platelet count; ICU, intensive care unit; LVAD, left ventricular assist device; MRCP, magnetic resonance cholangiopancreatography.

institution with the appropriate capabilities or transferred to such facility.[3,4] The tertiary care facility, in addition to providing direct patient care, provides training and educational opportunities for level I and II care centers.

Neonatal outcomes have improved through regionalization of care and transport of maternal patients to higher levels of care before delivery. One of the earliest reports authored by Harris and colleagues[5] in 1978 evaluated data on 239 consecutive infants who require NICU care following in utero maternal transport to a regional perinatal care center versus 642 infants who were born in outlying hospitals and then transported to regional intensive care units during the same 30-month time period in Arizona. Their data revealed a significant decrease in neonatal mortality for those infants transported through maternal transport versus newborn transport (23% vs 41%), particularly for infants weighing less than 1500 g and born before 34 weeks.[5] Reduction in neonatal morbidity and cost of neonatal care has also been demonstrated. Anderson and colleagues[6] evaluated transport data in a suburban population in Chicago and evaluated the efficacy of maternal transport in comparison with infants born in an outlying hospital and transported for NICU care. Their data revealed that complications of pregnancy (hypertension, diabetes, fetal growth restriction, and maternal heart disease) were more common in the transported mother and that preterm labor was more common in the infant who was transported after delivery in the referring hospital. Although they did not demonstrate a difference in the mean birth weight, gestational age, and survival rate for their study groups, they did see a difference in length of stay and, thereby, cost for care of the newborn (19 days for in utero transport and 27 days for infant transport with a cost difference of near $6000.00). The investigators concluded that there may be assumptions being made at outlying hospitals that spontaneous preterm birth is a lower risk than that of medically complicated maternal patients. The increased length of stay for the newborn delivered at the originating hospital and then transported for NICU care reveals the potential negative impact of not receiving immediate NICU care.[6] Similar findings have been noted in other countries capable of providing regionalized and higher levels of care.[7–9]

Prenatally diagnosed congenital malformations that require immediate neonatal interventions, such as certain cardiac lesions, obstructive masses, teratomas, and congenital diaphragmatic hernia cases, also benefit from transport and delivery in higher-level care settings. This point is particularly the case for the newborn who may need an EXIT (Ex Utero Intrapartum Treatment) procedure, extracorporeal membrane oxygenation, delivery to a cardiac catheterization, or other immediate surgical need.[10–13] Again, in utero transport with the mother being the best possible incubator reduces neonatal morbidity and mortality.

Recently, efforts have been focused on expanding levels of care to include maternal care concerns separate from neonatal care needs. The designations have expanded to include a level IV designation for women with complex medical and surgical needs.[14] This proposed designation was developed in response to mounting concerns regarding the increases in maternal morbidity and mortality in the United States. Hankins and colleagues[15] thoughtfully recommend a call to action for maternal regionalization of care, as had already been successfully done for neonatology. The highest level-of-care hospital would act as the central hub for maternal care providing the maximum level of resources and personnel to high-risk OB patients requiring that level of care. The referring hospitals would be satellites of care, which operate independently at their care levels but have a set of strict criteria by which a woman requires transfer to access a higher level of care. The relationship between these institutions would be enhanced by continued educational opportunities for OB care providers, ongoing training with evidence-based practices, and continuity of care through telemedicine and electronic records. Paramount to the organizational structure are the policies and guidelines of evidenced-based care that algorithmically support best practices in OB.[15]

The Society of Maternal Fetal Medicine and the American College of Obstetricians and Gynecologists, with the endorsement of 7 other nationally recognized organizations involved in OB care, developed an Obstetric Care Consensus, which defines the levels of maternal care described earlier. The goal of this publication is to reduce maternal morbidity and mortality with an equitable distribution of resources and capabilities within communities. Care definitions, capabilities, and OB personnel (nursing and OB providers) are defined for birth center, level I (basic care), level II (specialty care), level III (subspecialty care), and level IV (regional perinatal health care centers). The defined levels of care are a framework of best practice and allow for integration of hospital systems to improve overall maternal care of the community and region with appropriate allocation of resources (**Table 1**).[14] Levels of maternal care may differ from NICU levels of care based on available subspecialty care for the mother or NICU capabilities.

EMERGENCY MEDICAL TREATMENT AND ACTIVE LABOR ACT

A discussion regarding transport of OB patients involves an understanding of the Emergency Medical Treatment and Active Labor Act (EMTALA). EMTALA was enacted in 1986 as is commonly referred to as the antidumping law, as it requires a hospital's emergency department to provide a medical screening examination with stabilization of an emergency medical condition (including women in active labor) to any person who arrives at their facility for care regardless of their ability to pay, legal status, or citizenship. An emergency medical condition is defined as a condition manifesting itself by acute symptoms of sufficient severity (including severe pain) such that the absence of immediate medical attention could reasonably be expected to result in placing the individual's health (or the health of an unborn child) in serious jeopardy, serious impairment to bodily functions, or serious dysfunction of bodily organs. This definition includes any pregnant woman who presents in active labor. Under this law, she is required to receive care through delivery unless there is a reason for transfer to another facility. EMTALA applies to all hospitals that receive funds from the Centers for Medicare and Medicaid Services (CMS).[16]

Failures to comply with EMTALA can result in significant monetary penalties to both the hospital and the physician involved in the violation. The hospital can be fined up to $50,000 for each violation (up to $25,000 for hospitals with <100 beds), and the physician involved can also be penalized financially up to $50,000. Further, if the negligence is considered gross, flagrant, or repeated, then a withdrawal of CMS funding can occur as well as civil law suits.[16]

Under the framework of EMTALA, OB transports must be handled with care to provide the appropriate stabilizing medical services and evaluation. Transport can occur during labor if there is adequate time to transfer to a facility before delivery or if there is concern that a delivery in the originating institution will cause threat to the health or safety to the mother and her unborn child understanding the potential risk of an unstable transfer (ie, a woman in labor). The transferring physician is obligated to inform the mother of the need for transport explaining the risks and benefits of the transport with complete documentation of the reasons for transport, including benefits of transfer over the risks of remaining at the originating institution, and to obtain acceptance of transport from the receiving facility's physician that has services capable of providing the care with reduced risk of harm and adequate space and personnel to deliver the care. The transporting facility must provide all medical records for patients to the receiving facility. The mode of transportation and qualified EMS personnel with appropriate skills and equipment to monitor while en route are necessary for a successful transfer and to comply with EMTALA.[16] Transport is contraindicated when there is lack of an appropriate transport service available, inclement weather conditions making it hazardous for travel or known to pose potential risk from extended travel time,

Table 1
Maternal levels of care and capabilities

Level	Definition of Maternal Care	Capabilities	Nursing	OB Providers	Other Providers
Birth center	Uncomplicated OB care of low-risk woman with a singleton cephalic presenting fetus with delivery occurring at term	Low-risk maternal care with ability to initiate emergency procedures for stabilization and transport Relationship with hospital for transport, including available medical consultation Quality and patient safety program with guidelines and protocols of care Medical records	Capable of level I care with adequate staffing to care for mother and newborn	Qualified medical personnel licensed and recognized to provide maternal care: CNM, CPM, licensed midwives, OBs, family medicine physicians	
I	Uncomplicated OB care with the ability to detect, stabilize, and initiate appropriate care for patients requiring transport to a higher level of care	Birth center plus • Cesarean delivery capability • Resources: ultrasound, laboratory, and blood bank with ability to provide transfusion of blood and products • Relationship with hospital for transport, including medical consultation • Quality and patient safety program with guidelines and protocols of care • Medical records • Educational opportunities for continued OB learning	Capable of level I care with adequate staffing to care for mother and newborn and • Nursing leadership for perinatal care	Birth center, plus • OB provider who can perform cesarean delivery	Anesthesia provider capable of OB analgesia and surgical anesthesia

(continued on next page)

Table 1
(continued)

Level	Definition of Maternal Care	Capabilities	Nursing	OB Providers	Other Providers
II	Level I facility with extension of services to care for specific high-risk OB patients in the antepartum, intrapartum, and postpartum periods	Level I plus • Care of higher-risk antepartum, intrapartum, and postpartum OB complications as direct admission or acceptance of transport • Care of obese patients, including bariatric beds and long surgical equipment • Resources beyond level I center, including advanced diagnostic imaging with interpretation, including ultrasound, CT, and MRI • Ability to provide coordinated transport to a higher level of care	• Level II nursing capabilities with adequate staffing for mother and the newborn • Nursing leadership with experience in perinatal care and other administrative personnel capable of care integration with neonatal services	Level I plus • OB/gyn availability 24/7 • Board-certified medical director of OB care • MFM availability for direct or indirect consultation	• Anesthesia provider capable of OB analgesia and surgical anesthesia • Ability to consult OB specialty trained anesthesiologist • Medical and surgical specialists available for consultation to OB patients
III	Level II facility with extension of services for the medically complex, surgically complex, obstetrically complex maternal patients and fetal abnormalities	Level II plus • Advanced imaging modalities and interpretation available 24/7 • Blood bank with capability of massive transfusion protocols • Intensive care services with ability to provide MFM consultation as appropriate • Ability to provide educational outreach and training opportunities to level I–II care centers	• Level III nursing capabilities with adequate staffing for mother and the newborn • Nursing leadership with experience in perinatal care and other administrative personnel capable of care integration with neonatal services • Quality/patient safety personnel for program initiatives, data evaluation	Level II plus • Board-certified MFM director in addition to OB medical director • Director of OB anesthesia services	• OB anesthesiologist and anesthesia providers capable of OB analgesia and surgical anesthesia • Medical and surgical specialists available for consultation to OB patients • Intensive care physicians

| IV | Regional perinatal health care center extending services beyond level III to the most complex maternal conditions; critical-care OB services at all times of pregnancy, including antepartum, intrapartum, and postpartum | Level III plus • OB critical care capabilities and coordinated service care with a variety of subspecialty programs, including pulmonary intensive care, cardiac care, transplant, dialysis, medicine and surgical intensive care with unit capable of providing OB care in addition to the necessary medical/surgical care • Coordinated outreach activities with other hospital in the region with ability to synthesize and review transport data of OB patients, quality improvement programs, establishment of guidelines and protocols for perinatal care | Level III plus • Nursing leadership with expertise in maternal critical care • Director of OB nursing services | Level III plus • MFM available inpatient services 24/7 with expertise in critical care OB medicine | Level III plus • Specialists capable of multidisciplinary care |

Abbreviations: CNM, certified nurse midwife; CPM, certified professional midwife; CT, computed tomography; gyn, gynecology; MFM, maternal fetal medicine.
From American College of Obstetricians and Gynecologists and Society for Maternal–Fetal Medicine, Menard MK, Kilpatrick S, et al. Levels of maternal care. Am J Obstet Gynecol 2015;212(3):259–71; with permission.

maternal condition has not been stabilized (delivery is imminent, severe uncontrolled hypertension or hemorrhage with evidence of shock), unstable fetal condition (abnormal fetal heart rate tracing pattern that a delay in care/delivery would result in death or damage to the fetus/neonate), or patients' refusal to transport.

TRANSPORTATION AND EMERGENCY MEDICAL SERVICES

The business of medicine is competitive, with multiple hospital systems and transport companies existing in the same city, state, and region. Regionalization of perinatal care within a hospital system can occur within the same city from hospitals that offer basic OB services for healthy moms with term newborns to women requiring expanded OB and medical services and neonatal care for their newborns. Transport policies and agreements exist within the hospital system and external agreements when needing to transport to another hospital system with a higher level of care. Some of this is based on the level of service provided, locale, responsiveness of providers to facilitate care, third-party payers, and loyalties within the system and with providers themselves. Some of these economic pressures have led to a higher density of specialized care than potentially a region can support or needs.[17]

Perinatal transport services include transport of the gravid mother, neonate, or a delivered mother to a higher level of care than what is available at the originating facility. Transport, the process of moving from one location to another, in the medical field can be by ground transportation (ambulance or personal vehicle), air (rotor and fixed wing), or water vehicle. As the key intermediary between facilities, the manner of transport must occur in a timely and safe fashion with medical personnel capable of en route stabilization and care until arrival at the receiving facility. Interfacility transport can occur via one-way or 2-way transport. In a one-way transport, the originating hospital engages the transport team (which may be a hospital-based team) for the transport of patients from their facility to the referring facility. They maintain responsibility for patients until their arrival, and care is transferred to the receiving facility and physician. In a 2-way transport, the receiving facility either sends its hospital-based EMS crew or third-party contracted EMS transport team to pick up, assess, and assume responsibility for the care of those patients from the sending facility to the receiving facility.

Currently, 34 of the 50 states (68%) have an established state-level policy for neonatal transport. Six have a recommendation for the development of state-level policy for neonatal transport (Alabama, Arkansas, Indiana, Minnesota, Washington, and West Virginia); 5 have policies but not at a state level (Connecticut, Hawaii, Idaho, Oregon, and South Dakota); 4 have no policy (Kansas, Maine, New Hampshire, and Vermont). For maternal transport, only 60% of states have a policy.[18] These policies help to provide the timely provision of care, monitor efficiency in transfer and receipt of care, and ideally prepares for challenges of long-distance transport and competitive market forces.[17]

In addition to the organization structure that is provided by state policies on medical transport are the guidelines and accreditation of medical transport companies in the United States. The Commission on Accreditation of Medical Transport Systems, an independent nonprofit organization with 21 member organizations involved in medicine, transport, and emergency services, provides audit and accreditation for medical transport services. Although initially a voluntary process for the transport company, it has become more of a necessary accreditation, as many state regulatory bodies require it before they can have a license to operate. As of April 2016, 181 transport services have been accredited.[18] Accreditation standards with audits of measurable data for medical transport ensure patient care and safety while in transport by helicopter, fixed-wing plane, and ground transportation services. Accreditation occurs in 3-year cycles.[19]

Method of transport depends on the region, level of acuity, availability of transport services, and even the weather. Transport via airplane or helicopter over long distances may be common in states with large geographic distribution to move patients from a rural community hospital to a hospital with more resources. Helicopter transport may be more likely in urban, congested cities where ambulance transport could be particularly difficult during certain times of day (ie, rush hours) and ambulance transport more common for interfacility transfers over shorter distances and differing levels of acuity. The decision for ground versus air transport not only involves the time it takes for the transport and response time of the transport crew but also the level of acuity and concern for deterioration over time. For example, ground transportation may be appropriate for the evaluation of preterm labor in the early stages of labor versus the need for air transport in a more advanced stage of preterm labor. Air transport via airplane or helicopter may not be feasible in bad weather; therefore, the risks and benefits of ambulance transfer must be weighed against the potential delivery. It may be more beneficial to provide stabilization and care at the originating facility for safety of the mother and her baby.

In a prospective study of 51 American Society of Hospital-Based Emergency Air Medical Services member helicopter/ambulance services over a 6-month period, 472 maternal transports were initiated with 463 completed (9 were aborted when labor progressed rapidly and it was deemed safer to deliver at the transporting hospital than risk an in-flight delivery). Most transports were hospital to hospital at 449 of the 463, and the remaining 14 were from either a patient's home or highway. Helicopter transport was the most common method of transport at 77%, followed by 19% fixed wing, and 4% by ambulance transport. The overwhelming reason for transfer was to ensure that a premature infant delivered at a center with specialized neonatal facilities (ie, labor events, 71%), another 17% were transferred for OB hemorrhage, 9% for preeclampsia, and 2% for eclampsia. No deliveries occurred in the helicopter transports; there was one delivery in the airplane transport, and 1 for ambulance transport (the delivery actually occurred at the patient's home before ambulance arrival). These data overall show that most transports are successful in transferring pregnant patients to the accepting facility with minimal risk of a delivery event en route.[20]

Transport decisions at advanced cervical dilation and type of transport were evaluated in another retrospective review of maternal transports over a 21-month period in Arizona from January 1989 to September 1990. Transport of women in that program occur after independent evaluation of the mom and her condition at the time of transport by an experienced perinatal flight nurse who had at least 2 years of training on labor and delivery, with 10 weeks of didactic education and 25 flights performed with direct observation. Three percent of women who were evaluated for transport had a cervical dilation of 7 or greater (54% of them were at 10 cm). A decision was made to deliver 5 of these women at their referring facility. Most of the patients were transported by helicopter (mean transport time 15 minutes), one by fixed wing (transport time 91 minutes), and one by ambulance (transport time 27 minutes). None of the women transported delivered in route, and two-thirds of the women delivered within an hour of their transport to the tertiary care facility. This study shows the importance of time when considering a transport and the individualized assessment of women in labor by an experienced perinatal flight nurse with regard to the time it takes to move patients from the referring facility to the accepting facility.[20]

Table 2
Procedural guidelines for maternal transport

Timing	OB Complication		
	Premature Labor/PPROM	Preeclampsia/Eclampsia	Third-Trimester Bleeding

At sending facility	Medical screening examination
	• Medical, surgical, and OB history pertinent to the evaluation
	• Maternal vital signs (BP, temperature, pulse, respiratory rate)
	• Fetal heart rate evaluation
	• Assess contractions, frequency
	• Sterile vaginal examination/sterile speculum evaluation, determine fetal presentation
	Documentation/communication
	• Per hospital standards, flow sheet and electronic medical record
	• SBAR to managing provider for recommended course of care, orders
	• Managing provider contacts OB provider as receiving facility (typically a tertiary care center referral to perinatology services) with recommendations for transport
	  ○ SBAR communication with recommendation for transport
	  ○ Transport team notified (mutual decision-making, often at the direction of the receiving facility in a 2-way transport)
	  ○ Further recommendations for care/stabilization before transport
		Medical screening examination
		• Medical, surgical, and OB history pertinent to the evaluation
		• Maternal vital signs (BP, temperature, pulse, respiratory rate)
		• Focused maternal examination, including cardiac, pulmonary systems (pulmonary edema), abdominal examination (right upper quadrant/epigastric pain), neurologic examination for any focal deficits, deep tendon reflexes
		• Fetal heart rate evaluation
		• Assess contractions, frequency
		Documentation/communication
		• Per hospital standards, flow sheet and electronic medical record
		• SBAR to managing provider for recommended course of care, orders
		• Managing provider contacts OB provider as receiving facility (typically a tertiary care center referral to perinatology services) with recommendations for transport
		  ○ SBAR communication with recommendation for transport
		  ○ Transport team notified (mutual decision-making, often at the direction
			Medical screening examination
			• Medical, surgical, and OB history pertinent to the evaluation
			• Maternal vital signs (BP, temperature, pulse, respiratory rate)
			• Fetal heart rate evaluation
			• Assess contractions, frequency
			• Sterile vaginal examination/sterile speculum evaluation, determine fetal presentation
			• Ultrasound if possible to determine placenta location
			Documentation/communication
			• Per hospital standards, flow sheet and electronic medical record
			• SBAR to managing provider for recommended course of care, orders
			• Managing provider contacts OB provider as receiving facility (typically a tertiary care center referral to perinatology services) with recommendations for transport
			  ○ SBAR communication with recommendation for transport
			  ○ Transport team notified (mutual decision-making, often at the direction of the receiving facility in a 2-way transport)

Interventions
• IV access (best if 18 G or 16 G) with maintenance IV fluids
• Place urine catheter
• Laboratory tests: CBC, urine culture, infectious diseases
• Antenatal steroids if clinically indicated
• Magnesium sulfate for neuroprotection if <32 wk
• Tocolytic if appropriate (nifedipine, indomethacin)
• GBS prophylaxis per CDC's guidelines after GBS culture obtained for premature labor
• PPROM: antibiotics per hospital protocol (ampicillin 2 g IV [if not penicillin allergic] and erythromycin 250 mg IV (or some local protocols use azithromycin 250–500 mg IV)
• Pain management: fentanyl or morphine at the direction of the medical provider
• Communicate to patients and provide reassurance

of the receiving facility in a 2-way transport)
○ Further recommendations for care/stabilization before transport
Interventions
• IV access (best if 18 G or 16 G) with restricted maintenance IV fluids
• Place urine catheter
• Laboratory test: CBC, Cr, AST/ALT, urine protein (dip, P/C ratio)
• Treat severe range BP per established protocols
• Antenatal steroids if clinically indicated
• Magnesium sulfate for seizure prophylaxis (4–6 g IV load over 15–20 min, then 1–2 g/h continuous infusion)
• Communicate to patients and provide reassurance

○ Further recommendations for care/stabilization before transport
Interventions
• IV access, preferable (2) 16 G
• Place urine catheter
• Laboratory tests: CBC, T&S, and cross if transfusion indicated, DIC panel
• Maintenance IV fluids: LR or NS after initial fluid bolus of 500 mL to 1 L
• Blood transfusion as medically indicated
• Antenatal steroids if clinically indicated
• Care in the use of tocolytics and magnesium sulfate for neuroprotection as this may be contraindicated in the event on an ongoing abruption; consult receiving physician for advice
• Communicate to patients and provide reassurance

(continued on next page)

Table 2
(continued)

Timing	OB Complication		
	Premature Labor/PPROM	Preeclampsia/Eclampsia	Third-Trimester Bleeding

En route	Communication and assessment
	• SBAR and report of patients given by sending qualified medical personnel
	• Reassessment for stability of transfer to assure not at risk for imminent delivery, maternal and/or fetal compromise
	• Documentation of lines, maternal and fetal status
	• Obtain all pertinent prenatal records, laboratory test results, and studies performed (OB ultrasound) to hand off to receiving facility
	• Report given to dispatch for further communication to receiving facility
	• Document per guidelines patient status en route
	• Communicate to patients and provide reassurance
	Medical evaluation
	• Maternal positioning with leftward tilt
	• Maternal cardiac monitoring and pulse oximetry, if IV magnesium infusing
	  ○ Evaluate respiratory rate, deep tendon reflexes, urine output
	• Maternal vital signs and fetal heart rate evaluation every 15 min
	• Assure maintenance of IV access
	Emergency procedures
		Communication and assessment
		• SBAR and patient report given by sending qualified medical personnel
		• Reassessment for stability of transfer to assure not at risk for imminent delivery, maternal and/or fetal compromise
		• Documentation of lines, maternal and fetal status
		• Obtain all pertinent prenatal records, laboratory test results, and studies performed (OB ultrasound) to handoff to receiving facility
		• Report given to dispatch for further communication to receiving facility
		• Document per guidelines patient status en route
		• Communicate to patients and provide reassurance
		Medical evaluation
		• Maternal positioning with leftward tilt
		• Maternal cardiac monitoring and pulse oximetry, if IV magnesium infusing
		  ○ Evaluate respiratory rate, deep tendon reflexes, urine output
		• Maternal vital signs and fetal heart rate evaluation every 15 min
		• Assure maintenance of IV access
		• O₂ 6–12 L by nonrebreather, prn
		Emergency procedures
			Communication and assessment
			• SBAR and report of patient given by sending qualified medical personnel
			• Reassessment for stability of transfer to assure not at risk for imminent delivery, maternal and/or fetal compromise
			• Documentation of lines, maternal and fetal status
			• Obtain all pertinent prenatal records, laboratory test results, and studies performed (OB ultrasound) to handoff to receiving facility
			• Report given to dispatch for further communication to receiving facility
			• Document per guidelines patient status en route
			• Communicate to patients and provide reassurance
			Medical evaluation
			• Maternal position with leftward tilt
			• Maternal cardiac monitoring and pulse oximetry
			• Maternal vital signs, urine outputs, and fetal heart rate every 15 min
			• O₂ 6–12 L by nonrebreather, prn
			• Assure maintenance of IV lines
			Emergency procedures
			• Shock/hypoperfusion

- Magnesium sulfate toxicity: calcium gluconate 1 g IV push slowly over 3 min with careful evaluation of maternal vital signs

- Magnesium sulfate toxicity: calcium gluconate 1 g IV push slowly over 3 min with careful evaluation of maternal vital signs
- Severe range BP (initiated within 30–60 min of the severe range BP with goals of 140–160/90 mm Hg):
  ○ Hydralazine: 2–10 mg IV push every 15–20 min, or
  ○ Labetalol 10–20 mg IV for the first dose every 10 min, and if BP not effective, double dose at next administration
  ○ Nifedipine 10 mg orally; may repeat in 30 min
- Pulmonary edema
  ○ Morphine 2–5 mg slow IV push
  ○ Furosemide 20–40 mg slow IV push over 2–3 min
- Eclampsia
  ○ Establish and protect airway
  ○ If not on magnesium, bolus 4–6 g IV over 10–15 min
  ○ If on magnesium, bolus 2–4 g IV over 5–10 min for a total of 8 g
  ○ Recurrent seizures: diazepam 5–10 mg IV slow push (can repeat every 15 min up to 30 mg); assure secure airway for respiratory depression

  ○ If blood is with patients, continue infusion
  ○ Increase IV fluid administration
  ○ Elevate legs and apply military antishock trousers
  ○ Increase O_2 to 12 L nonrebreather
  ○ Call medical director to administer ephedrine 5–25 mg slow IV with care to evaluate BP on cycle
  ○ If related to immediate delivery, provide uterotonics
    ■ Oxytocin: 20–30 u/L NS, 125–150 mL/h
    ■ Methylergonovine 0.2 mg IM
    ■ Hemabate 0.25 IM; contraindicated in presence of maternal asthma or pulmonary hyeprtension

(continued on next page)

Table 2
(continued)

Timing	OB Complication		
	Premature Labor/PPROM	**Preeclampsia/Eclampsia**	**Third-Trimester Bleeding**
At receiving facility	Communication and assessment • SBAR communication and handoff with clear communication of events that may have occurred en route, stability of mothers and fetuses, including fetal heart rate tracing abnormalities • Receive sending facilities paperwork/medical records • Obtain transport paperwork from EMS team • Begin maternal/fetal evaluation for the next set of interventions/stabilization • Communicate to referring provider patients' arrival, stability, and plan of care, including potential length of stay with plan for ongoing communication during their hospitalization; when discharged, send discharge summary and, if delivered, delivery summary for neonates	Communication and assessment • SBAR communication and handoff with clear communication of events that may have occurred en route, stability of mothers and her fetuses, including fetal heart rate tracing abnormalities • Receive sending facilities paperwork/medical records • Obtain transport paperwork from EMS team • Begin maternal/fetal evaluation for the next set of interventions/stabilization • Communicate to referring provider patients' arrival, stability and plan of care, including potential length of stay with plan for ongoing communication during their hospitalization; when discharged, send discharge summary and, if delivered, delivery summary for neonates	Communication and assessment • SBAR communication and handoff with clear communication of events that may have occurred en route, stability of mothers and fetuses, including fetal heart rate tracing abnormalities • Receive sending facilities paperwork/medical records • Obtain transport paperwork from EMS team • Begin maternal/fetal evaluation for the next set of interventions/stabilization • Communicate to referring provider patients' arrival, stability, and plan of care, including potential length of stay with plan for ongoing communication during their hospitalization; when discharged, send discharge summary and, if delivered, delivery summary for neonates

Abbreviations: ALT, alanine transaminase; AST, aspartate transaminase; BP, blood pressure; CBC, complete blood count; CDC, Centers for Disease Control and Prevention; Cr, creatinine; DIC, disseminated intravascular coagulation; GBS, group B strep; IM, intramuscular; LR, lactated ringers; NS, normal saline; O₂, oxygen; P/C, protein to creatinine ratio; T&S, type & screen.

EMS personnel who provide care during maternal transport should have specialty skills in the care of OB patients and neonates. Some transport service companies have teams specifically designed for high-risk OB transport for both air and ground transport.[21] The qualifications and skills should include the ability to perform a vaginal examination and delivery if needed, certification in advanced cardiovascular life support with the ability to intubate, experience in OB nursing in a tertiary care center, and successful completion of the flight program certification process. In a survey of more than 200 air medical programs that belonged to the Association of Air Medical Services (133 respondent programs), 76% of their transport crews were made up of a nurse/paramedic team, with many programs requiring the nurse to be a certified paramedic in addition to their license as a nurse. Eleven percent had nurses only for their EMS team, and 5% had physician and nurse/paramedic teams, with the remainder of the team makeup being nurse, paramedic, and respiratory therapist combinations.[22] Three out of 4 air transport programs required crew orientation materials for the management of high-risk OB patients, but only half were required to have a current certification for neonatal resuscitation.[21] More importantly and revealing of limitations, only half of the aircraft had pelvic access in the normal configuration for patient loading. For those who did not have this access and it was deemed important for evaluation, the aircraft would have to land in order to do so. In this survey, 80% of the programs transported less than 50 high-risk OB patients annually out of a median of 800 (96–4500) medical transports. For the crew, the greatest concern they had about high-risk OB transport was the risk of an in-flight delivery.[22]

COMMUNICATION, PROTOCOLS, AND EQUIPMENT

Communication and patient care guidelines are crucial to a successful maternal transport. Communication is initiated when the call from the referring provider (person qualified to perform the medical screening examination) contacts the accepting provider with a desire to transfer OB patients from their facility. Important in this communication is an indication for transfer, pertinent medical and OB history with gestational age and presentation of symptoms, findings of the examination including maternal vital signs, cervical examination, and fetal heart rate evaluation/ultrasound findings. Situation, Background, Assessment, and Recommendation (SBAR) is one of the leading communication tools used in health care today to promote quality and safety in patient care with a shared set of expectations.[23] This form of direct communication is particularly important in the transport setting where not only do patients' conditions need to be communicated but also the expected mode of transport and any pretransport recommendations for medications, procedures, and evaluations.

Hospitals typically have a centralized access center (bed control and transport department) to help facilitate phone calls from transporting and accepting medical providers and may have the capabilities to further assist in the arrangement of transport, including notification of the transport team. A further delegated responsibility is to provide direct communication of when a transport leaves the sending facility and communicating patient status on arrival to the receiving facility. Additionally, many are equipped to record the phone calls, which may be important in a review/audit process for transports and quality of the communication process. The OB providers (sending and receiving) should also clearly document the content of the discussion, including reason for transport; arrangements made for transport; and all pertinent medical and OB history, including maternal weight, gestational age of the fetus, stabilization, and pretransport care; medications; laboratory and radiologic studies performed; fetal monitoring; and cervical examination.

Table 3
Equipment and medications for maternal transport

General	OB Delivery Kit	Maternal Resuscitation Kit	Neonatal Resuscitation Kit	Medications/IV Fluids	Other
EMS 12-lead cardiac monitor and cardiac electrodes	Sterile speculum	Oral airways	Pediatric stethoscope	Lactated ringers, normal saline or dextrose solutions	Transport/charting paperwork
Bag valve mask/self-inflating bag valve mask	Bulb syringe	ET tubes and connectors	Neonatal laryngoscope	Sterile KY gel	Flashlight
Blood pressure cuff (sphygmomanometer)	Suction trap	Stylet	ET tubes and connectors	Albuterol, unit dose (2.5 mg)	Batteries
Laryngoscope handle and blade	Cord clamp × 2	End-tidal CO_2 detector	Stylet	Atropine (1 mg)	Blankets both maternal and pediatric
Suction equipment	Curved Kelly clamp		End-tidal CO_2 detector	Ammonium salts	Infant hat
Electronic fetal monitor	Short ring forceps		Microdrip extension tubing set	Calcium gluconate (10%)	IV starting kits
Fetal Doppler	Scissors			Dextrose 50% (50 mL)	Mainline tubing
Stethoscope	Plastic placenta bag			Diazepam (10 mg)	Blood tubing with pump
Thermometer	Perineum pads			Diphenhydramine (25 mg)	IV catheters (16 G, 18 G, 24 G, 23 G) butterfly
Sterile gloves	Towels			Ephedrine (50 mg)	Tourniquet
Red biohazard bags				Epinephrine 1:10,000	Band-Aids (Johnson & Johnson, New Brunswick, NJ)
Emesis bag/basin				Furosemide (20 mg)	Plastic bags
Reflex hammer				Hemabate (0.25 mg)	Vacutainer and blood tubes (purple and red)
O_2 tank, tubing, and mask				Hydralazine (20 mg)	Alcohol prep pads
Syringes (1 mL, 5 mL, and 10 mL)				Labetalol (20 mg)	Tape
Foley catheter				Lidocaine 1 g/50 mL	
Benzoin				Magnesium sulfate (10 g)	
Antiseptic solution/wipes				Methergine (0.2 mg)	
				Misoprostol (100 mcg)	
				Morphine (10 mg)	
				Naloxone (0.4 mg)	
				Oxytocin (10 U)	
				Promethazine (25 mg)	
				Verapamil (5 mg)	
				Xylocaine gel	

Abbreviations: CO_2, carbon dioxide; ET, endotracheal; O_2, oxygen.
Data from Foley MR, Strong Jr TH, Garite TJ, editors. Transport of the critically ill obstetric patient in obstetric intensive care manual. 2nd edition. New York: McGraw Hill Co, Inc; 2004. p. 249–56.

Labor and delivery units have guidelines and standard order sets for the management of certain complications of pregnancy, including preterm labor, preterm premature rupture of the membranes (PPROM), third-trimester bleeding, preeclampsia/eclampsia, and trauma (**Table 2**). Often, these care procedures have been implemented as a part of the stabilization of OB patients. Routinely, this would include assessment of maternal vital signs and for maternal stability and an assessment of fetal status regardless of the presenting complaint. Often, checklists are developed along with the protocols to assure uniformity in the assessment and delivery of care while limiting the chance for oversights in care.

Notification and activation of the transport team occurs through EMS dispatch services. Engagement of the team via established guidelines for crew makeup and preparedness then takes place. Transport teams commonly use checklists to prepare for transport, including a review and check of equipment needed for specialty transports, such as OB patients.

Equipment and medication needs for an OB transport should include the necessary items to provide en route care of maternal patients and, in the rare circumstance of a delivery, care of the neonate. These items would include an OB delivery kit, infant resuscitation equipment, and, for OB emergencies not related to delivery, cardiac monitoring equipment and adult airway and resuscitation equipment. IV access is critical and should be secure and in place before transport should IV medications be required en route (**Table 3**).[24]

SUMMARY

Perinatal regionalization of care with a distinct level of neonatal and maternal services provides the descriptive classification to guide providers toward OB and neonatal care settings that are risk appropriate for OB patients. When gravid patients arrive to a hospital where resources are limited, then transport from that facility is necessary. These actions will decrease maternal morbidity and mortality for the newborn and, in the setting of severe maternal illness, the mothers' own morbidities and mortality. A decision to transport accepts the very small risk of deterioration during transport with the desired goal of achieving the appropriate level of care for the maternal/fetal unit. For the neonate, in utero transport has proven to reduce morbidities and mortality and is preferred when possible over delivery, stabilization, and then neonatal transport. Additionally, maternal/fetal transport fosters family and patient-centered care so that the maternal-newborn unit remains in continuity. Successful transports require direct communication, preparation, timeliness, and skilled EMS personnel capable of acting in unpredictable circumstances. Development of guidelines, procedures, and policies with compliance to EMTALA regulations and state/local statutes helps ensure organizational structure to the transport of OB patients.

REFERENCES

1. Barkley KT. The ambulance. The story of emergency transportation of sick and wounded through the centuries. Kiamesha Lake (NY): Load N Go Press; 1990.
2. Shah MN. The formation of the emergency medical services system. Am J Public Health 2006;96:414–23.
3. Ryan GM. Toward improving the outcome of pregnancy: recommendations for the regional development of perinatal health services. Obstet Gynecol 1975; 46(4):375–84.
4. Little GA, Horbar JD, Watchel JS, et al. Chapter 2: evolution in quality improvement in perinatal care in toward improving the outcome of pregnancy

III: enhancing perinatal health through quality, safety and performance initiatives. White Plains (NY): March of Dimes National Foundation; 2010.

5. Harris TR, Isaman J, Giles HR. Improved neonatal survival through maternal transport. Obstet Gynecol 1978;52(3):294–300.

6. Anderson CL, Aladjem S, Ayuste O, et al. An analysis of maternal transport within a suburban metropolitan region. Am J Obstet Gynecol 1981;140(5):499–504.

7. Kaneko M, Yamashita R, Kai K, et al. Perinatal morbidity and mortality for extremely low-birthweight infants: a population based study of regionalized maternal and neonatal transport. J Obstet Gynaecol Res 2015;41(7):1056–66.

8. Hohlagschwandtner M, Husslein P, Klebermass K, et al. Perinatal mortality and morbidity. Comparison between maternal transport, neonatal transport and inpatient antenatal treatment. Arch Gynecol Obstet 2001;265:113–8.

9. Kollee LA, Brand R, Schreuder AM, et al. Five-year outcome of preterm and very low birth weight infants: a comparison between maternal and neonatal transport. Obstet Gynecol 1992;80(4):635–8.

10. Aly H, Bianco-Battles D, Mohamed MA, et al. Mortality in infants with congenital diaphragmatic hernia: a study of the United States National Database. J Perinatol 2010;30:553–7.

11. Adzick NS, Harrison MR, Crombleholme TM, et al. Fetal lung lesions: management and outcomes. Am J Obstet Gynecol 1998;179(4):884–9.

12. Carlan SJ, Knuppel RA, Perez J, et al. Antenatal fetal diagnosis and maternal transport gastroschisis-a maternal infant case report. Clin Pediatr 1990;29(7):378–81.

13. Jowett VC, Sankaran S, Rollings SL, et al. Foetal congenital heart disease: obstetric management and time to first cardiac intervention in babies delivered at a tertiary centre. Cardiol Young 2014;24(3):494–502.

14. American College of Obstetricians and Gynecologists. Levels of maternal care. Obstetric care consensus No. 2. Obstet Gynecol 2015;125:502–15.

15. Hankins GD, Clark SL, Pacheco LD, et al. Maternal mortality, near misses and severe morbidity lowering rates through designated levels of maternity care. Obstet Gynecol 2012;120(4):929–34.

16. US Code Title 42 Chapter VII Subchapter VXIII Part E SS1395dd Examination and Treatment of Emergency Medical Conditions and Women in Labor.

17. Richardson DK, Reed K, Cutler C, et al. Perinatal regionalization versus hospital competition: the Hartford example. Pediatrics 1995;96:417–23.

18. Okoroh EM, Droelinger CD, Lasswell SM, et al. United States and territory policies supporting maternal and neonatal transfer: review of transport and reimbursement. J Perinatol 2016;36:30–4.

19. Available at: http://www.camts.org/. Accessed April 30, 2016.

20. Low RB, Martin D, Brown C. Emergency air transport or pregnant patients: the national experience. J Emerg Med 1988;6:41–8.

21. Elliott JP, Sipp TL, Balazs KT. Maternal transport of patients with advanced cervical dilation-to fly or not to fly? Obstet Gynecol 1992;79(3):380–2.

22. Jones AE, Summers RL, Deschamp C, et al. A national survey of the air medical transport of high-risk obstetric patients. Air Med J 2001;20(2):17–20.

23. O'Daniel M, Rosenstein AH. Chapter 33 professional communication and team collaboration. In: Hughes RG, editor. Patient safety and quality: an evidence-based handbook for nurses. Rockville (MD): Agency for Healthcare Research and Quality (US); 2008. p. 271–84.

24. Elliott JP. Chapter 19: transport of the critically ill obstetric patient. In: Foley MR, Strong TH Jr, Garite TJ, editors. Obstetric intensive care manual. 2nd edition. New York: McGraw Hill Co, Inc; 2004. p. 249–56.

Index

Note: Page numbers of article titles are in **boldface** type.

Obstet Gynecol Clin N Am 43 (2016) 841–854
http://dx.doi.org/10.1016/S0889-8545(16)30076-6
0889-8545/16/$ – see front matter

obgyn.theclinics.com

UNITED STATES POSTAL SERVICE ®

Statement of Ownership, Management, and Circulation
(All Periodicals Publications Except Requester Publications)

1. Publication Title	2. Publication Number	3. Filing Date
OBSTETRICS AND GYNECOLOGY CLINICS OF NORTH AMERICA	000 – 276	9/18/2016

4. Issue Frequency	5. Number of Issues Published Annually	6. Annual Subscription Price
MAR, JUN, SEP, DEC	4	$310.00

7. Complete Mailing Address of Known Office of Publication (Not printer) (Street, city, county, state, and ZIP+4®)

ELSEVIER INC.
360 PARK AVENUE SOUTH
NEW YORK, NY 10010-1710

Contact Person
STEPHEN R. BUSHING

Telephone (Include area code)
215-239-3688

8. Complete Mailing Address of Headquarters or General Business Office of Publisher (Not printer)

ELSEVIER INC.
360 PARK AVENUE SOUTH
NEW YORK, NY 10010-1710

9. Full Names and Complete Mailing Addresses of Publisher, Editor, and Managing Editor (Do not leave blank)

Publisher (Name and complete mailing address)

ADRIANNE BRIGIDO, ELSEVIER INC.
1600 JOHN F KENNEDY BLVD. SUITE 1800
PHILADELPHIA, PA 19103-2899

Editor (Name and complete mailing address)

KERRY HOLLAND, ELSEVIER INC.
1600 JOHN F KENNEDY BLVD. SUITE 1800
PHILADELPHIA, PA 19103-2899

Managing Editor (Name and complete mailing address)

PATRICK MANLEY, ELSEVIER INC.
1600 JOHN F KENNEDY BLVD. SUITE 1800
PHILADELPHIA, PA 19103-2899

10. Owner (Do not leave blank. If the publication is owned by a corporation, give the name and address of the corporation immediately followed by the names and addresses of all stockholders owning or holding 1 percent or more of the total amount of stock. If not owned by a corporation, give the names and addresses of the individual owners. If owned by a partnership or other unincorporated firm, give its name and address as well as those of each individual owner. If the publication is published by a nonprofit organization, give its name and address.)

Full Name	Complete Mailing Address
WHOLLY OWNED SUBSIDIARY OF REED/ELSEVIER, US HOLDINGS	1600 JOHN F KENNEDY BLVD. SUITE 1800 PHILADELPHIA, PA 19103-2899

11. Known Bondholders, Mortgagees, and Other Security Holders Owning or Holding 1 Percent or More of Total Amount of Bonds, Mortgages, or Other Securities. If none, check box ▶ ☐ None

Full Name	Complete Mailing Address
N/A	

12. Tax Status (For completion by nonprofit organizations authorized to mail at nonprofit rates) (Check one)
The purpose, function, and nonprofit status of this organization and the exempt status for federal income tax purposes:
☐ Has Not Changed During Preceding 12 Months
☐ Has Changed During Preceding 12 Months (Publisher must submit explanation of change with this statement)

13. Publication Title	14. Issue Date for Circulation Data Below
OBSTETRICS AND GYNECOLOGY CLINICS OF NORTH AMERICA	JUNE 2016

PS Form **3526**, July 2014 [Page 1 of 4 (see instructions page 4)] PSN: 7530-01-000-9931   PRIVACY NOTICE: See our privacy policy on www.usps.com

---

15. Extent and Nature of Circulation			Average No. Copies Each Issue During Preceding 12 Months	No. Copies of Single Issue Published Nearest to Filing Date
a. Total Number of Copies (Net press run)			458	386
b. Paid Circulation (By Mail and Outside the Mail)	(1)	Mailed Outside-County Paid Subscriptions Stated on PS Form 3541 (Include paid distribution above nominal rate, advertiser's proof copies, and exchange copies)	104	107
	(2)	Mailed In-County Paid Subscriptions Stated on PS Form 3541 (Include paid distribution above nominal rate, advertiser's proof copies, and exchange copies)	0	0
	(3)	Paid Distribution Outside the Mails Including Sales Through Dealers and Carriers, Street Vendors, Counter Sales, and Other Paid Distribution Outside USPS®	145	163
	(4)	Paid Distribution by Other Classes of Mail Through the USPS (e.g. First-Class Mail®)	0	0
c. Total Paid Distribution (Sum of 15b (1), (2), (3), and (4))			249	270
d. Free or Nominal Rate Distribution (By Mail and Outside the Mail)	(1)	Free or Nominal Rate Outside-County Copies included on PS Form 3541	37	71
	(2)	Free or Nominal Rate In-County Copies included on PS Form 3541	0	0
	(3)	Free or Nominal Rate Copies Mailed at Other Classes Through the USPS (e.g. First-Class Mail)	0	0
	(4)	Free or Nominal Rate Distribution Outside the Mail (Carriers or other means)	0	0
e. Total Free or Nominal Rate Distribution (Sum of 15d (1), (2), (3) and (4))			37	71
f. Total Distribution (Sum of 15c and 15e)			286	341
g. Copies not Distributed (See Instructions to Publishers #4 (page #3))			172	45
h. Total (Sum of 15f and g)			458	386
i. Percent Paid (15c divided by 15f times 100)			87%	79%

* If you are claiming electronic copies, go to line 16 on page 3. If you are not claiming electronic copies, skip to line 17 on page 3.

PS Form **3526**, July 2014 (Page 2 of 4)

16. Electronic Copy Circulation	Average No. Copies Each Issue During Preceding 12 Months	No. Copies of Single Issue Published Nearest to Filing Date
a. Paid Electronic Copies ▶	0	0
b. Total Paid Print Copies (Line 15c) + Paid Electronic Copies (Line 16a) ▶	249	270
c. Total Print Distribution (Line 15f) + Paid Electronic Copies (Line 16a) ▶	286	341
d. Percent Paid (Both Print & Electronic Copies) (16b divided by 16c × 100) ▶	87%	79%

☒ I certify that 50% of all my distributed copies (electronic and print) are paid above a nominal price.

17. Publication of Statement of Ownership
☒ If the publication is a general publication, publication of this statement is required. Will be printed
in the DECEMBER 2016 issue of this publication. ☐ Publication not required.

18. Signature and Title of Editor, Publisher, Business Manager, or Owner   Date

Stephen R. Bushing   9/18/2016

STEPHEN R. BUSHING - INVENTORY DISTRIBUTION CONTROL MANAGER

I certify that all information furnished on this form is true and complete. I understand that anyone who furnishes false or misleading information on this form or who omits material or information requested on the form may be subject to criminal sanctions (including fines and imprisonment) and/or civil sanctions (including civil penalties).

PS Form **3526**, July 2014 (Page 3 of 4)   PRIVACY NOTICE: See our privacy policy on www.usps.com

Moving?

Make sure your subscription moves with you!

To notify us of your new address, find your **Clinics Account Number** (located on your mailing label above your name), and contact customer service at:

Email: journalscustomerservice-usa@elsevier.com

800-654-2452 (subscribers in the U.S. & Canada)
314-447-8871 (subscribers outside of the U.S. & Canada)

Fax number: 314-447-8029

Elsevier Health Sciences Division
Subscription Customer Service
3251 Riverport Lane
Maryland Heights, MO 63043

*To ensure uninterrupted delivery of your subscription, please notify us at least 4 weeks in advance of move.

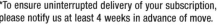

Printed and bound by CPI Group (UK) Ltd, Croydon, CR0 4YY

07/10/2024

01040504-0008